Dr. M's

Seven-X Plan for Digestive Health

Acid Reflux, Ulcers, Hiatal Hernia, Probiotics,
Leaky Gut, Gluten-free, Gastroparesis,
Constipation, Colitis, Irritable Bowel, Gas,
Colon Cleanse/Detox & More

Anil Minocha MD

Professor of Medicine

Certified, Physician Nutrition Support Specialist

Fellow, American College of Physicians

Fellow, American College of Gastroenterology

Fellow, American Gastroenterological Association

Praise for Dr. M's Seven-X Plan for Digestive health

"Dr Minocha's Seven-X Plan for Digestive Health is a valuable contribution to the field of gastroenterology. If you are looking for a holistic whole-body solution to your digestive ailments, then this is the book for you!"

> -**Dr. Robynne Chutkan**, Founder of *the Digestive Center for Women*, Author of *Gutbliss - A 10-Day Plan to Ban Bloat, Flush Toxins, and Dump Your Digestive Baggage*

"A treasure trove of key information on probiotics, intestinal infections and everything you ever could want to know about the digestive system."

> -**Chris Adamec**, Co-author of *Fibromyalgia for Dummies*

"If the proverbial 'cast iron' describes only other people's stomachs, you'll be fascinated by this accessible and infinitely helpful guide to your own GI system and how to keep it healthy -- information that just might cause you to start feeling good all over."

> -**Victoria Moran**, author of *Main Street Vegan*

"Hooray! Thanks to Dr. Minocha, we finally have a book that explains complementary and alternative medicine therapies as they relate to a wide swath of digestive diseases, all written in an easy to read format and in layman's terms. In particular, I found the information on the role of bacteria is in gut health as well as GI disease and dysfunction, a subject that often leaves many healthcare providers scratching their heads, very helpful and his description of his practical Seven-X Plan is easy to understand and follow. This is a great addition to the library of anyone who struggles with a digestive condition, especially those who have not found relief from traditional medicine!"

> -**Jill Sklar**, author of *The First Year: Crohn's Disease and Ulcerative Colitis*

Other books by Dr. Minocha

Encyclopedia of Digestive System and Digestive Disorders

Handbook of Digestive Diseases

Guide to Alternative Medicine and the Digestive System

LOGOS Enterprises LLC

Shreveport, LA, 71115, USA

ISBN: 978-0-9915031-1-7

Library of Congress Control Number: 2014902722

This work is meant for informational use only and by no means represents recommendations for diagnosis or treatment of any reader. Neither the publisher nor the author is engaged in rendering medical advice or services to any individual reader. Nothing in this book is intended to be a substitute for consultation with a licensed physician. All matters of health require medical supervision. Only your licensed medical provider can determine what remedies are in the best interest of your health and what to do about your illness. Never implement any health information from a book without discussing with your physician.

The procedures, treatments, and practices described in this book should be implemented only by a licensed physician and only in a manner consistent with the professional standards set for the circumstances that apply in each specific situation. Neither the publisher nor the author is responsible for your specific health or allergy needs that may require. The author, editor, and publisher cannot accept responsibility for errors, exclusions, or the outcome of the application of the material presented herein. There is no expressed or implied warranty of this book or the information imparted by it.

Neither the publisher nor the author has financial interest in the pharmaceuticals, commercial products, or equipment mentioned in this book.

PREFACE

Medicine is an art, not a science, and our already-vast knowledge is increasing exponentially. This book fulfills the need for a quick, concise source of practical clinical information, allowing the reader to better understand illness and be a better-informed consumer of health information, especially during a visit to the physician.

A highlight of the book is a generous coverage of natural treatment and alternative medicine therapies, especially coverage of topics like gut bacteria and dysbiosis, leaky gut syndrome, inflammation, probiotics, gluten-free diet, colon cleanse and flush, and body detox for digestive tune-up.

To achieve the goal of providing a condensed version of the state of knowledge for a broad audience, I have presented mainstream consensus as well as controversial positions. In my opinion, the gut plays a critical role in health and sickness. Digestive immune processes including gut psychology play a critical role not just in GI illnesses (morning sickness, acid reflux, food allergies, gastroparesis, irritable bowel syndrome or spastic colon, ulcerative colitis, Crohn's, constipation), but also in neurobehavioral disorders (autism, ADHD, OCD), chronic pain syndromes (fibromyalgia, chronic fatigue syndrome, restless leg syndrome, temporomandibular joint disorder [TMJD], migraine headache), autoimmune conditions (rheumatoid arthritis, ankylosing spondylitis), and skin disorders like allergies, skin eczema, acne, and psoriasis. The gut has a brain of its own, and the term gut psychology has been used to describe the role of gut in anxiety and depression. In fact, unhealthy gut bacteria linked to depression have been called "melancholic microbes."

Evidence indicates that the digestion connection to your overall health is real. Trust your gut! The use of terms like optimal or perfect digestion, healthy digestion, good gut, and gutbliss by experts highlights the importance our gut plays in overall health. Likewise, there is a plethora of diet strategies including Paleo diet,

Mediterranean diet, DASH diet, and GAPS diet. While goals are similar – including but not limited to perfect digestion – the strategies of the various experts vary.

The integrative gastroenterology approach outlined in Dr. M's Seven-X Plan will promote digestive and immune functioning inside the GI tract and allow you to attain digestive wellness. Just as an example – natural treatment for leaky gut is provided.

I have at times sacrificed finer detail for the sake of brevity and clarity. This book should not be used to make a diagnosis or initiate any treatment. All illness requires medical supervision by a licensed physician.

Knowledge is broad-based, and each person is unique. It is critical that no one adopt any changes based on this book without discussing with a physician.

As for myself, this book has been several years of hard work, but it has been a lot more fun!

TABLE OF CONTENTS

SECTION I
Your Body Needs Seven-X
Digestive Problem Solution

CHAPTER 1

Rising Tide of Digestive Illnesses

KEY POINTS

- Digestive illness is widespread.
- Damage to the gastrointestinal system has potential for illness throughout the body.
- Diagnostic and therapeutic frustrations abound, pushing patients to seek answers from not just their own physicians but also practitioners of Eastern systems of medicine.
- Alternative medicine therapies are becoming increasingly popular. There is concern and criticism about the safety of complementary and alternative therapeutic formulations available on market.
- Gut offers an attractive therapeutic for healing of the multisystem disorders, e.g. use of probiotics for brain dysfunction in liver disease.

"Man is a food-dependent creature; if you don't feed him he will die. If you feed him improperly, part of him will die." ...Emanuel Cheraskin MD

Some things to chew on before we get started:

- People are talking about "leaky gut." Do you know what it is? What is its significance in health and sickness?
- Did you know that there is a lot of published research on foods that protect against cancer? How much do you know about foods that protect against or promote cancer?
- A pregnant woman with nausea and vomiting refuses all pharmaceutical medications and wishes to use natural remedies. What are her options? Do they help?

- You have heard that yogurt with its bacteria is good for health. Do you know what kind or brand of yogurt to buy? Are all yogurts the same?
- You are planning a trip to Mexico and are concerned about traveler's diarrhea. Antibiotics prevent traveler's diarrhea but are not routinely recommended. Are there any other options to prevent traveler's diarrhea?
- You have heard that probiotics are healthy bacteria. Do you know which ones actually are beneficial? Are all probiotics helpful for all or most health problems?
- Did you know that medical treatment of ulcerative colitis is suboptimal and even the most expensive and toxic biologic drugs do not help many patients? What can you do?
- Have you read about fecal transplantation in the news recently? Do you know what it is?

When was the last time your doctor discussed things like this with you during your visit? Does he or she even have time to do that? If thinking about the above has piqued your curiosity and whet your appetite to read more of what I have to say, read on.

WHY I WROTE THIS BOOK

As a practicing gastroenterologist and nutritionist who is also involved in training future physicians, I have frequently been frustrated as well as saddened by the lack of knowledge (or desire to learn) among healthcare providers about the vast variety of "medicines" used by patients. As a physician scientist, I have been intrigued by the demand for a much higher level of evidence from complementary and alternative medicine therapies than we demand from mainstream modern Western medicine prior to accepting its use.

A comparison of studies related to mainstream modern Western medicine and alternative medicine therapies has consistently demonstrated that there is no significant difference in quality between the two kinds of studies.

Let it not be forgotten that physicians use mainstream medications for unapproved uses about half the time! The majority of the expensive devices and procedures go into mainstream practice long before controlled trials have demonstrated any benefit!

THE ANCIENT WISDOM

There is a good rational basis for the ancient saying: All sickness and all health begins in the stomach.

Most cultures, both modern and ancient, believe that maintaining a healthy digestive system is critical for well-being. We don't have to go too far to find out the truth – when our digestive system is functioning well, we feel better.

WHAT IS DIFFERENT NOW?

OUR DIGESTIVE SYSTEM AND NUTRITION IS NOT WHAT IT USED TO BE

- Many complex changes have occurred in our lifestyle, nutrition, and environment in recent decades.
- Modern agriculture farming and raising of farm animals bears no resemblance to the ancient jungle life or the medieval country life.
- There has been a rapid urbanization from country to city to suburbia and a speeding-up of our culture. Americans now have fast-paced lifestyles, with a heavy emphasis on eating out, fast food, and stored, canned and processed food.

What we currently consume bears no nutritional resemblance to what our forefathers did.

HOW IS OUR DIET AND GUT DIFFERENT?

- Our food has a very high glycemic load, including high fats with changes in nutrient density, micronutrient concentration, and acid-base balance.
- Generally, food has high sodium, low potassium, low magnesium, and low fiber.
- We intake high amounts of high glycemic sugar-laden empty calories and the wrong sweeteners.
- One-third of our diet is not cooked at home. Much of it is processed and canned. The Food and Drug Administration is only now asking that trans-fats be banned from cooking.
- The number of calories consumed from snacks has increased by over 50 percent.
- There has been an exponential increase in salty snacks, pizza, baked goods, cereals, and carbonated beverages across the world, even in countries like India, which suffered frequent famine only a few decades ago.
- There has been an exponential increase in food additives and preservatives.
- We have increased consumption of low-calorie sweeteners, especially in beverages. Research evidence indicates that such a use actually leads to more weight gain!
- There is a rising intake of alcohol.
- We have increased the use of antibiotics and pain-killing non-steroidal anti-inflammatory drugs (NSAIDs). Frequently, they are not needed and only damage the gut – increasing its permeability and altering gut bacteria.

These alterations in lifestyle and nutrition over time have modified our digestive system physiology and the gut bacteria; this may be at the heart of many of the chronic diseases suffered today.

To add gasoline to the fire, the government dietary guidelines are frequently based not just on science but also by business and political interests. For example, pizza is deemed to be part of vegetables in school-sanctioned lunches.

DIGESTIVE DISTRESS IS WIDESPREAD

Gastrointestinal illness, whether induced by ulcers, gastritis, abnormal functioning, *H. pylori* bacteria, or infections, is a common problem, affecting hundreds of millions of people worldwide. GI illness is a part of the overall problem in many other disorders.

In fact, a disordered gut likely plays a critical role in causation and persistence of a wide range of diverse disorders like GI and liver diseases, chronic pain syndromes (fibromyalgia, chronic fatigue syndrome, migraine headache, restless leg syndrome, TMJD), and neurobehavioral dysfunction like autism and ADHD, also known as ADD. Arthritis, allergies, skin eczema, acne, and psoriasis are widespread. Many patients just use over-the-counter (OTC) medications, while a small fraction actually sees a doctor.

I personally know a police officer working the night shift who carries around a bottle of antacids in his patrol car, takes several antacid pills every day, but has never seen a physician about this.

REFERENCES

1. Cordain L, Eaton SB, Sebastian A, Mann N, Lindeberg S, Watkins BA, O'Keefe JH, Brand-Miller J. Origins and evolution of the Western diet: health implications for the 21st century. *Am J Clin Nutr.* 2005 Feb; 81(2):341-54.
2. Wang CK, Myunghae Hah J, Carroll I. Factors contributing to pain chronicity. *Curr Pain Headache Rep.* 2009 Feb; 13(1):7-11.
3. Shaheen NJ, Hansen RA, Morgan DR et al. The burden of gastrointestinal and liver diseases, 2006. *Am J Gastroenterol.* 2006 Sep; 101(9):2128-38.
4. Lightfoot E, Slaus M, O'Connell TC. Changing cultures, changing cuisines: Cultural transitions and dietary change in

Iron Age, Roman, and Early Medieval Croatia. *Am J Phys Anthropol*. 2012 Aug; 148(4):543-56.

CHAPTER 2

Why Are Patients Frustrated?

KEY POINTS

- Diagnostic frustrations abound because testing reveals positive diagnosis only in a minority of patients.
- The majority of patients with functional bowel disorders, chronic pain, and inflammatory bowel disease do not get sustained relief from mostly currently available medicines.

A wide variety of factors contribute to frustrations among patients as well as healthcare providers.

DIAGNOSTIC FRUSTRATIONS

Despite advances in medicine, less than a quarter of patients with indigestion symptoms can be documented to have ulcers or gastroparesis (slow stomach). Similarly, the lower GI problems yield a precise diagnosis only in a minority of patients.

Most of the patients have normal results on routine testing and get labeled with such "waste paper basket" diagnoses as dyspepsia, gastritis, spastic colon, or irritable bowel syndrome etc. We are usually unable to offer a precise diagnosis, much less an effective, reliable treatment plan to such patients. Despite the lack of diagnosis in many of the patients, they are treated with drugs like acid-blocking proton pump inhibitors (PPIs) and even perhaps antidepressants, despite conflicting evidence of clinical efficacy.

Almost half of the patients complaining of heartburn and diagnosed as gastroesophageal reflux disease (GERD) have a normal upper GI scope and normal pressures on manometry testing, the testing of pressure waves of contractions and coordination of the esophagus. Some even have acid reflux within the normal range, based on monitoring of pH in the esophagus.

Despite this, they still continue to be treated with high-dose acid blockers, even though there is increasing evidence that these drugs are inappropriately used in majority of cases. In fact, the majority of patients with GERD have to continue taking their anti-GERD medications long after the anti-reflux surgery, which corrects the muscle problems at the junction of the esophagus and stomach.

For a while, especially in the 1990s, many diverse ailments were attributed to *Helicobacter pylori* (Hp) infection. It was not unusual for experts to show slides announcing, "The only good *H. pylori* is dead *H. pylori*." We still don't understand all the implications of the presence of *H. pylori* fully, since it appears to be related to dyspepsia in a small fraction of patients, but its presence has been shown to be helpful against GERD. Yet we keep looking for it and killing it in many cases, even without ulcers or cancer.

Do we understand fully the potential ramifications of eradication of *H. pylori* on the body? Few people appreciate the fact that *H. pylori* has been here as long as mankind itself, and the history of *H. pylori* bacteria in the human stomach parallels the history and migration of humans, starting in Africa and then on to the rest of the world.

We don't yet have full and clear understanding of what causes stomach ulcers. Oxidative stress, infection with *H. pylori*, use of NSAIDs, and lowering of stomach wall defense are some of the mechanisms involved. Increasingly, we are finding that a large fraction of ulcers are non-Hp, non-NSAID related. About half of the patients continue to have stomach pain long after the ulcer heals. Symptoms of indigestion improve in less than 15 percent of patients after eradicating Hp infection.

We should, at the same time, be alert to the critical differences between functional and organic diseases. Functional disorders are characterized by the absence or paucity of abnormalities on structural or laboratory testing. A classic example is irritable bowel syndrome (IBS), wherein while endoscopic exam is normal, biochemical, physiological, and biopsy changes can be found in many patients.

> The diagnostic criteria of IBS are clinical and change every few years based on "expert consensus," while the patient continues to suffer. However, given the economic environment and how physicians are paid, many procedural specialist physicians spend more time doing procedures that carry higher reimbursement. This in turn reduces the time they have to spend face-to-face with their patients, helping them understand the situation and cope with it better.

THERAPEUTIC FRUSTRATIONS

Disease states associated with chronic pain form a major component of this category. Why is it that the patients don't always get better with modern medicine? The answer probably lies at least in part in the fact that most of the modern-day ailments are multifactorial in causation and involve a multitude of interactions between the biological systems in the body, including the central nervous system (CNS), and environmental factors.

> The modern medicines frequently rely on a single specific molecule or a combination of few discrete molecules to cure a disease that is actually based on disturbance of biological pathways that are full of redundancies. When one pathway is blocked, the other one takes over to sustain the disease process. Thus blocking one pathway by a single discrete drug may not necessarily relieve the illness. In many instances, the treatment response is no more than 10 to 25 percent above the placebo.

Ancient systems of medicine were usually holistic, taking into account the whole body system and not just a component.

Incorporating that idea into modern medicine could benefit patients significantly.

For example, disaster-related environmental exposures like 9/11 have been shown to contribute to the development of GERD reflux symptoms, which may be potentiated by concomitant asthma and post-traumatic stress disorder (PTSD). How does a prescription of strong acid blocker drugs help target the cause of the problem in such cases?

It's no wonder that many of the chemically-defined treatments frequently gain a limited superiority over placebo. At the same time, the power of modern medicine cannot be underestimated. An ideal situation is a combination of the best of everything, including conventional and complementary medicine that is available.

PEOPLE ARE SPENDING MORE AND MORE ON ALTERNATIVE MEDICINE OPTIONS

Complementary and alternative medicine (CAM) has been growing in popularity in western countries and has gathered increasing recognition in recent years with regard to both treatment options and health hazards. The variety of systems present a wide range of therapeutic approaches including diet, herbs, metals, minerals, and precious stones.

CAM stems from knowledge based on centuries of experience, observations, empiricism, and intuition handed down through generations through word-of-mouth and treatises. Most CAM diagnoses are based on symptoms and follow the holistic or whole body treatment pattern.

For example, Ayurveda, most commonly practiced in India, is the oldest system of medicine in the world. The written documentation of diagnostic and healing acumen of Ayurveda predates the advent of modern medicine by thousands of years.

Ayurveda is an ancient Indian system of medicine. The word Ayurveda is derived from two Sanskrit words: *ayus,* meaning life, and *veda,* meaning science. Ill-health is not natural and represents a disrupted homeostatic balance and disharmony. It is a therapeutic strategy involving multidimensional strategies, including nutrition and digestion. Ayurveda is directed at restoring the balance needed for healthy state. Healthy digestion is fundamental to a healthy body. Nourishment is derived not just from ingested food, but also from the mind-body system, like what we hear, feel, and smell. Each person's constitution is based on one of three *doshas*. They are Vata (movement), Pitta (metabolic processes), and kappa (body structure). An excess or deficiency of one or more doshas leads to sickness.

Many of the traditional remedies have been passed down through families for generations. The patient's familiarity with the system breeds more trust, especially when the modern medicine is failing him or her.

WHY DO PATIENTS FLOCK TO ALTERNATIVE MEDICINE THERAPIES?

Patients are more interested in relief and less interested in what may be causing the problem. The diagnosis may be ulcer or gastritis based on modern medicine, or a disharmony of the body systems of Vata, Pita, or Kappa based on Ayurveda, but the patient's goal remains the same. Practitioners of modern medicine rarely shy away from making a diagnosis, even though there may not be enough scientific knowledge to precisely support the diagnosis or a treatment plan.

The treatments of gastrointestinal pain, whether it is IBS, functional heartburn, or dyspepsia, also continue to be based on strategic trial and error or a "step wise" approach, despite all the "medical advances."

CRITICISM OF ALTERNATIVE THERAPIES

The increasing use of natural and non-medicinal therapies, as well as the rapid growth of "natural health foods" and the herbal product industry, is being viewed with increasing concern at several levels, including:

- The potential for complications
- The use of possible contraindicated treatments
- Potential delays in getting proven and potentially more effective treatment
- Wasting precious time and money trying possibly ineffective treatments for serious illnesses like cancer
- A sub-optimal regulatory environment
- Placebo effect without any actual efficacy

> There is and likely always will be an inherent conflict between the CAM practitioners and the purists demanding evidence for safety and efficacy. Ultimately, there is only one medicine—the medicine that works. The need of the current times is for the practitioners to work together to optimize the best possible benefit for the ailing patient.

STATUS OF ALTERNATIVE MEDICINE THERAPIES

There is a dire need to look at the active principles of herbal medicines, as well as the mechanisms involved in non-herbal therapies. While there are only limited head-to-head comparisons of herbal remedies and conventional chemically-defined pharmaceuticals, the combination of herbal extracts and multiple bioactive ingredients appears to be advantageous for conditions such as non-ulcer dyspepsia, IBS, and inflammatory bowel disease. However, proof shall only be in the pudding!

REFERENCES

1. London F. Take the frustration out of patient education. *Home Health Nurse*. 2001 Mar; 19(3):158-63.

2. Li J, Brackbill RM, Stellman SD et al. Gastroesophageal reflux symptoms and comorbid asthma and posttraumatic stress disorder following the 9/11 terrorist attacks on World Trade Center in New York City. *Am J Gastroenterol*. 2011; Nov; 106(11):1933-41.

3. Posadzki P, Alotaibi A, Ernst E. Prevalence of use of complementary and alternative medicine (CAM) by physicians in the UK: a systematic review of surveys. *Clin Med*. 2012 Dec; 12(6):505-12.

CHAPTER 3

Pivotal Role of Digestive System in Your Health

KEY POINTS

- Damage to the gut can cause sickness throughout the body. Classic examples include celiac disease and inflammatory bowel disease, both of which affect organs far beyond the gut.
- The gastrointestinal system offers an appealing target for interventions, with the goal of healing of the multi-system diseases (e.g. use of probiotics for hepatic encephalopathy).

HEALTHY DIGESTIVE SYSTEM

From the moment you take a gulp to the time undigested matter is expelled, the culinary journey through your alimentary canal is nothing short of a wild roller coaster ride. A healthy digestive system allows optimal processing of ingested food matter and efficient absorption of nutrients, while ignoring unneeded substances or bacteria and fighting off potentially noxious ones. When healthy, our bodies get rid of GI waste matter efficiently and rather effortlessly. The very complex intestinal barrier, while well-conserved during the course of evolution, is not perfect.

Simple examples include celiac disease and Crohn's disease, where the net effect is not just a dysfunctional gut (with its diarrhea and malnutrition), but also a variety of body-wide disorders, including increased incidence of skin diseases and cancers.

An imbalanced state leads to disease when persons who are genetically predisposed to certain illnesses are exposed to a toxic environmental milieu. When this "perfect storm" occurs, the body's ability to repair the diseased components is impaired. Such a state can manifest changes in different parts of the body that are seemingly unrelated to the digestive system itself. This concept also explains why everyone exposed to similar circumstances does not get sick.

FUTURE OF NUTRITION IN HEALTH

The role of interconnections and interactions between what is in the gut (including food) and the genetic predispositions for optimal health is being increasingly appreciated. In this context, I have included a full chapter, Chapter 25, on different foods involved in protecting against or promoting cancer.

This has led to the new science of nutrigenomic or nutrigenetic approaches to individualizing nutrition, with the goals of disease prevention, health maintenance, and strengthening repair pathways to heal the body during periods of sickness.

Studies with the use of pre- and probiotic therapies have been promising. Genetically-modified novel foods may be artificially developed to conform to unique genotypes. This, however, raises a host of ethical challenges. Efforts to harness the full potential of human gut bacteria are in its infancy. According to Dr. Kau and colleagues from the Washington University School of Medicine in St Louis, Missouri, understanding how our diet affects the composition and dynamic functioning of our gut bacteria – and its interactions with our immune system – represents an area of future opportunity and challenge.

REFERENCES

1. Flint HJ, Scott KP, Louis P, Duncan SH. The role of the gut microbiota in nutrition and health. *Nat Rev Gastroenterol Hepatol*. 2012 Oct; 9(10):577-89.

CHAPTER 4

Laying the Foundation of the Seven-X Plan

KEY POINTS

- The gut plays a critical role in your overall health.
- Just as important as what we eat is what we avoid eating.
- Due to redundancy in the biologic metabolic systems, a multi-pronged strategy is critical to achieving a state of positive health.

Over decades of my exposure to Eastern and Western medicine, as well as treating thousands of patients and educating thousands of medical students, interns, residents, and gastroenterology fellows, I have come to the conclusion that not only are the core elements of most GI illnesses the same, but also that Hippocrates was correct when he stated, "All illness begins in the gut."

It is like hitting the knee with a baseball bat or a crow bar: the injuries, while different, are also rather similar. Although a forensic specialist can discern the causative factor, it looks and feels the same to most of us – red, swollen, and painful. Many (not all) of the elements of the treatment of a busted knee are similar, irrespective of what caused it.

The same is true for the gut. Much of the appearance and symptoms of GI disorders are the same, irrespective of the cause. The Seven-X plan strikes at the core of the common critical elements involved in causation (and, as such, in prevention) and healing of unhealthy gut and digestion.

For example, I am making no news with recognizing and accepting the critical role that our diet plays in our health and sickness. For example, our original gut-brain axis as God intended may have been transformed into a nightmare of a grain brain. Some of us just can't handle so much gluten!

I have devoted a whole section, Section VI, to "Healing Nutrition." This includes chapters on the role of elimination and exclusion diets (gluten-free, casein-free), the role of breast and cow's milk in our health and sickness, and foods that prevent cancer.

Still another section, Section III, of the book is devoted to intestinal bacteria, and how they affect health and contribute to disease. Separate chapters in the section discuss the role that probiotics play in "resetting" the unhealthy bacteria to the right balance for healing the damaged gut and impaired digestion. The discussion of probiotics makes it abundantly clear that all probiotics are not created equal. Probiotics are like antibiotics: they are tailored to treat particular infection. In fact, there is a wide variation in the number and kind of bacteria in any formulation. Some are single-strain formulations while others have multiple strains. The book provides tips on what to look for to pick a particular probiotic brand, depending on what health issue needs to be addressed.

I could go on and on.

In a nutshell, the book goes through the description of the multitude of elements involved in GI sickness and then describes common complaints and disorders along with their modern as well as natural/alternative medicine options.

The book winds down with a section condensing the information provided in the preceding chapters of the book into the components of the Seven-X Plan required for healing the unhealthy gut and the maintenance program for future. This includes Dr. M's Plan for Weekly Colon Cleanse and Body Detox in Chapter 48.

Why do I go through the lengthy description of the issues involved in preceding chapters before getting into the actual seven components? The answer is simple. The reader is likely to adopt the measures in the plan if she understands the reasoning behind it and the research it is based on.

Another question one might ask: Why do I go into description of some common GI disorders that people might suffer from? Again, knowledge is power. The reader is likely to get the most out of their doctor's visit if he knows what to ask about. In addition, some of the elements of the Seven-X Plan may uniquely apply to certain conditions. For example, the reader can identify which particular strains of probiotics may be uniquely helpful for IBS, constipation, or ulcerative colitis.

Likewise, for the reader whose focus is cancer prevention through proper diet, I have devoted Chapter 25 to this issue.

The Seven-X Plan for Digestive Health treatise is one single source that provides answers to questions about our GI health and illness we encounter on an everyday basis, and many more. The *raison d'être* for this book is my conviction that there is a conspicuous need for a systematic approach to address the sick gut at the core of any illnesses.

While the book outlines both the modern and complementary and alternative medicine therapies, the book by design is heavy on prevention and alternative therapies. Let's be candid: The source of continued education for healthcare providers is coming increasingly from pharmaceutical representatives and company-sponsored conferences in exotic locales. Awareness of vast research on complementary and alternative therapies has fallen behind. That holds true for both physicians and patients.

Dr. M's Seven-X Plan heals the gut dysbiosis and the gut leakiness, resulting in a healed gut-immune-skin-brain axis that makes the body disease-proof. This, in turn, tames the imperfections and powers up your grain brain to an improved body and better brain. The result just may be a new and better YOU!

The extra-emphasis on the holistic approach with alternative medicine therapies is meant to correct the imbalance of knowledge of healthcare providers as well as patients. The goal is purely to provide information; it is not meant as medical advice for anyone with any disorder. Knowledge is power!

As a physician-scientist-teacher, the Seven-X Plan for Digestive Health has been my most ambitious and rewarding professional undertaking to date. This incredible journey has taken me into the wonderlands of diverse and myriad ancient cultures and systems of medicine. It has indeed been an enlightening, intriguing, and humbling experience.

My big regret has been that I did not have this knowledge when I needed it. It's come with lots of experiences, both personal and professional. And no, I have not kept the best of health. But there is a silver lining to it. My challenges with health helped me reflect and crystallize the sum total of my knowledge and experiences into a well-defined framework that I am calling the Seven-X Plan for Digestive Health. Putting it into a book form allows me to share what I have learned so others may benefit from it at much earlier stages of life.

 I do not profess to have covered each and every thing; that would be a profound exercise in ignorance and arrogance. I sincerely hope that readers will find this book helpful and informative, ultimately leading not just to healing the primary GI illness, but also identifying GI symptoms that may be part of illness in patients with less-understood disorders.

Finally, the state of medicine is never perfect and is always evolving. Cure is always a worthy goal, but one should not let the search for perfection get in the way of good. If the Seven-X Plan outlined in the book makes the person feel better than other therapeutic strategies have, well, that in itself is a giant leap in the right direction.

As for me, the research and writing involved has been a labor of love and a lot more of fun.

Cheers!

SECTION II
Your Gut Feelings Need to Be Part of Any Gut Plan

CHAPTER 5

Stress and Your Gut Psychology

KEY POINTS

- The gut has a brain of its own, literally. It is in constant communication with our big brain.
- Stress plays a role in many GI and non-GI diseases.

Stress is all around and within us. All of us, no matter how rich and mighty, encounter it in our daily lives.

TYPES OF STRESS

Broadly speaking, stress may be physical or psychological. Irrespective of the type, it promptly arouses the body's defensive mechanisms to ward off the danger to its "normal balance" of bodily structure and functioning in order to ensure its survival.

BIG BRAIN-LITTLE BRAIN CONCEPT

When we think of our nervous system, we automatically think of our brain in the head. Well, that is the big brain. Our body also has the enteric nervous system – the "little brain" –which is constantly communicating with our big brain in a bidirectional manner.

Think of our big brain exercising the overall control over the body for its well-being, whereas the little brain represents the local control of the gut.

Bidirectional gut-brain communications control the GI function during health as well as sickness. These interactions occur via complex messaging signals including the nervous, immune, and endocrine messaging systems.

BODY SYSTEMS REACTING TO STRESS

We always think of immune responses as well as physical defense reactions (like a racing heart or sweating) as responses to actual or perceived stress.

Our gastrointestinal system is not immune to the stressful provocation and actually participates in numerous ways, including but not limited to its own gut-associated immune system. For example, we have all heard or suffered through diarrhea during exam days or heartburn during stressful conversations.

EFFECT OF STRESS ON GUT FUNCTION

- Altered gastrointestinal secretions
- Altered GI movements
- Increased leakiness of the gut
- Changes in blood flow to the gut
- Altered gastrointestinal bacterial patterns, which can make the body more vulnerable to infection, inflammation, and disorders associated to them

HOW DOES STRESS AFFECT GUT

The lining of the gut wall and its mucous layer represents a vast communication environment for our body, brain, and the trillions of bacteria in our gut. It acts as a barrier against bacterial infection.

The gut's normal bacterial inhabitants, as well as "bad" bacteria, talk to the gut wall and affect the body's reactions, including immune responses.

Nerve components in the gut wall provide pathways for bacterial messaging to nerve circuits that play a vital role in controlling pain response, immune reaction, modulation, emotions, and other bodily functions.

As we all know, stressful situations can evoke a wide variety of symptoms, including heartburn, bloating, gas, and diarrhea. These symptoms don't occur without any basis. For example, simple situations like a heated argument increase gastric acid secretion.

Any disturbance of the brain-gut axis may affect even simple functions like appetite and eating behavior, resulting in increased food consumption. The expression "comfort foods" just did not arise out of thin air.

BRAIN-GUT AXIS

The components of this axis include the big brain, the autonomic nervous system (ANS), the enteric nervous system (ENS), and a variety of hormones and neurotransmitters.

The brain-gut axis is also involved in the "Gut-Clock" (sometimes called circadian rhythm), disruption of which has been implicated in many gastrointestinal disorders including GERD, stomach ulcers, inflammatory bowel disease, and irritable bowel syndrome.

Melatonin, used frequently as a sleeping aid, also improves symptoms in patients with irritable bowel syndrome (IBS), inflammatory bowel disease (IBD), and gastroesophageal reflux disease (GERD).

HOW DOES STRESS AFFECT HEALTH AND CAUSE GI DISEASE?

Stress with roots in the brain produces alterations in the nerves in the gut; this activation of the immune system disturbs the healthy balance of pro- and anti-inflammatory factors, hormones, and other biochemicals leading to disease.

According to Dr. Lyte and colleagues from the Texas Tech University in Lubbock, Texas, stress messengers like norepinephrine, at the critical crossroad of above factors not only affect the protective cell lining of the gut but also the bacteria, especially along the gut wall.

BRAIN-GUT-BACTERIA AXIS

The better term for the brain-gut axis might be the brain-gut-bacteria axis, since intestinal bacteria, even though it is technically not part of our bodies, actively participates in brain-gut communications and brings about changes in the body.

Brain signals, including stress, alter intestinal bacteria via modulation of gastrointestinal motility and secretion. They also alter intestinal permeability directly via neurochemical signals released into the gut lumen from nerve (neuronal message) and immune cells (immune message) in the gut wall.

The neuronal, immune, and hormonal messages modulate the balance of pro- and anti-inflammatory cytokines. Stress-induced hormonal changes potentiate the virulence of potentially disease-producing bacteria like E. coli.

Conversely, the intestinal bacteria interact with our body via the lining of the gut wall (hormonal message) and impact gastrointestinal secretions, movements, and pain sensitivity.

Interference in the bidirectional interactions between the gut bacteria and the brain has been incriminated in the causation of several GI diseases, including irritable bowel syndrome and inflammatory bowel disorders.

CRF AT THE CROSSROADS OF BRAIN-GUT AND STRESS

Corticotropin Releasing Factor (CRF) receptors are present in both the brain and the gut. CRF is a neurochemical signal involved in the endocrine, nervous, and immune systems.

CRF-mediated interactions play a vital role in GI movements, leakiness, secretions, and inflammation. For example, CRF is involved in stress-induced contradictory functions, such as the stomach slowing down while the colon speeds up.

According to Drs. Tache and Bonaz from the Digestive Diseases Research Center at the University of California, Los Angeles, the CRF messaging system is the main coordinator of hormonal, interactive, and immune reactions to stress.

EXAMPLES OF GI DISEASES ASSOCIATED WITH STRESS
- Chronic heartburn, GERD
- Peptic ulcer disease
- Functional dyspepsia
- Irritable bowel syndrome
- Inflammatory bowel disease
- Pelvic dyssynergia

REFERENCES

1. Konturek PC, Brzozowski T, Konturek SJ. Stress and the gut: pathophysiology, clinical consequences, diagnostic approach and treatment options. *J Physiol Pharmacol*. 2011 Dec; 62(6):591-9.
2. Bravo JA, Julio-Pieper M, Forsythe P et al. Communication between gastrointestinal bacteria and the nervous system. *Curr Opin Pharmacol*. 2012 Dec; 12(6):667-72.

3. Peacock J, Whang W. Psychological distress and arrhythmia: risk prediction and potential modifiers. *Prog Cardiovasc Dis.* 2013 May-Jun; 55(6):582-9.

SECTION III
Healthy Bacterial Balance in Gut is Decisive

CHAPTER 6

You Are Not Alone: The Bacterial Universe Inside Your Gut

KEY POINTS

- A single layer of cells separates the human body from trillions of bacteria.
- Gut bacteria are in constant contact directly with the gut and indirectly with the rest of the body – they have potential to affect our health.
- Different bodies establish different relationships with bacteria. These bacterial patterns, once established, persist throughout life.
- The human body combined with its intestinal bacteria may represent a composite super-organism that needs to be considered as a whole when considering a disease.
- Use of pro- and prebiotics can help alter a disturbed microbial pattern and the abnormal interaction resulting in not just healing but also better health.
- Knowledge about the bacterial universe inside the body is important to understand overall health and sickness.

WHY DO WE NEED TO KNOW?

While we are always aware of the "outside" environmental influences affecting our body, we seldom think of the even bigger universe inside in our gut that may be affecting our physical and mental being every second of the day and night.

> Mammals, including human beings, are super-organisms, a composite of mammalian and bacterial cells existing in a peaceful and mutually-beneficial relationship.

The number of normal bacterial inhabitants in the gut is several times greater than the number of cells lining our gut. In fact, they exceed the number of human cells by as many as 10 to one. The gut wall is in constant contact with trillions of bacteria, comprised of over 1,000 different species.

This realization has led to a proliferation of bacterial and yeast products also known as probiotics. They come in the form of different kinds of yogurt (healthy and otherwise) or in capsules. There are also butters, infant formulas, skin lotions, and creams fortified with probiotics. The commercial market for probiotics exceeds $120 million per month.

GUT BACTERIA

The intestinal bacteria provide a humungous amount of microbial stimulation and interactions that can help or harm the human body. The gut bacteria are not just essential for normal life, they are critical for a normal state of health. Interactions between normal gut bacteria and intestinal cells are vital for the maturation of our immune system.

A normal, peaceful balance between the human gut and the gut bacteria is maintained by complex interactions and biochemical bidirectional messaging. This interplay plays a vital role in protection against a variety of diseases.

> Epidemiological data suggests that changes in the intestinal bacteria over decades may be a link between the modern lifestyle and the increased prevalence of certain autoimmune and allergic diseases. Restoration of healthy bacteria in the gut may occur as a result of natural progression or by use of probiotics.

THE BACTERIAL FINGERPRINT IN THE GUT

While 1,000 or so species have been identified, most of the bacteria in our bodies are derived from about 40 or 50 species.

Our unique bacterial fingerprint is established early in life and stays constant. Identical twins even present similar patterns.

Each person's unique bacterial fingerprint can be disrupted as a result of infection or medication use, particularly antibiotics. On occasion, these alterations become permanent and cause chronic disease, like post-infectious IBS.

FACTORS AFFECTING GUT BACTERIA

GUT BACTERIA IN THE FIRST FEW WEEKS OF LIFE

The bacterial pattern in a baby depends on multiple factors, including where the baby was born. It can be different if he was born at home or in a hospital, in an urban or rural area, or in a developed or developing country. Whether the baby was delivered vaginally or by C-section also has a profound effect.

EFFECT OF FAMILY, HOME, AND SURROUNDINGS

Family size and maternal diet have an impact on intestinal bacterial pattern. As such, there are often similarities in bacterial patterns among family members. This may in part explain the prevalence of certain diseases within a family, especially when no identified genes can be demonstrated.

EFFECT OF "ROUTINE" ANTIBIOTICS

Antibiotics disrupt the gut bacterial pattern by indiscriminately killing many of them. Use of antibiotic treatments changes the delicate intestinal bacterial balance. Such occasions provide an opportunity for silent, opportunistic bacteria to launch an attack and cause disease.

A glaring example is that of *Clostridium difficile*, which is normally present in many of us. It can cause colitis when subjects are treated with antibiotics.

> Lack of exposure to certain bacteria at critical times of maturation of the immune system (generally in infancy and early childhood) may be a critical factor in numerous autoimmune, allergic, and neuro-behavioral disorders, as well as chronic pain.

EFFECT OF SICKNESS AND STRESS

- The gut flora is also altered during stress and disease.
- Pancreatitis in experimental animal (animal models) demonstrates that good bacteria disappear within four to six hours of a stressful situation. Within four hours, there is overgrowth of disease-producing bacteria and a migration of these bacteria from our gut into our body.
- Patients lose their beneficial lactic acid bacteria after even a short stay in a hospital's critical care unit.
- Astronauts returning to earth are found to have absent or reduced beneficial lactobacilli bacteria, along with an overgrowth of disease-producing bacteria.
- The local release of biochemical signals such as noradrenaline by the body has an effect not only on the composition of the intestinal bacteria, but also on the ability of the beneficial ones to stick to the gut wall and carry out their protective functions.

MISCELLANEOUS FACTORS

Other factors documented to affect the intestinal bacterial patterns include:

- In a baby, whether he is breast- or formula-fed
- Use of drugs, including NSAIDS or antibiotics during early life
- Vegetarian or non-vegetarian diet
- Use of fresh or canned foods
- Use of additives and preservatives

▪ Type of cooking (predominantly boiled/broiled or fried)

> An unhealthy imbalance in our gut frequently occurs because of changes in the intestinal barrier, also known as intestinal hyperpermeability or leaky gut. The leakiness is a result of dysfunctional tight junctions (like joints between cells) in the barrier, bacterial toxins, anti-bacterial chemicals secreted by bacteria, or biochemical substances involved in inflammation.

The unhealthy imbalanced state between human and intestinal bacteria makes us vulnerable not just to intestinal infections but also to infections at other distant sites, including the lungs, and may lead to development of chronic inflammatory, autoimmune, and allergic diseases. (See Chapter Nine for details.)

FORGET THE MYTHS – HERE ARE SOME FACTS ABOUT OUR GUT BACTERIA

▪ Not all detected bacteria in feces are normal inhabitants. They may just be transiently passing through the gut. For example, food-associated species (found in things like yogurt) may just pass through the body and cannot be called permanent inhabitants.

▪ The bacteria in feces may or may not represent the bacteria actually in contact with the gut wall. The ones in contact are more likely to affect us than those in the middle of the intestinal lumen – the hollow part of the tube that is the human gut.

▪ A mismatch as a result of fewer beneficial bacteria or more disease-producing bacteria in the gut allows the disease-producing bacteria to assert their negative influence and cause disease.

Intestinal bacteria do not affect only the gut. These bacteria can impact distant organs, such as the brain. In fact, there is a bi-directional interaction and exchange of biochemical messaging signals between gut bacteria and the nerve cells in the gut, which in turn communicate with our nerve cells in the spinal cord and the brain.

Gut bacteria can cause functional bowel disorders (such as IBS) where the brain-gut connections are intimately involved. There is potential to affect the chronic pain syndromes (eg fibromyalgia) as well neuropsychiatric disorders (e.g. depression, schizophrenia, autism, ADHD or ADD) as well.

ACTIONS OF GUT BACTERIA

Gut bacteria have effects on numerous elements of the body and our health, including:

- The intestinal structure, function, and related biochemical interactions
- Immune cells and their secretions
- Maturation of blood vessels
- Activating or suppressing gene function
- Releasing a variety of chemicals participating in the inflammation process
- The release of intestinal hormonal factors
- Producing short chain fatty acids (SCFAs) via the fermentation of undigested food in the colon. These SCFAs are a source of nutrition for the colon and play a role in the healthy functioning of the gut.
- Reducing or eliminating bad bacteria, toxins, and cancer-producing biochemicals
- Synthesizing vitamins like the vitamin B group, vitamin K, and folic acid

REFERENCES

1. Cerf-Bensussan N, Gaboriau-Routhiau V. The immune system and the gut microbiota: friends or foes? *Nat Rev Immunol.* 2010 Oct; 10(10):735-44.

2. Fujimura KE, Slusher NA, Cabana MD, Lynch SV. Role of the gut microbiota in defining human health. *Expert Rev Anti Infect Ther.* 2010 Apr; 8(4):435-54.

3. Lee YK, Mazmanian SK. Has the microbiota played a critical role in the evolution of the adaptive immune system? *Science.* 2010 Dec 24; 330(6012):1768-73.

4. Sekirov I et al. Gut microbiota in health and disease. *Physiol Rev.* 2010 Jul; 90(3):859-904.

5. Cryan JF, O'Mahony SM. The microbiome-gut-brain axis: from bowel to behavior. *Neurogastroenterol Motil.* 2011 Mar; 23(3):187-92.

6. Raison CL, Lowry CA, Rook GA. Inflammation, sanitation, and consternation: loss of contact with coevolved, tolerogenic microorganisms and the pathophysiology and treatment of major depression. *Arch Gen Psychiatry.* 2010 Dec; 67(12):1211-24.

CHAPTER 7

Bacteria Help the Gut Attack the Bad and Tolerate the Good

KEY POINTS

- The intestinal bacteria imprint upon our biological and immune systems at or shortly after birth; this imprint establishes a template that affects our body systems throughout life.
- The cells lining the gut wall do not disregard the normal bacterial inhabitants. These non-disease-producing bacteria play an important role in growth and development. In fact, cells of the intestinal wall rely upon them to repair and maintain integrity of the gut wall.
- The human gut wall learns to recognize and tolerate the normal, healthy bacterial inhabitants, while at the same time reacting with defensive inflammation to disease-producing bacteria.

PROTECTOR ROLE OF BACTERIA ON IMMUNE SYSTEM

The cell lining of the gut wall is the largest surface area by which the body comes into direct contact with the external environment. This single-cell lining limits our body's contact with foreign proteins that can cause allergic reactions and thwarts the entry of potentially disease-producing bacteria into the body.

- Bacterial sensors in our gut are the "tip of the spear" against invading pathogens. Bacterial sensors allow the gut wall not just to sense, but also to differentiate between disease-producing bacteria and beneficial bacteria, based on their structural patterns.

- The normal bacterial inhabitants of the gut help in the development of a baby's immunity. They prevent disease-producing bacteria from taking hold in the gut. The bacterial signals in the gut merge with the mother's white blood cells, which are transported to the breast milk to help fight infections during this most vulnerable period.
- All bacteria in the gut are not equally involved in the protection mechanisms. Specific patterns of gut bacteria are responsible for induction of specific immune cells.

NORMAL GUT BACTERIA DO NOT CAUSE INFLAMMATION

There is a critical need for a healthy balance between tolerating normal inhabitants and launching defenses against disease. This poses a unique challenge to our intestinal immune system. Any agitation of a key mechanism involved in inflammation or repair processes results in a disorderly and unhealthy biological balance, leading to chronic uncontrolled inflammation.

A variety of cells and mechanisms are involved in maintaining this healthy delicate balance.

OUR DENDRITIC CELLS

These are involved in a variety of seemingly opposing mechanisms of inflammation, including:

- Orchestrating protective immunity and tolerance in the gut
- Activating the immune system by capturing foreign proteins (from food) and bacteria and presenting them to T-cells of our immune system
- Developing a "knack" for differentiating between normal gut inhabitants and foreign particles, including things we may be allergic to

- Differentiating between dangerous disease-producing bacteria and trillions of harmless ones

The dendritic cells can activate or suppress the immune system. These seemingly contrasting actions appear chaotic but are actually highly organized, allowing for a peaceful gut.

This is comparable to the peace between the West and the Soviet Union during the Cold War. This efficient system of maintaining peace between opposing forces involved in inflammation, injury, and repair is known as immune tolerance. A breakdown in any of the mechanisms involved in immune tolerance results in chronic intestinal inflammation and can cause a variety of chronic diseases throughout the body.

OUR INTESTINAL EPITHELIAL CELLS, BACTERIA AND INFLAMMATION

Intestinal epithelial cells (IEC) are also essential for the maintenance of a healthy balance of inflammatory processes. They facilitate recognition and differentiation between gut bacteria, disease-producing bacteria, and human feedback mechanisms.

THE DELICATE EQUILIBRIUM BETWEEN THE INTESTINAL BACTERIA AND INTESTINAL IMMUNE SYSTEM

The gut-bacterial interactions help maintain a healthy balanced state for maintaining the structural and functional integrity of the intestinal wall and healthy digestion. The intestinal barrier maintains a local healthy response to the intestinal bacteria, while protecting us against disease producing organisms.

DIFFERENTIATING PATHOGENS FROM COMMENSALS

The bacteria whether normal inhabitants or disease producing have binding sites that let them attach to the gut wall and interact. Recognition of a contact with bacteria sets off a defensive inflammatory reaction needed to alert and protect the host.

> In contrast to the disease-producing bacteria, normal inhabitants from a healthy gut develop different chemical signals for a totally opposite response that maintains a healthy state. These signals which have been conserved during the course of evolution are recognized by the host immune system.

This recognition leads to the normal inhabitants being recognized as nonthreatening resulting in suppression of the inflammation and disease producing surge of events or perhaps even shut them out completely. This constant signaling system enhances the ability of the gut wall cope with the injury, while at the same time and also primes the gut for its repair response.

HOW INTESTINAL BACTERIAL IMBALANCE OCCURS

The intestinal epithelium represents a highly selective barrier between the harsh gut environment with bacteria, foreign proteins and toxins and the intestinal immune cells. Yet, it is a porous wall. The entrance of the foreign proteins and bacteria across the gut wall into the human body has potential to initiate and/or perpetuate chronic inflammation. Various mechanisms are involved.

- Biochemical messages are constantly exchanged between the gut and the bacteria thus regulating and controlling the inflammation. These delicate signaling biochemicals are released by the bacteria as well as the immune cells allowing the interchange of information between them. Of course, these delicately balanced interactions are complex and vulnerable to disruption.

- Above bidirectional communication pathways are important for induction of the immune system responses as well the opposite, i.e. initiating and perpetuating chronic inflammation.

GUT BACTERIA VERSUS PROBIOTICS

- The gut bacteria as well as the probiotics utilize the same bacterial recognition and signaling systems
- Probiotics modify and readjust abnormal intestinal function and immune reactions. Read more about probiotics in Chapter Ten.

REFERENCES

1. Ronald PC, Beutler B. Plant and animal sensors of conserved microbial signatures. *Science.* 2010 Nov 19; 330(6007):1061-4.

2. Hajishengallis G, Lambris JD. Microbial manipulation of receptor crosstalk in innate immunity. *Nat Rev Immunol.* 2011 Mar; 11(3):187-200.

3. Salzman NH. Microbiota-immune system interaction: an uneasy alliance. *Curr Opin Microbiol.* 2011 Feb; 14(1):99-105.

4. Sansonetti PJ. To be or not to be a pathogen: that is the mucosally relevant question. *Mucosal Immunol.* 2011 Jan; 4(1):8-14.

CHAPTER 8

Gut Bacteria Sow Seeds of Future Health During Pregnancy

KEY POINTS

- Selective bacterial exposure of a fetus during pregnancy can affect important organs in the body during the early developmental phase, contributing to health later on in life.
- The use of probiotics by pregnant mothers presents an attractive therapeutic target that can affect the baby's health after birth.
- The maternal intestinal bacteria affect the fetus's health, even though it is frequently assumed that the baby in the womb lives in a sterile environment.

THE ROLE OF CONTROLLED BACTERIAL EXPOSURE AND ITS SOURCES

While the maternal environment protects the fetus against a barrage of bacteria when it is not capable of handling such an attack, the developing fetus is actually selectively exposed to intestinal bacteria and bacterial products.

> The growing baby in the womb is provided with a controlled exposure to the outside environment, including a low level of selective contact with bacteria. This helps to develop organs and prime the baby's body for the eventual mother lode of bacteria waiting upon birth. These concepts are supported by the fact that maternal exposure to farm animals reduces the risk of skin eczema and allergies in infants.

These bacteria can affect important organs in the body during early development, when babies are vulnerable or "naïve," thus determining health and sickness later on in life – even into adulthood.

BACTERIA - FROM MOTHER'S GUT TO FETUS

- The passage of bacteria across the gut wall is a normal phenomenon, which significantly increases during pregnancy and nursing.
- The growing baby in the womb is exposed to her mom's gut bacteria via the placenta and the amniotic fluid. Vaginal delivery exposes the newborn to a massive amount of bacteria.
- Bacteria may pass across the mom's intestinal wall to a fetus or to a baby via breast milk. The maternal bacteria are further transferred to the baby via skin-to-skin contact.
- According to Dr. Mold and colleagues from the University of California, San Francisco, a large number of maternal cells cross the placenta and enter the lymph nodes of the fetus. They activate the regulatory immune cells that prevent a fetus from launching an immune reaction against its mother.

POTENTIAL MODES OF ENTRY OF BACTERIA INTO THE WOMB

- Ascending through the birth canal
- Via blood through the placenta
- Retrograde entry from fallopian tubes

HYGIENE HYPOTHESIS (OLD FRIENDS HYPOTHESIS) SUPPORTING BACTERIA-FETUS CONNECTION

- Maternal exposure to farms, a bacteria-rich environment, modifies inborn natural immunity and protects against allergic sensitization in babies. According to Dr. Ege and colleagues, the changes of allergic sensitization can be seen in umbilical cord blood during pregnancy.

- Cat exposure during pregnancy has similar protective effects against the risk of eczema in the child.
- Dr. Conrad and colleagues from the Philipps University of Marburg in Marburg, Germany, conducted a study of maternal exposure to cowshed bacteria during pregnancy. The investigators demonstrated that such an exposure to a farming-related bacterial environment protects against the development of allergic diseases in the child after birth and into adult life.

DIRECT EVIDENCE FOR BACTERIAL CONTACT WITH FETUS

- The human uterus is not sterile but contains bacteria.
- DNA from the normal inhabitants of the human gut like *Bifidobacterium* and *Lactobacillus* can be identified in most human placenta.
- Studies by Dr. Bearfield and colleagues from the Queen Mary School of Medicine and Dentistry in London indicate that certain bacteria (like *Streptococci*) seen in the uterus may come from the mother's mouth. Bacterial invasion of the uterus by species like *P. gingivalis* suggest that harmful bacteria can be found in the uterus as well. The presence of these bacteria from the mouth brings into focus the importance of teeth in health and sickness.
- Dr. Andrews and colleagues have shown that many as 82 percent of women have at least one species of bacteria in uterus approximately three months after delivery. As such, the presence of bacteria in uterus is not necessarily harmful.

Women who test positive for bacteria in uterus have higher levels of inflammatory biochemicals and suffer greater number of pregnancy- and delivery-related complications.

EFFECTS ON IMMUNE SYSTEM

- Mom's infections and passage of her antibodies across the placenta causes immune reactions in the fetus. Maternal antibodies also alter the composition of the initial load of bacteria presented to the newborn, as well as defensive substances in the breast milk.

- The modification of the immune system after the delivery depends on the type of bacteria. This in turn affects whether there is an increase or decrease in inflammation. The presence of *Lactobacillus* is associated with reduced inflammation.

EVOLUTION FROM INITIAL TO FINAL INTESTINAL BACTERIAL IMPRINT

The maturation of the initial bacterial "fingerprint" to the final imprint after birth develops in a logical fashion. The first contact and impact is the mother lode of bacteria from the birth canal, followed by breastfeeding, the weaning process, and snowballing contact with the environment.

Babies born vaginally and breastfed have predominantly beneficial *Bifidobacterium* bacteria. In contrast, formula-fed babies have more diverse bacteria that can include disease-producing bacteria. One study indicated that diverse forms of *Bifidobacteria* species comprised much of the intestinal bacteria in exclusively breastfed infants, but only half that in formula-fed babies.

The difference in *Bifidobacterium* tends to continue after weaning over to formula feeding. By the age of one year, the infant's bacterial profile starts to evolve to an adult form, with the final establishment of an adult intestinal bacterial fingerprint by two to three years of age.

NOT ALL COMMON INTESTINAL BACTERIA ARE ABUNDANT IN THE ENVIRONMENT

It should be noted that not all normal inhabitants of the gut are widely prevalent in the environment. *Bifidobacterium* bacteria are seen in infants' guts, suggesting that these are acquired from the early environment, primarily from the mother. This pattern has been present throughout evolution, suggesting that it has a beneficial role for the baby.

PRETERM INFANTS

Not much is known about gut colonization and the composition and evolution of bacteria in preterm babies.

> Factors involved in disruption of normal intestinal bacterial development include Caesarian section, frequent use of antibiotics, intravenous feeding instead of breastfeeding and minimal skin-to-skin contact for bacterial transfer when a baby is in neonatal intensive care.

There is a delayed appearance of beneficial *Bifidobacteria* bacteria, along with diminished variability of bacteria types, in the intestines of very-preterm infants.

BACTERIAL EXPOSURE DURING BIRTH AND THE RELATED RISK OF ILLNESS

- Passage of *U. urealyticum* from mom to the preterm infant carries a high risk of lung disease in infants.
- Low-virulence bacteria isolated from the uterus are associated with evidence of brain lesions and cerebral palsy in very-preterm infants.

> The ORACLE II trial has shown that giving antibiotics to women in spontaneous preterm labor with intact membranes results in an increase in functional challenges among their children at age seven, along with an increased risk of cerebral palsy.

THERAPEUTIC IMPLICATIONS

Manipulation of the maternal bacterial environment offers an attractive therapeutic target. Providing probiotics during pregnancy provides a unique opportunity to reduce the risk of diverse immune, allergic, and inflammatory diseases in later life.

BACTERIA: BOTH GOOD A ND BAD

We now know that bacteria cannot just be understood in terms of infections, but also positive beneficial interactions that have a significant impact on bodily function, especially the immune system. There is increasing evidence that early environmental and bacterial influences have impact far beyond just the gut – they can affect a person's overall immune system.

REBOOTING THE BODY'S HARD DRIVE

Analogous to many computer problems, the ability to "reboot" dysfunctional interactions during pregnancy and soon after delivery has the potential to affect body metabolism and the immune system. Using specific probiotics can accomplish this and affect long-term health of the baby. As mentioned later on, probiotics reduce the risk of certain diseases in babies at risk and may have an effect on growth.

CONCLUSIONS

A fetus is exposed to bacterial influences which are moderated by the mother's defense mechanisms. The type of bacterial influences (pro- or anti-inflammatory), nutrition, medication intake (for example antibiotics), and toxin exposure (such as mercury or alcohol) all have potential to impact human health long after birth.

One potential therapeutic target in this complex maze of interactions is the use of probiotics, which may reset the entire body system and contribute to health.

REFERENCES

1. Rautava S, Luoto R, Salminen S, Isolauri E. Microbial contact during pregnancy, intestinal colonization and human disease. *Nat Rev Gastroenterol Hepatol.* 2012 Oct; 9(10):565-76.

2. Sanz Y. Gut microbiota and probiotics in maternal and infant health. *Am J Clin Nutr.* 2011 Dec; 94(6 Suppl):2000S-2005S.

CHAPTER 9

The Role of Abnormal Intestinal Bacteria or Dysbiosis in Chronic Diseases

KEY POINTS

- Any disruption of the normal healthy balance between the gut and the bacteria can create uncontrolled and self-perpetuating inflammation, not only in the gut but across the various systems of the body.
- These changes have been incriminated in the causation of a wide variety of seemingly dissimilar diseases such as irritable bowel syndrome, inflammatory bowel disease, brain dysfunction due to liver disease, skin eczema, asthma, fibromyalgia, and growth retardation.

SCIENTIFIC RATIONALE

The human immune system is a sort of sensory system that takes in and integrates vital information. It is capable of learning and remembering data, recognizing pathogens and the dangers they might pose.

Intestinal bacteria are critical for the initiation and perpetuation of chronic intestinal inflammation. Modern lifestyle choices, including eating canned and processed foods, can reduce the variety of bacteria within the gut and alter bacterial input for sensory education for the human immune system.

> Altered abnormal bacterial patterns or dysbiosis in infancy and early childhood can disrupt the mutually beneficial human-bacterial interactions. A lack of anti-inflammatory feedback signals alters the body's biological defense function. The effect of antibiotics on the bacteria and indirectly on our immune system depends not just on the number but also the specific kind of bacteria or flora involved.

Under such circumstances, even some normal bacterial inhabitants can stimulate specific immune cells and put them into an uncontrolled overdrive. This initiates a cascade leading to uncontrolled chronic inflammatory and allergic diseases in later life, particularly in people who are genetically vulnerable.

SMALL INTESTINAL BACTERIAL OVERGROWTH (SIBO)

An abnormal increase of bacteria in the small intestine is called small intestinal bacterial overgrowth (SIBO). The implications of SIBO are increasingly coming under the microscope. SIBO has been incriminated in numerous diseases, such as severe acute pancreatitis, IBS, inflammatory bowel disease, brain dysfunction due to liver disease, and fibromyalgia.

SIBO is amenable to antibiotic treatment. Gut-selective antibiotics are preferred over broad-spectrum antibiotics. In addition to measures to strengthen the intestinal barrier outlined in other chapters, SIBO may be treated with:

- Probiotics
- Prokinetic agents (drugs to promote movements of the gut), although there is a lack of effective and safe prokinetic drugs in the market
- Herbal microbials (Dysbiocide, FC Cidal, and ADP)
- Dietary modifications like trial of avoidance of fermentable oligo-di-monosaccharides and polyols (FODMAPs)

The important role of dietary modifications should not be underestimated. FODMAPs in the gut undergo fast fermentation by the bacteria and create biochemical substances that promote leakiness of the gut and SIBO.

FODMAPs include:

- Fructose (fruits, honey, high fructose corn syrup)
- Lactose (dairy products)
- Fructo-oligosaccharides or fructans (wheat, onions)
- Galacto-oligosaccharides or galactans (legumes, beans, cabbage, onions)
- Polyols (apples, pears, plums, low calorie sweeteners)
- Polydextrose and isomalt (artificial sweeteners)
- Read more in Chapter 21 on elimination diets.

INFLAMMATORY BOWEL DISEASE (IBD)

Gastrointestinal bacteria are key to the development and persistence of chronic inflammation. Numerous genes have been implicated in inflammatory bowel disease. However, even in identical twins with a genetic predisposition, Crohn's disease and ulcerative colitis do not always occur, suggesting the important role of environmental factors like intestinal bacteria.

Specific bacteria or bacterial clusters are needed to induce chronic inflammation.

- Inflammatory bowel disease and functional bowel disorder have distinct patterns of intestinal bacteria.
- There is reduced bacterial diversity in patients with inflammatory bowel disease, including reductions in the specific anti-inflammatory normal inhabitants.
- Our immune status has a profound impact on the bacterial composition of the gut and subsequent risk for disease.
- The hygiene hypothesis also known as the "old friends" hypothesis is based on the fact that unsanitary conditions appear to protect against chronic inflammatory bowel disease.

- Evidence suggests that probiotics that reorganize the balance of healthy bacteria have therapeutic benefits in IBD.

ALLERGIC DISEASES

Allergic sensitization appears to be preceded by changes in the person's unique fingerprint of gut bacteria or bacterial clusters. While skin barrier dysfunction is involved in the causation of skin eczema, an intestinal barrier dysfunction appears to play a key role by allowing antigen migration through the gut mucosal barrier. Evidence indicates that probiotics can help prevent allergic skin eczema.

HEPATIC ENCEPHALOPAHY

Liver dysfunction impairs the ability of the liver to eliminate toxins. First-line treatment for hepatic encephalopathy is the use of laxatives followed by antibiotics. These management strategies have stood the test of time, suggesting a bidirectional messaging between the gut bacteria and the brain, albeit in unhealthy state. The mechanism of action of both these treatments is via their actions on the intestinal bacteria.

Probiotics to reset the healthy bacterial balance have been recognized by some professional medical societies as a treatment option for liver-induced brain dysfunction.

PSYCHO-NEUROLOGICAL DISORDERS

There is bidirectional biochemical messaging between the brain and normal bacterial inhabitants of the gut. This plays a critical role in maintaining a healthy biological balance, which maintains stability within the intestinal bacterial patterns. These bacterial patterns in the gut and their exchange with the brain have the potential to modify brain function and behavior.

Studies also show that changes in established behavioral patterns can change GI biological function and the composition of normal intestinal bacteria inhabitants.

Intestinal bacteria produce neurotransmitters in our body. These include serotonin, melatonin, histamine, and acetylcholine. These neurotransmitters of bacterial origin communicate with nerve cells in the gut (enteric nervous system), which then communicates with the brain and affects brain function.

Intestinal bacteria ferment undigested food, producing several gases like carbon monoxide, hydrogen sulfide, and nitric oxide. These gases can also act as neurotransmitters. For instance, when the brain is under stress, intestinal bacteria produce specific biochemicals like putrescine, spermidine, spermine and cadaverine.

Intestinal bacteria not only affect the brain's response to stress, but also the normal thinking function. In studies, when harmful bacteria are introduced into an animal's gut, they activate the brain stem region, producing an anxiety-like feeling. Other bacteria, though, had the power to decrease anxiety in mice and enhance memory.

Some experts have invoked the hygiene hypothesis in the pathogenesis of disorders such as depression. The evidence supporting this concept includes the following:

- There is a high prevalence of depression in patients with chronic inflammatory bowel diseases, such as Crohn's disease. The number may be as high as 60 percent.
- Medication-induced depression in mice results in an increased risk of colitis.
- Some data indicates beneficial bacteria in the form of probiotics benefits psychological dysfunction.
- Reducing sugar in the diet improves behavior in some patients with depression. This probably happens through alteration in bacterial fermentation patterns of sugars.

- Studies suggest that consuming beneficial bacteria (probiotics) reduces anxiety in patients with chronic fatigue syndrome.

CHRONIC PAIN SYNDROMES

Multiple sources support the concept that intestinal bacteria are involved in chronic pain disorders.

- Use of antibiotics disrupts the normal bacterial imprint in animals, resulting in increased levels of certain neurochemicals in intestinal nerve cells associated with pain.
- Animals raised in a germ-free environment have a higher threshold of somatic pain perception, compared to conventional mice. When bacteria are introduced into the gut of such germ-free animals, it reverses the increased threshold for pain back to normal levels.
- The numbers of beneficial bifidobacterium bacteria are decreased in patients with chronic fatigue syndrome and fibromyalgia.

Drs. Othman and colleagues from the New Mexico Veterans Affairs Healthcare System in Albuquerque, New Mexico, point out the association of small intestinal bacterial overgrowth and fibromyalgia and irritable bowel syndrome, as well as potential implications of such changes. According to Drs. Wallace and Hallequa from the University of California, Los Angeles School of Medicine, SIBO associated with increased pain is common in fibromyalgia and responds at least transiently to antibiotic treatment.

INFECTO-OBESITY

Biological signals from the intestinal bacteria affect fat storage in our bodies. There are differences between the intestinal bacteria of obese and lean animals. Intestinal bacteria of obese animals harvest more energy from ingested food. This is a transmissible feature: introduction of bacteria from obese mice into the lean mice results in an increase in body fat in the lean mice. Bacteria do not just affect the quantity of fat but also the *types* of body fat.

ACNE

Increasing evidence suggests that abnormal intestinal bacteria and leaky gut are involved in causing acne. According to the gut-brain-skin axis theory, intestinal bacterial and the use of probiotics for healing is based on their effect on mental depression, anxiety, inflammation, oxidative stress, body fat, even mood and temperament. According to Dr. Bowe and colleagues from the State University of New York Downstate Medical Center in Brooklyn, NY, "This intricate relationship between gut microbiota and the skin may also be influenced by diet."

ANKYLOSING SPONDYLITIS

Klebsiella bacteria have been implicated in the pathogenesis of IBD as well as ankylosing spondylitis. These bacteria preferentially grow in starch-rich environments. Dr. Rashid and colleagues from the prestigious King's College in London suggest the use of antibiotics and low-starch diet for treatment of such arthritic processes. In fact, the use of low starch diet has been shown to ameliorate inflammation in this disorder.

MISCELLANEOUS

Several other diseases associated with changes in intestinal bacteria include:

- Asthma and allergies
- Atherosclerosis
- Autism
- Autoimmune diseases like rheumatoid arthritis
- Cancer
- Diabetes mellitus

- Nonalcoholic fatty liver disease
- Restless leg syndrome

REFERENCES

1. Noor SO, Ridgway K, Scovell L et al. Ulcerative colitis and irritable bowel patients exhibit distinct abnormalities of the gut microbiota. *BMC Gastroenterol.* 2010 Nov 12; 10:134.

2. Forsythe P, Sudo N, Dinan T et al. Mood and gut feelings. *Brain Behav Immun.* 2010 Jan; 24(1):9-16.

3. O'Mahony SM, Marchesi JR, Scully P et al. Early life stress alters behavior, immunity, and microbiota in rats: implications for irritable bowel syndrome and psychiatric illnesses. *Biol Psychiatry.* 2009 Feb 1; 65(3):263-7.

4. Pasarica M, Dhurandhar NV. Infectobesity: obesity of infectious origin. *Adv Food Nutr* Res. 2007; 52:61-102.

5. McLoughlin RM, Mills KH. Influence of gastrointestinal commensal bacteria on the immune responses that mediate allergy and asthma. *J Allergy Clin Immunol.* 2011 May; 127(5):1097-107.

6. Erridge C. Diet, commensals and the intestine as sources of pathogen-associated molecular patterns in atherosclerosis, type 2 diabetes and non-alcoholic fatty liver disease. *Atherosclerosis.* 2011 May; 216(1):1-6.

7. Tlaskalová-Hogenová H, Stěpánková R, Kozáková H et al. The role of gut microbiota (commensal bacteria) and the mucosal barrier in the pathogenesis of inflammatory and autoimmune diseases and cancer: contribution of germ-free and genotobiotic animal models of human diseases. *Cell Mol Immunol.* 2011 Mar; 8(2):110-20.

8. Vaahtovuo J, Munukka E, Korkeamäki M et al. Fecal microbiota in early rheumatoid arthritis. *J Rheumatol.* 2008 Aug; 35(8):1500-5.

9. Wallace DJ, Hallegua DS. Fibromyalgia: the gastrointestinal link. *Curr Pain Headache Rep.* 2004 Oct; 8(5):364-8.

10. Weinstock LB, Fern SE, Duntley SP. Restless legs syndrome in patients with irritable bowel syndrome: response to small intestinal bacterial overgrowth therapy. *Dig Dis Sci.* 2008 May; 53(5):1252-6.

CHAPTER 10

Probiotics: Poop for Thought

KEY POINTS

- All probiotics are not the same, and the benefits are strain-specific.
- Probiotic administration can play an important role in health maintenance and prevention of disease.
- Probiotics help multiple disorders including irritable bowel syndrome, infectious diarrhea, constipation, and inflammatory bowel disease.
- Despite widespread use, reports of side effects related to probiotics have been exceedingly rare.

The Roman historian *Plinio* promoted the use of fermented milk for GI infections. In the early 20th century, Russian-born microbiologist Dr. Metchnikoff observed longevity in certain Bulgarians who consumed significant amounts of fermented products. He theorized that fermented foods seed the gut with healthy bacteria, suppressing the harmful ones and preventing illness and healing the body systems.

> The intestinal bacteria are the largest source of bacterial stimulation. This has potential for both harmful and beneficial impact on human health. As much as 85 percent of immune system elements can be found in the gut. Low levels of intestinal inflammation may have far-reaching effects on our bodies, including the heart and brain.

In recent years, much attention has been paid to the role of probiotics in protecting against infections and preventing or treating chronic inflammatory diseases and allergic disorders. Many integrative medicine practitioners recommend this for use in patients with neurobehavioral dysfunction like autism. While controversial, many (including me) believe that the gut plays a critical role not just in GI problems in these patients (which are common), but also mental issues. These have a tendency to improve upon probiotic treatment, since studies suggest that severity of neurological problems correlates with severity of GI problems. Again, this is controversial, but most parents of autistic children that I know have their kids on probiotics.

MECHANISM OF ACTION OF PROBIOTICS

- Inhibiting growth of and invasion by disease-producing bacteria
- Strengthening the leaky intestinal barrier, making it less porous for undesirable proteins, bacteria, and toxins to pass through
- Promoting protective biochemicals while suppressing those that promote unrestricted inflammation
- Altering sensitivity to pain

The above actions occur in part by modifying the intestinal bacterial balance towards healthy patterns.

LIVE OR KILLED PROBIOTIC BACTERIA?

While the general consensus is that probiotic bacteria have to be alive to have beneficial effects, there is evidence that elements of probiotic bacteria that have been killed may inhibit inflammation and programmed cell death. Such actions have been shown to heal animal colitis.

NOT ALL PROBIOTICS ARE THE SAME

The effect of any probiotic depends upon the particular strain used. Use of each probiotic strain results in a unique profile of biochemicals secreted by immune as well as intestinal cells interacting with those particular bacteria. Research suggests a broad gamut of influence than is commonly attributed to these unique biochemicals.

IRRITABLE BOWEL SYNDROME

Multiple trials have examined the role of pre- and probiotics in irritable bowel syndrome. Overwhelming data suggests that probiotics are beneficial. Please refer to Chapter 37 on Irritable Bowel Syndrome for details.

LACTOSE INTOLERANCE

Multiple studies have examined the effect of probiotics in patients with lactose intolerance. Most persons with lactose intolerance can handle 12 grams per day if given as a single dose and as high as 25 grams per day when given in divided doses with food.

Results of the studies on the role of probiotics have been mixed. A systematic expert review in 2010 on treatments of lactose intolerance concluded that there is insufficient evidence of the beneficial role of probiotics.

BOOSTING IMMUNITY AGAINST INFECTIONS

Any imbalance in the "Cold War" between good and bad bacteria provides a greater opportunity for the bad bacteria to assert themselves and cause disease. The number of beneficial bacteria can be boosted by probiotic supplementation to enhance defenses against infections.

Numerous animal studies have documented the immune-boosting properties of probiotics. For example, baby formula fortified with the probiotic *Lactococcus lactis* provides superior protection against bad respiratory and GI bacteria in rabbits.

EFFECT ON IMMUNE SYSTEM AND INFECTIONS DURING INFANCY

Some studies have shown benefits of probiotics in infants. Dr. Ortiz-Andrellucchi and colleagues conducted a double-blind trial to determine if a mom's probiotic intake can modify the immune system in her baby. The probiotic treatment (*L. casei*) was undertaken for six weeks, and then the infants were followed for six months. Probiotic treatment resulted in fewer GI disturbances in the breastfed child of the mothers who consumed the probiotic.

INFECTIONS IN KIDS AT RISK FOR ALLERGIES

A double-blind trial examined the effect of feeding a synbiotic mixture of four probiotic species (*L. rhamnosus GG* and *LC705, B. breve Bb99,* and *Propionibacterium freudenreichii ssp shermanii*) plus prebiotic galactooligosaccharides to pregnant moms for allergy prevention in high-risk infants. The moms were given the synbiotic mixture during the last four weeks of pregnancy; after delivery, the infants were given the same synbiotic mixture for six months. Over the two years of infancy, respiratory infections occurred less frequently in the kids treated with synbiotic.

INFECTIONS IN KIDS ATTENDING DAY CARE FACILITIES

Use of probiotics in kids attending day care reduces the number of infections among kids, suggesting they have an impact on the spread of infections. For example, Dr. Weizman and colleagues investigated the effect of two different probiotics in preventing infections in infants attending day care centers. Healthy infants received formula supplemented with *Bifidobacterium lactis (BB-12), Lactobacillus reuteri,* or no probiotics for 12 weeks. Kids who did not get probiotics suffered significantly more fevers and diarrheal episodes than kids on probiotics.

INFECTIONS IN THE ELDERLY

Aging is generally associated with lowered immunity and greater vulnerability to infections. A controlled trial examined the effect of milk fermented with yogurt cultures and probiotic *L. casei DN-*

114001 over a period of three weeks. There was a 20 percent reduction in the duration of winter infections in the elderly as a result of preventative probiotic treatment. Similar beneficial results have been found with the use of probiotic *Lactobacillus johnsonii La1* in tube-fed elderly patients.

INFECTIONS IN HEALTHY ADULTS

Regular intake of probiotics can reduce potentially pathogenic bacteria in the upper respiratory tract, suggesting a linkage of the lymphoid tissue between the gut and the upper respiratory tract. In one study, healthy subjects given the probiotic *L. reuteri* needed fewer sick days than those on placebo.

A probiotic combination of *L. gasseri PA 16/8, B. longum SP 07/3, and B. bifidum MF 20/5* reduces the severity of cold symptoms during winter months.

VULVO-VAGINAL INFECTIONS

A crossover trial conducted by Dr. Hilton and colleagues from the Long Island Jewish Medical Center over one year examined the effect of daily consumption of yogurt containing *Lactobacillus acidophilus* for prevention of vulvo-vaginal candida infections in women. Consumption of probiotic yogurt resulted in a threefold reduction in infections. The average number of infections over six months was 2.54 in the control subjects and only 0.38 in the yogurt group.

SMALL INTESTINAL BACTERIAL OVERGROWTH (SIBO)

Dr. Gabrielli and colleagues from the Catholic University of the Sacred Heart examined the effect of probiotic *Bacillus clausii* in patients diagnosed with SIBO, based on hydrogen breath test. Hydrogen breath test normalized after the probiotic treatment in 47 percent of the patients at the end of one month. This success rate is comparable to that achieved with many antibiotics used in clinical practice.

In contrast, another trial failed to document beneficial effect of probiotics (*L. rhamnosus and L. acidophilus*) in reducing the risk of SIBO in kids. However, the above two studies may not be comparable since different probiotic treatments were used.

CONCLUSION ABOUT ROLE OF PROBIOTICS FOR INFECTIONS

While many of the studies on using probiotics to boost immunity and fight infections appear convincing, it is difficult to make a sweeping call in favor of any particular individual probiotic or combination. As far as probiotics being used singly, *L. casei* or *L. reuteri* appear to be promising.

PREVENTION AND TREATMENT OF ALLERGIC DISEASES

The composition of the intestinal bacteria may be different in patients with allergic diseases, compared to healthy controls. Such differences may precede the development of the condition. Probiotics differentially change the peripheral immune factors in healthy persons and patients with allergic disorders like skin eczema.

ECZEMA IN KIDS

Results of the clinical studies in atopic dermatitis have been mixed. A recent expert review by Dr. Foolad and colleagues from the University of California, Davis reported their findings in the prestigious *Journal of American Medical Association*.

Dr. Foolad's team concluded that "the best evidence lies with probiotics supplementation in mothers and infants in preventing development [of] and reducing" skin eczema. They also found supplementation with prebiotics and black currant seed oil to be beneficial.

FOOD ALLERGIES

The interest in modifying intestinal bacteria with pre- and probiotics to prevent and treat food allergies has multiplied in recent years. Modification of intestinal bacteria with probiotics has been shown to modify the immune system and has potential to prevent and treat food allergy. However, much of the literature stems from experiments in animals and is contradictory.

Most recently, VSL#3, a very potent probiotic blend, has been shown to heal inflammation due to food allergy in mice.

RESPIRATORY ALLERGIES

Studies examining the role of pre- and probiotics in allergic rhinitis (inflammation of the nose) have been yielding promising results. While data on use of probiotics for allergic disorders is somewhat mixed, *L. casei*, *L. reuteri*, and *L. Lactobacillus rhamnosus strain GG (ATCC 53103)* show promise for prevention.

ENHANCING GROWTH AND DEVELOPMENT

Infants and children who have fewer infections, feeding problems, orodental sickness, and allergies during the formative years are likely to develop better than their sicker counterparts. Probiotics enhance immunity and prevent allergies and inflammation.

Dr. Saran and colleagues from the Centre for Research on Nutrition Support Systems in New Delhi, India, investigated the effect of probiotic supplementation on poor children with growth retardation. The study group received yogurt containing *L. acidophilus* while the control group received a supplement without probiotic daily for a period of six months. There was a significant increase in weight and height in the probiotic group as compared to the control group, and this was associated with fewer cases of diarrhea and fever. Another trial demonstrated that the children receiving the probiotic-supplemented formula had superior changes in their height and weight compared to those receiving regular formula.

It should be noted that some studies have also shown no effect of probiotics on growth and development in kids. Data, although promising, is too preliminary to make specific recommendations.

INFLAMMATORY BOWEL DISEASE (IBD)

Intestinal bacteria play an important role in the causation of inflammatory bowel disease. Bacterial patterns are also different between the active and inactive disease in patients. Probiotics have the potential to alter the intestinal flora in favor of beneficial bacteria, affecting the immune and inflammatory response.

While probiotics have been shown to be helpful in fighting ulcerative colitis, the results in Crohn's disease have yielded mixed results and have largely been disappointing. See Chapter 40 on Crohn's disease for details.

DIARRHEA

Multiple randomized controlled trials have documented the beneficial effect of probiotics in various kinds of diarrhea, especially infectious diarrhea and traveler's diarrhea. Similarly, probiotics help in recurrent *C. difficile* colitis.

BRAIN DYSFUNTION DUE TO LIVER DISEASE (HEPATIC ENCEPHALOPATHY)

A decrease in the detoxification capacity of the body can cause brain dysfunction, especially in patients with chronic liver disease. Probiotics are effective in ameliorating mental dysfunction, especially in mild cases.

NEUROPSYCHOLOGICAL DYSFUNCTION

L. casei reduces anxiety in patients with chronic fatigue syndrome. *L. helveticus* administered healthy subjects reduces psychological distress, whereas *B. longum* reduces anxiety as compared to placebo.

Probiotic mixture of *Lactobacillus acidophilus, Bifidobacterium lactis* plus *Lactobacillus fermentum* has been shown to reverse impaired brain dysfunction and improve spatial memory and performance brain functions in in rats.

The term "melancholic microbes" has been coined to describe the connection between unhealthy gut bacteria and depression.

Dr. Dinan and colleagues from the University College Cork describe the term "psychobiotics" as the healthy bacteria of benefit in psychiatric illnesses. Examples of psychobiotics include *B. infantis*. It produces gamma-aminobutyric acid (GABA), which is an important neurotransmitter involved in regulation of anxiety and depression in the brain.

B. infantis administered to depressed animals normalizes their behavior. The bacterial GABA from the gut may impact the brain via the gut-brain axis. In humans, *B. infantis* is effective in treating irritable bowel syndrome by multiple mechanisms, including favorably modifying the pro-inflammatory to anti-inflammatory chemical ratio.

OBESITY

Have you wondered why, despite dieting and cutting down calories, you are unable to lose weight and be thin? Unhealthy gut bacteria and the inflammation are to blame, at least in part. Now you can do something about it.

According to Dr. Luoto and colleagues from the Turku University Hospital in Finland, the "potential of gut microbiota modulation with specific probiotics and prebiotics lies in the normalization of aberrant microbiota, improved gut barrier function and creation of an anti-inflammatory milieu. This would suggest a role for probiotic/prebiotic interventions in the search for preventive and therapeutic applications in weight management." Dr. M's Seven-X Plan targets all these factors and more.

Specifically with respect to probiotics, it should be pointed out that there is a high degree of functional variability even among the *Lactobacilli*. While one species may reduce weight, another might result in actual weight gain. There can be variability in the effects of different strains of the same species. In addition, a particular probiotic bacteria may have one effect in one species, and exactly the opposite in another.

Based on the limited literature available, the probiotics with anti-obesity effects in humans include *Lactobacillus gasseri, L. plantarum, L. amylovorus* and L. *fermentum.*

CANCER

Multiple studies have documented the benefit of probiotics in reducing the risk of cancer recurrence in patients with transitional cell carcinoma of the bladder following resection.

LIMITED EVIDENCE OF THE BENEFITS OF PROBIOTICS

Probiotics may have an effect on the following conditions:

- Preventing orodental disorders like dental caries, gingivitis, plaque, and bad breath
- Decreasing intestinal colic in babies
- Reducing cholesterol
- Improving recovery from fatigue in athletes
- Chronic pain disorders like restless leg syndrome, fibromyalgia, and chronic fatigue syndrome
- Neuropsychological dysfunction like manic depressive disorder, attention deficit hyperactivity disorder (ADHD), and autism
- Ageing processes
- Psoriasis

SAFETY OF PROBIOTICS

While complications have rarely been reported, probiotics are safe in immune-compromised patients and even have potential to boost immunity in such patients.

Dr. Whelan and colleagues from King's College in London performed a systematic expert review of literature to examine the safety of probiotics in patients receiving nutritional support. The authors found that most trials showed either no effect or a positive effect of probiotics on outcomes related to safety, like mortality and infections.

CONCLUSIONS

Probiotics have beneficial effects in preventing diseases and improving health. Not only do they act as a digestive aid and boost the immune reaction, they restore the gut barrier function by modifying the bacterial balance in favor of the beneficial ones.

Expert working groups have given probiotics a grade "A" recommendation for treating acute diarrhea in kids, reducing the risk of antibiotic-associated diarrhea, averting and sustaining remission in pouchitis, and treating and preventing atopic eczema associated with cow's milk allergy. Experts have also determined "B" grade recommendations in several other areas of treating inflammatory bowel disease and irritable bowel syndrome.

> The probiotics with perhaps the greatest number of proven benefits are *Lactobacillus rhamnosus strain GG* and *Saccharomyces boulardii*. Use of multi-strain formulations is more likely to be beneficial than single-strain formulations.

Results from meta-analyses and systematic reviews that lump all probiotic bacteria together to examine the effects in any disease should be interpreted with a grain of salt. Specific strains are effective against specific disease states. We should not expect reproducible results from studies that employ a variety of species or strains, different formulations, and diverse dosing schedules.

Read about Dr. M's Probiotic Tips to Defeat Bad Gut-Bacteria in Chapter 44.

REFERENCES

1. Minocha A: Probiotics for Preventive Health. Nutr Clin Pract. 2009 Apr-May; 24(2):227-41

2. Whelan K and Myers CE Safety of probiotics in patients receiving nutritional support: a systematic review of case reports, randomized controlled trials, and nonrandomized trials. Am J Clin Nutr. 2010 Mar; 91(3):687-703.

3. Balakrishnan M, Floch MH. Prebiotics, probiotics and digestive health. *Curr Opin Clin Nutr Metab Care.* 2012 Nov; 15(6):580-5.

4. Ortiz-Andrellucchi A, Sánchez-Villegas A, Rodríguez-Gallego C et al. Immunomodulatory effects of the intake of fermented milk with Lactobacillus casei DN114001 in lactating mothers and their children. *Br J Nutr.* 2008 Oct; 100(4):834-45.

5. Saran S, Gopalan S, Krishna TP. Use of fermented foods to combat stunting and failure to thrive. *Nutrition.* 2002 May; 18(5):393-6.

CHAPTER 11

Prebiotics and Synbiotics

KEY POINTS

- Prebiotics serve as food for the large intestine.
- Prebiotics stimulate growth of beneficial intestinal flora.

PREBIOTIC VERSUS SYNBIOTIC

Prebiotics (also known as "colonic food") are acted upon and fermented by the intestinal bacteria. It allows specific changes, both in the composition and activity of the gut bacteria, benefiting our well-being and health.

A synbiotic is a combination of prebiotic and probiotic. The combination has potential to provide at least additive and possibly synergistic beneficial effect.

PROPERTIES OF A SUCCESSFUL PREBIOTIC

- Not destroyed or absorbed in the gut on its journey from the mouth to the colon
- Undergoes bacterial fermentation in the gut
- Selectively promotes the activity and/or number of the beneficial normal inhabitants like *bifidobacteria* and *lactobacilli* to provide health benefits
- Develops prebiotics targeted to specific health situations

FUNCTIONS OF PREBIOTICS IN THE INTESTINES

- Maintain structural and functional integrity of the gut wall
- Regulate water and electrolyte balance
- Provide energy and nutrients for bacteria and the body

TYPES OF PREBIOTICS

Fiber in our diet is the most common prebiotic. Fructo-oligosaccharides (FOS) are promising prebiotics because they are selective towards the more healthy gut bacteria. Galacto-oligosaccharides (GOS) are used in infant formula foods. Inulin-type fructans also have positive prebiotic effects.

Other products with possible prebiotic potential include soybean oligosaccharides from soybean whey. Isomalto-oligosaccharides may be considered a quasi-prebiotic since they are partially metabolized in human gut.

POSSIBLE HEALTH BENEFITS OF PREBIOTICS

- Improved lactose tolerance
- Improved resistance to infectious agents, decreasing gastrointestinal and respiratory infections
- Decrease in cholesterol
- Treating weight- and obesity-related disorders
- Increased bacterial synthesis of vitamins
- Protection against allergies by reducing inflammation
- Improved absorption of nutrients like calcium and magnesium
- Improved glucose control

TYPES OF PREBIOTIC PRODUCTS ON MARKET

Products available on the market that may be strengthened with prebiotics include dairy products, health drinks, infant formula, cereal, dried foods, canned foods, and pet foods.

Always consider health benefits of prebiotics in the context of the FODMAP hypothesis. Optimizing the mix of different types of non-digestible carbohydrates may yield best results.

REFERENCES

1. Roberfroid M, Gibson GR, Hoyles L et al. Prebiotic effects: metabolic and health benefits. *Br J Nutr*. 2010 Aug;104 Suppl 2:S1-63.

2. Gourbeyre P, Denery S, Bodinier M. Probiotics, prebiotics, and synbiotics: impact on the gut immune system and allergic reactions. *J Leukoc Biol*. 2011 May; 89(5):685-95.

3. Vitali B, Ndagijimana M, Cruciani F et al. et al. Impact of a synbiotic food on the gut microbial ecology and metabolic profiles. *BMC Microbiol*. 2010 Jan 7; 10:4.

SECTION IV
Leaky Gut Syndrome is Critical to Seven-X Plan

CHAPTER 12

What is Leaky Gut Syndrome?

KEY POINTS

- The human body is constantly being subjected to a barrage of chemical, physical and biological insults from inside the gut. The body is also protected by the so-called intestinal barrier.
- The intestinal barrier is highly selective and semi-porous.
- A disruption of the intestinal barrier exposes the gut (and, indirectly, the rest of the body) to trillions of bacteria, potentially harmful foreign proteins, and other toxins.
- Contact between noxious substances and the gut immune system via a leaky barrier can create abnormal stimulation, leading to infection or uncontrolled inflammation at distant sites in the body.
- The integrity of the intestinal barrier is affected by numerous internal factors, as well as by intestinal bacteria, diet, lifestyle, and stress.

A single microscopic layer of intestinal cells separates a vastly complex assortment of contents of the gut from the human body – the intestinal immune system, blood vessels, and the sterile core of the body.

The intestinal barrier is composed of antibodies, antibacterial proteins, and *tight junctions* that bind the cells of the barrier to each other. This selectively permeable arrangement permits the intestinal bacteria to exchange signals with the immune cells and nerve cells. This signal exchange then can communicate with distant sites in the body, including the brain.

POTENTIAL CHRONIC CONSEQUENCES OF LEAKY GUT

Disruption of healthy patterns of intestinal bacteria in early life can lead to a disorder of the gut's ability to differentiate between normal bacterial inhabitants and the unhealthy, disease-producing bacteria. This can trigger uncontrolled inflammation, setting the stage for further leakiness in a vicious cycle. This creates a perfect environment for the person to suffer from chronic allergic and autoimmune diseases.

TIGHT JUNCTIONS (TJS)

Structural and functional integrity of dynamic tight junctions is critical for maintaining a healthy balance of selective intestinal penetrability. Inflammation disrupts these tight junctions, increasing intestinal permeability and creating a so-called "leaky gut." This allows toxins and foreign proteins to cross the intestinal barrier and interact with our internal tissues.

FACTORS AFFECTING GUT PERMEABILITY

Normal factors in a healthy person

- Programmed cell death
- Inflammation
- Intestinal bacteria
- Biochemicals involved in nerve signaling and inflammation
- Immune cells

Abnormal factors

- Intestinal obstruction
- Poor or lack of blood supply to the gut
- Jaundice
- Inflammatory bowel disease
- Cancer
- Trauma, including surgery

- Infections
- Slow gut
- Small intestinal bacterial overgrowth

THE GUT DEPENDS ON NORMAL BACTERIAL INHABITANTS FOR BARRIER INTEGRITY

- A delicate equilibrium between the intestinal bacteria and immune cells in the gut must exist in order to maintain reliability and normal function of the intestine. Multiple interactions are involved in immune cells tolerating normal bacterial inhabitants and food proteins while reacting to toxins and disease-producing bacteria.
- The intestinal cells and its resident immune cells do not simply tolerate normal bacterial inhabitants – they depend on them.
- Some passage of bacteria across the gut wall occurs all the time for "checking up." This allows the body to sample intestinal bacteria and proteins so the gut can mount a controlled immune reaction to foreign proteins and bad bacteria.

EFFECT OF CHANGES IN INTESTINAL BACTERIA

Selectively getting rid of intestinal bacteria reduces respiratory infections in critically ill patients. Probiotics may reduce the prevalence of disease-producing bacteria in the gut and help reduce infections after surgical operations.

EFFECT OF DISEASE-PRODUCING BACTERIA ON BARRIER INTEGRITY

The complex interactions between bad intestinal bacteria and the intestinal wall epithelium can disrupt the intestinal barrier, alter fluid and electrolyte absorption pathways, and provoke an inflammatory reaction.

Functional abnormalities in tight junctions can cause several inflammatory diseases, including inflammatory bowel disease, Type I diabetes, and celiac disease.

HUMAN, DIETARY, AND ENVIRONMENTAL FACTORS

Age: Intestinal leakiness is higher at infancy and old age. The leakiness is especially high in premature babies.

Pregnancy: High stress is a risk factor for spontaneous abortion. Stress increases intestinal leakiness, allowing passage of bacteria and toxins into the body and provoking abnormal activation of the immune system and inflammation. This affects a pregnant woman's adaptation to pregnancy, and the baby in the womb is then perceived as foreign. Strengthening the intestinal barrier and restoration of immune tolerance by use of probiotics may offer a new therapeutic target in such cases.

Exercise: Exercise-heat stress causes a decrease in blood flow to the gut since blood goes preferentially to exercising muscles. This disrupts the intestinal barrier. Dr. Smetanka and colleagues from the University of Iowa studied marathon runners who take ibuprofen prior to and during running. These runners developed intestinal leakiness, demonstrated by increased urinary lactulose excretion and increased presence of tested sugars in the blood. Half of the runners also developed GI infection symptoms.

Farm environment: Contact with farm animals contributes to the protective "farm effect" and strengthens the gut barrier. A pregnant woman's exposure to animal sheds during pregnancy offers a protective benefit for the baby. The umbilical cord in such cases has higher levels of antibodies, as well as other protective interferons.

Diet: The diet affects tight junctions as well as immune functions.

- The intestinal barrier is impaired in patients with kidney failure, but it can be restored to normal when patients eat a low-protein diet.

- Potato skins worsen intestinal permeability and aggravate inflammatory bowel disease in animals. Avoid a high-potato diet, especially fried potatoes.
- Consumption of formula diet with pre-digested proteins improves Crohn's disease symptoms.
- Low-mineral water improves intestinal leakiness in patients with skin eczema.
- Rapid fermentation of high FODMAPs diet produces excess acids, gases (hydrogen, carbon dioxide, methane and hydrogen sulfide), and surfactants that reduce surface tension. These factors mess up the intestinal barrier. FODMAPs have been implicated in the rising tide of a variety of conditions, like Crohn's disease, celiac disease, IBS, chronic fatigue syndrome, and autism.
- Milk fat has adverse affects in animal colitis, whereas fermented milk is beneficial. Infants consuming only formula show 2.8 times more leakiness compared to those receiving some human milk.
- Consumption of unprocessed cow's milk protects against disruption of intestinal barrier. This protection can also be seen in non-farm kids ingesting unpasteurized cow's milk. (I am not advocating drinking unpasteurized milk.)
- Hot spices like black and red pepper have digestive stimulant action and heal digestive disorders. Inflammation is a pivotal component of numerous diverse diseases, such as atherosclerosis and cancer. Studies suggest possible strengthening of intestinal barrier by hot peppers. However, the effects in damaged epithelium may be quite the opposite.
- Dehydration increases intestinal leakiness. The increase in permeability is subdued in subjects receiving fluids during exercise.
- Prolonged fasting combined with stress leads to intestinal damage as well as passage of bacteria and toxins from the gut into the body across a leaky gut. Fasting for a couple of days with adequate hydration should not be a problem in adequately

nourished persons. Maintain adequate hydration, even during a short fast.

Gliadin: Celiac disease happens as a result of a breakdown of tight junctions with increased leakiness of the food protein gliadin. Gliadin has also been implicated in the pathogenesis of a variety of other autoimmune disorders.

Food surfactants: Food-grade surfactants are common additives in foods we buy from the grocery store. These surfactants cause separation of the tight junctions and allow increased passage of harmful protein breakdown products across the gut wall into the body.

Fats: Excessive dietary fat causes an increase in intestinal leakiness. Genetic obesity does not play a role. While certain fats dilate the tight junctions, omega-3 fatty acids actually strengthen the barrier via their anti-inflammatory action. Likewise, butyrate, a short chain fatty acid, enhances the barrier function.

Alcohol: Alcohol intake, both acute and chronic, disrupts intestinal barrier via multiple actions, including inflammation, oxidative stress, and histamines. Alcoholic subjects have five times higher levels of bacterial toxins in their blood than healthy controls. Acute consumption of alcohol also causes gastrointestinal ulcers. The alcohol-induced intestinal permeability promotes abnormal passage of bacterial toxin across the gut wall and into the blood stream, causing damage to distant organs. This is thought to be a big factor in causing alcoholic liver disease.

The above notwithstanding, moderate drinking, especially red wine, has been associated with positive health outcomes. Data on the effect of smoking on the intestinal barrier is mixed.

Surgery

In addition to the effects of fasting, handling of the gut during surgery itself affects the intestinal barrier. For example, gallbladder surgery, when using tiny incisions during laparoscopic cholecystectomy, causes much less of an increase in intestinal permeability and increase in blood levels of bacterial endotoxin, as compared to the open surgical approach using one big incision.

Iron

Taking iron pills increases intestinal leakiness. This could be one of the mechanisms explaining the negative effects of medicinal iron supplementation on health.

Nonsteroidal anti-inflammatory drugs (NSAIDs)

NSAIDs cause abnormalities of the intestinal barrier._NSAIDs reduce energy production by the cells, thus impairing the tight junctions. Chronic use of NSAIDs causes ulcers and bleeding, along with precipitating relapses in patients with inflammatory bowel disease.

Stress/anxiety

Stress alters the fluid and electrolyte balance, mucus secretion, and structural and functional changes of gut barrier making the gut leaky. Alterations in intestinal barrier function are seen in animal models of acute as well as chronic stress.

Rats separated from their mothers show increased sensitivity to pain and increased bowel movements, suggesting disrupted intestinal barrier.

Stress worsens colitis in animal models of inflammatory bowel disease. Stress and anxiety are involved in causation and worsening of functional bowel disorders like IBS. Stressed patients are more likely to suffer relapses of functional and inflammatory disorders.

The intestinal barrier is a highly complex structure that allows for selective permeability. Intestinal contents including diet, drugs, and intestinal bacteria interact with the gut barrier and, indirectly, with the body's immune cells and nerve cells. These processes play a critical role in health and sickness. Simple things, like being fed on breast milk or formula milk during infancy, may have long-term consequences.

REFERENCES

1. Catalioto RM, Maggi CA, Giuliani S. Intestinal epithelial barrier dysfunction in disease and possible therapeutical interventions. *Curr Med Chem.* 2011; 18(3):398-426.

2. Cario E. Heads up! How the intestinal epithelium safeguards mucosal barrier immunity through the inflammasome and beyond. *Curr Opin Gastroenterol.* 2010 Nov; 26(6):583-90.

CHAPTER 13

Diseases Associated with Leaky Gut

KEY POINTS

- While the evidence of a cause-effect relationship is evolving, clinical and experimental data suggests that leaky gut is involved in causing and perpetuating many GI and non-GI diseases.
- While celiac disease is a classic example, leaky gut may be seen in GI disorders like inflammatory bowel disease, irritable bowel syndrome, food allergies, liver disorders, and neurobehavioral disorders like fibromyalgia and autism.
- The leaky barrier abnormalities may be seen before or may occur after onset of the disease.
- Apparently, different diseases occur when the interaction of leaky barrier, abnormal gut bacteria, and abnormal immune reactions in genetically-vulnerable patients creates a "perfect storm" critical to the disease.
- Evidence suggests that leaky gut is just one part of the overall disease-causing mechanisms of various diseases. Other external factors, including abnormal bacterial patterns, are involved.

Although abnormal intestinal barrier function or leaky gut may be an effect of a disease, mounting evidence points to its involvement in *causing* the disease.

A disrupted barrier allows for bacteria and toxins to enter the body, provoke inflammation, and a torrent of reactions ensues, depending upon the person's genes and environmental factors.

CELIAC DISEASE

Celiac disease is a classic example where leaky gut syndrome is involved. There is an abnormal immune reaction, and a variety of body systems are involved, causing variable clinical features in different persons.

The offending toxin in gluten is gliadin. Genes are also involved.

HOW DOES IT OCCUR?

The gut barrier is leaky because of abnormal tight junctions, as well as increased absorption of unwanted material through the cells into the body.

This permits gliadin contained in gluten to be absorbed, enter the body, and trigger an immune response.

Abnormalities of the intestinal barrier are seen even in celiac disease patients without symptoms while on a gluten-free diet, suggesting that leaky gut is a cause and not an effect. Healthy relatives of the celiac disease patients can even have leaky gut.

Celiac disease patients have varied symptoms beyond the gut, including liver disease. Such distant manifestations may be due to shared genes or the complex effects of abnormal intestinal leakiness, inflammation, and antibodies occurring due to the abnormal immune reaction.

TYPE-1 DIABETES MELLITUS

The interaction of various discrete factors creates a "perfect storm" critical to the development of Type-1 diabetes. Leaky gut, abnormal gut bacteria, an abnormal immune system, and abnormal genes appear to play a central role in causing Type-1 diabetes.

Abnormal function of the gut barrier is seen in the BioBreeding diabetes-prone rat, which develops diabetes spontaneously on exposure to normal diet. The altered intestinal barrier is seen in such animals prior to the onset of disease, suggesting that leaky gut is a cause and not an effect of the disease.

HUMAN DATA

- Changes in tight junctions of the gut barrier and increase in space between the cells of the barrier are seen in diabetic patients.
- Type-1 diabetes is common in patients with celiac disease, and both disorders involve a leaky gut. Thus, leaky gut may be a common denominator in the cause of these two disorders.
- The gliadin component of gluten that is involved in celiac disease is also involved in Type-1 diabetes.
- Prediabetic subjects with normal glucose levels show increased leakiness. The increase in leakiness is at the highest just prior to development of disease symptoms.
- Many cases of Type-1 diabetes are preceded by infection. Loss of intestinal barrier integrity by infection causes activation of the cells that cause diabetes.

According to Dr. Skogg and colleagues of Uppsala University in Sweden, the rapid increase in diabetes argues against a critical role for genes and for the involvement of infectious agents entering the pancreas, leading to the development of diabetes.

AGING-ASSOCIATED DEMENTIA

While controlled data of aging in humans shows no differences in usual intestinal parameters, data from animals suggests otherwise.

- Puppies and large dogs have higher intestinal permeability than adult and small dogs.
- Elderly patients may suffer increased leakiness due to impaired blood flow and the increased use of gut-toxic medications,

especially NSAIDs. Some experts have speculated that this may contribute to cognitive decline.

According to Dr. Brenner at the St. Louis Veterans Affairs Medical Center, a leaky gut would allow intestinal contents into the body. They may then reach the brain via the blood and create abnormalities of brain cells and cognitive decline.

INFLAMMATORY BOWEL DISEASE (IBD)

Studies suggest that a leaky gut barrier is critical to the development of IBD (Crohn's disease and ulcerative colitis). The disrupted barrier results in an exaggerated immune reaction and inflammation. However, it should be noted that while disrupted intestinal barrier function is central to the development of IBD, it by itself is not sufficient to cause IBD.

Patients with IBD have abnormal tight junctions, making them discontinuous and leaky. In addition to an increase in inflammatory cells, there is increased programmed cells death seen in the cells of the gut barrier. There is a case of a child with increased leakiness who developed Crohn's disease eight years later.

- Experimental models of IBD first develop increased intestinal leakiness, which is then followed by the development of colitis.
- Certain breeds of mice are prone to developing Crohn's disease. Increased gut leakiness in these animals is documented before the development of Crohn's.
- There is increased intestinal leakiness in patients with active Crohn's disease in both the damaged areas of gut as well as non-damaged ones.
- Subjects at familial risk for IBD have increased gut leakiness long before development of the disease. For example, increased permeability can be seen in as many as 25 percent of healthy first-degree relatives of patients with IBD.

IBD is associated with involvement of other organs like arthritis. Mechanisms common to multiple organ involvement include an enhanced intestinal permeability. Drugs like Remicade not only suppress uncontrolled inflammation but also reduce the accompanying gut leakiness.

NSAID-INDUCED GUT DISEASE (ENTEROPATHY)

Non-steroidal anti-inflammatory drugs (like aspirin and ibuprofen) cause damage to the gut. The damage can occur even if the drug is given by injection rather than as a pill. Increased gut leakiness is the central mechanism that converts the biochemical damage to tissue damage in the gut. Use of human lactoferrin (five grams per day for two days) by mouth diminishes the leakiness caused by the NSAID indomethacin.

LIVER DISEASES

LIVER CIRRHOSIS

Liver cirrhosis is associated with increased intestinal leakiness as well as leakiness of the blood vessels. This leakiness can be documented prior to the appearance of bacterial DNA in the blood and body fluids in patients with cirrhosis. The increasing intestinal leakiness correlates with increasing severity of the liver disease.

Spontaneous infections of body fluids occur in such patients, most likely due to passage of gut bacteria across the leaky gut wall into the body. Antibiotics are frequently used in cirrhotic patients on an ongoing basis to prevent such infections.

HEPATIC ENCEPHALOPATHY (BRAIN DYSFUNCTION OF LIVER DISEASE)

Hepatic encephalopathy (HE) is more likely in patients with liver cirrhosis if they have small intestinal bacterial overgrowth as well.

Symptoms of HE may be mild, such as altered behavior, confusion, slurred speech, and sleep problems, to more severe, such as sleeping much of the time, all the way to coma and unresponsiveness to pain. Antibiotics that are poorly absorbed and work only on the gut are effective for the treatment and prevention of hepatic encephalopathy.

Some liver societies recommend probiotics (beneficial bacteria) to manage this disorder.

ALCOHOLIC LIVER DISEASE

Alcohol causes damage to the intestinal wall, rendering the gut leaky. This, in turn, is one of the mechanisms involved in causing alcoholic liver disease.

- The toxin of the gut bacteria passes through the leaky gut into the body and causes inflammation, including in the liver.
- The increased bacterial toxin in the body also causes changes in the hormonal balance in the body. This increases the pressure in veins of the stomach and esophagus. These veins can then rupture and cause life-threatening bleeding.
- Preventative use of antibiotics in patients with bleeding reduces the risk of death. This suggests that antibiotics are acting on intestinal bacteria that may be passing across the gut wall.

FATTY LIVER DISEASE

Intestinal leakiness is involved as a factor in causing fatty liver disease due to obesity, drugs, toxins, alcohol, and other elements.

Probiotic treatment with the beneficial *Lactobacillus GG* bacteria diminishes oxidative stress, intestinal leakiness, and liver damage in animals with fatty liver disease caused by alcohol.

PRIMARY BILIARY CIRRHOSIS (PBC)

There is increased stomach and intestinal leakiness in patients with primary biliary cirrhosis. The disrupted gut barrier exposes immune cells of the gut to the gut bacteria, and there is a subsequent immune reaction including antibody formation. This is evident from the fact that the anti-mitochondrial antibodies commonly seen in patients with PBC also react with proteins from intestinal bacteria.

INTRAHEPATIC CHOLESTASIS OF PREGNANCY (ICP)

Intrahepatic cholestasis of pregnancy is a liver condition that may occur during late pregnancy and resolve after the delivery. The complications include damage to the growing fetus, still birth, and premature deliveries.

> Dr. Reyes and colleagues from Universidad de Chile compared the severity of gut leakiness in 22 normal pregnant and 29 non-pregnant women. Intestinal permeability was higher in women with ICP, and these abnormalities persisted long past pregnancy. The investigators concluded that leaky gut may be a factor causing this disease by increasing the passage of bacterial toxin from the gut into the woman's body, causing liver damage.

IRRITABLE BOWEL SYNDROME (IBS)

IBS, frequently labeled as a "functional disorder," is being increasingly recognized as an abnormal activation of the immune system, causing low-grade inflammation in the gut. Leaky gut allows an increased amount of bad intestinal contents, including bacteria, to cross. This in turn activates the intestinal immune system responses, resulting in IBS symptoms. The following facts support this hypothesis:

- There is increased intestinal leakiness in patients with IBS.
- An increased number of immune-related cells are seen in the gut wall of IBS patients.
- Patients with self-reported food allergies have a prevalence of IBS and other allergic disorders.
- There is a subgroup of patients with IBS who have typical IBS symptoms in association with allergic symptoms; this may be

called atopic IBS. Allergies are associated with leaky gut. If IBS is associated with allergies, it would suggest that leaky gut is the common denominator.

CONGESTIVE HEART FAILURE (CHF)

CHF is being increasingly recognized as a disease involving multiple systems in the body. Dr. Sandek and colleagues studied 22 patients with CHF and compared them to healthy controls. They found a 35 percent increase in gut leakiness in CHF patients, as well as a decreased absorption of nutrients.

Authors concluded that congestive heart failure is a multi-system disorder that includes hormonal imbalance, abnormal blood vessel function, and increased gut leakiness with a decreased absorption of nutrients. This may sound like a contradiction, but it can occur because leakiness and nutrient absorption involve different pathways.

The disruption of the intestinal barrier results in increased passage of intestinal bacterial toxins to enter the body, causing inflammation, which further worsens heart dysfunction.

> The above evidence suggests that intestinal dysfunction and leaky intestinal barrier may underlie the chronic low-grade inflammation and the resulting malnutrition. The gut offers an attractive target for therapeutic interventions in congestive heart failure.

FOOD ALLERGIES

Most cases of childhood food allergy do not persist into adulthood. In contrast, once a food allergy is established in an adult, it is rarely cured. Leaky gut barrier allows abnormal/allergenic proteins from the food to cross the gut, inciting the immune cells in the gut wall to react and produce abnormal antibodies.

Healthy feeding practices during early infancy promote tolerance to different foods and reduce risk of allergies.

STEPS IN CAUSATION

- The initial critical step is exposure of the gut immune cells to the offending food protein through the disrupted gut barrier.
- The offending food protein passes between the cells of the barrier into the gut wall and interacts with immune cells.
- The immune activation disrupts tight junctions of the barrier, increasing leakiness.
- Once sensitized, increased leakiness persists, even if the offending food is excluded from the diet, suggesting that abnormal gut leakiness is a causative factor in food allergies.

HUMAN DATA

- Infants with a food allergy have increased intestinal leakiness as shown by the lactulose/mannitol ratio test for sugar absorption. The severity of symptoms is directly proportional to the severity of the abnormal gut barrier.
- Food protein-induced enterocolitis syndrome occurs in kids up to age three. Usually, cow's milk and soy are the offending factors, although grains (rice, oat, and barley), vegetables, chicken, and fish may be involved.
- Foods causing allergies can also trigger skin eczema. A defective skin barrier and defective intestinal barrier allow abnormal reactions to allergens to occur.
- Liver transplant patients have increased gut leakiness. The increased intestinal leakiness correlates with increased incidence of new food allergies starting in patients after the transplantation surgery. This occurs even if the donor of transplant organ did not have history of food allergies.

SKIN ALLERGIES

There is potential for absorption of food antigens in persons with unhealthy genes during periods of increased permeability like acute sickness. This can lead to skin diseases, including allergies.

Distinct foods may trigger skin symptoms in about 30 percent of patients. Symptoms may occur within minutes of consuming food, without any skin eczema itself. Some patients suffer from worsening of skin eczema.

> Disruption of both the skin and intestinal barrier are involved. Probiotics can help treat skin eczema. Multiple studies have documented the beneficial effect of probiotics in reversing the increased intestinal leakiness and reducing the risk of skin eczema in high-risk infants whose parents have history of allergies.

MAJOR DEPRESSION

Psychiatric factors may determine gastrointestinal health outcomes and vice versa. Evidence suggests that depression is associated with increased oxidative stress, inflammation, and an abnormally active immune system.

Intestinal bacteria and leaky gut play a role in depression. In fact, injection of bacterial toxin can induce symptoms of depression.

> An interplay of multiple discrete factors, like increased gut leakiness and increased inflammation with abnormal immune system, compounded by stress can kick up a "perfect storm," leading to several symptoms of major depression involving multiple body systems.

ANIMAL DATA

- Mice separated from their mothers develop structural changes in the intestine. This is associated with increased gut leakiness along with an increased risk of colitis.
- Presence of depression reactivates inflammation in mice with healed colitis.

HUMAN DATA

Dr. Maes and colleagues examined whether an increase in passage of toxins from gut bacteria across the gut and into the blood plays a role in causing major depression. They found that the antibody levels to these bacterial toxins are much higher than those seen in healthy controls. The increase in antibody levels correlates with the severity of intestinal leakiness.

This suggests that disrupted intestinal wall function plays a role in causing inflammation and subsequent symptoms of depression (such as sadness, loss of energy, and changes in weight). The authors suggested that such patients should be assessed for leaky gut by testing for an antibody panel and treated accordingly.

Studies conducted by Dr. O'Donovan and colleagues from the School of Medicine in Dublin, Ireland, have documented that suicidal thoughts in depressed patients is associated with increased levels of inflammation.

But what is the source of this increased inflammation?

According to Dr. Berk and colleagues from IMPACT Strategic Research Centre, Deakin University in Geelong Australia, most of the factors involved in inflammation associated with depression are not carved in stone and are potentially modifiable. These include increased psychological stress, unhealthy diet, sedentary lifestyle, obesity, smoking, increased gut permeability, allergies, dental cavities, sleep, and vitamin deficiency, especially Vitamin D.

CHRONIC FATIGUE SYNDROME (CFS)

Evidence suggests that chronic fatigue syndrome (CFS) is associated with abnormalities of the immune system, along with increased oxidative stress and increased intestinal leakiness.

Drs. Ferraro and Kilman from the New York Psychiatric Institute said in 1933, "We must not forget here the possibility that in the future more appropriate and more delicate biochemical methods may allow us to detect [circulating gut-derived toxins] in an easier and more accurate way than we are now able to do." That has thus far remained a pipe dream.

- The prevalence and levels of antibodies against the intestinal bacterial toxins are significantly increased in patients with CFS compared to normal volunteers. Levels of antibodies correlate with symptoms of CFS as measured on the FibroFatigue scale. This suggests that the gut bacteria and toxins enter the body and provoke immune reaction and inflammation.
- The levels of antibodies against cow albumin also correlate with antibody levels against intestinal bacterial toxin suggesting that leaky gut allows passage of cow's albumin as well as bacterial toxins into the body.
- Normalization of leaky gut and levels of antibodies against the bacterial toxin in patients with CFS results in clinical improvement.

> Dr. Maes reported a case of a 13-year-old girl with CFS who showed very high levels of gut leakiness and inflammation. The patient was treated with antioxidants and put on a "leaky gut diet," resulting in normalization of the passage of bacterial toxin accompanied by a "complete remission" of the CFS symptoms.

According to Dr. Bested and colleagues from the Complex Chronic Diseases Program at BC Women's Hospital and Health Centre in Vancouver, Canada, "It seems vital to underscore the fact that any discussion of microbiota and mental health, or probiotics as an intervention in behavioral medicine, is not akin to discussions" of antidepressant drugs. They argue that there are numerous ways in which the gut bacteria may interact with environmental factors, including the person's diet.

FIBROMYALGIA

Evidence supporting the concept of leaky gut in fibromyalgia comes from studies by Dr. Goebel and colleagues from the University Hospital in Wuerzburg, Germany. These investigators studied patients with fibromyalgia, patients with complex regional pain syndrome (CRPS), and healthy control patients. Intestinal leakiness was examined using a standardized three-sugar test.

The authors found that the intestinal permeability is increased both in patients with fibromyalgia and CRPS, compared to healthy controls.

The pain intensity of fibromyalgia correlates with the degree of small intestinal bacterial overgrowth, which in turn is associated with increased intestinal leakiness.

AUTISM

While many children with autism demonstrate increased gut leakiness, the involvement of gastrointestinal dysfunction in the pathogenesis is controversial.

HYPOTHESIS

Leaky gut allows the breakdown products of food in the gut to cross the gut wall and enter the blood circulation. These extrinsic compounds can then interact with brain.

Dr. Theoharides and colleagues from the Tufts University School of Medicine in Boston suggest that non-allergic activation of intestinal and brain immune cells could provide unique targets for autism therapy.

DATA IMPLICATING LEAKY GUT

- Increased reaction of immune system to food proteins
- Greater degree of inflammation in the gut wall of autistic kids
- 70 percent of kids with an autistic spectrum disorder (ASD) have a history of gastrointestinal problems, compared with 28 percent of controls and 42 percent of kids with other developmental abnormalities
- One-third of patients with an ASD have a history of cow's milk and/or soy protein intolerance during infancy

Studies by Dr. Lau and colleagues from Columbia University have shown that children with autism have higher levels of antibodies against gliadin from gluten compared with unrelated healthy controls. These investigators concluded that the underlying mechanism may involve abnormalities of the immune system and/or leaky gut.

Some studies have reported beneficial effects from dietary intervention with a gluten-free and casein-free diet. A Cochrane database review found that dietary intervention has significant effects on overall autistic traits, social remoteness and overall ability to interconnect and interact.

Dr. Heberling and colleagues have proposed that a "circular model" is involved in causing autism. This includes oxidative stress, metabolic defects causing changes in intestinal bacterial balance, and environmental bacterial contaminants further causing increased oxidative stress in individuals. These factors are involved in a circular cascade, where treatments targeting one single factor would have limited utility.

These authors proposed a multi-pronged treatment to target leaky gut, abnormal intestinal bacterial patterns, and metabolic defects as a treatment for autism.

PSORIASIS

Abnormalities of intestinal structure and function have been implicated in causing psoriasis. Emotional stress is a trigger for psoriasis. As many as 78 percent of patients indicate that stress affects their disease.

SUPPORTIVE EVIDENCE

- Genetic abnormalities known to be risk factors for gastrointestinal diseases (inflammatory bowel disease, celiac disease) are also related to Type-1 diabetes mellitus and psoriasis.
- Abnormalities of tight junctions of the intestinal wall are seen not only in inflammatory bowel disease but also in some types of psoriasis.
- Dr. Humbert and colleagues studied intestinal permeability in psoriatic patients and healthy controls using the EDTA absorption test. The 24-hour urine excretion of EDTA from psoriatic patients was significantly higher than in controls, suggesting that leaky gut is involved.
- Microscopic abnormalities of the colon are seen in patients with psoriasis, even when the intestinal wall appears normal.
- Psoriasis is common in patients with celiac disease.

ASTHMA

Patients suffering from asthma have heightened intestinal leakiness as compared to patients with chronic obstructive pulmonary disease (COPD) and healthy controls.

Boosting airway immune cells by stimulation of intestinal immune cells has been advocated as a strategy for better control of asthma.

HIV

Increased gut permeability is seen in HIV infection. Passage of intestinal bacteria across the gut wall occurs, as demonstrated by increased levels of bacterial toxin in the blood. The levels decline in patients on anti-HIV treatment.

Dr. Leite and colleagues from Brazil conducted a randomized, controlled trial and found that glutamine administration helps improve intestinal permeability problems in HIV patients.

ARTHRITIS

Gut and joint arthritis appear to be connected closely. Over the course of evolution, certain kinds bacteria like *Shigella, Yersinia,* and *Salmonella* have become smarter and use the normal transport systems in the gut to infect the gut wall and then spread infection to the entire body.

Although usually such a bacterial exposure results in the body learning to tolerate the bacterial proteins as its own, sometimes the tolerance can be lost, resulting in an immune reaction and uncontrolled inflammation.

Leaky gut barrier and inflammation of gut as seen in inflammatory bowel disease (IBD) and celiac disease are associated with arthritis. Both bacterial and dietary proteins can gain access into the body through a leaky gut. Arthritis is the most common form of manifestation of IBD outside of the gut. Various types of joint involvement are seen. A prototype is ankylosing spondylitis.

The reverse may also occur. For example, inflammation of the gut wall is seen in ankylosing spondylitis without GI problems but can later on become full-blown IBD.

Not just the bacterial proteins, dietary proteins absorbed past the barrier cause immune reaction resulting in arthritis. An example is drinking cow's milk by rats results in the development of arthritis.

This fact may be a consideration in patients with difficult to manage arthritis.

MISCELLANEOUS CONDITIONS

Leaky gut has been implicated as a causative factor in a variety of other diseases, including severe pancreatitis, collagenous colitis, sepsis syndrome, multi-organ failure, schizophrenia, and cancer.

While the relationship between leaky gut and sickness is ripe for further exploration, depending upon clinical context, it may be prudent to adopt a strategy against leaky gut by implementing measures to strengthen the intestinal barrier, including a "leaky-gut diet."

Read about Dr. M's Approach to Healing Leaky Gut in Chapter 43.

REFERENCES

1. Fasano A. Leaky gut and autoimmune diseases. *Clin Rev Allergy Immunol*. 2012 Feb; 42(1):71-8.
2. Seo YS, Shah VH. The role of gut-liver axis in the pathogenesis of liver cirrhosis and portal hypertension. *Clin Mol Hepatol*. 2012 Dec; 18(4):337-46.
3. Vaarala O. Leaking gut in type 1 diabetes. *Curr Opin Gastroenterol*. 2008 Nov; 24(6):701-6.
4. Brenner SR. Hypothesis: intestinal barrier permeability may contribute to cognitive dysfunction and dementia. *Age Ageing*. 2010 Mar; 39(2):278-9.
5. Salim SY, Söderholm JD. Importance of disrupted intestinal barrier in inflammatory bowel diseases. *Inflamm Bowel Dis*. 2011 Jan; 17(1):362-81.
6. Reyes H, Zapata R, Hernández I et al. Is a leaky gut involved in the pathogenesis of intrahepatic cholestasis of pregnancy? *Hepatology*. 2006 Apr; 43(4):715-22.

7. Sandek A, Bauditz J, Swidsinski A et al. Altered intestinal function in patients with chronic heart failure. *J Am Coll Cardiol*. 2007 Oct 16; 50(16):1561-9.
8. Perrier C, Corthésy B. Gut permeability and food allergies. *Clin Exp Allergy*. 2011 Jan; 41(1):20-8.
9. Maes M, Kubera M, Leunis JC. The gut-brain barrier in major depression: intestinal mucosal dysfunction with an increased translocation of LPS from gram negative enterobacteria (leaky gut) plays a role in the inflammatory pathophysiology of depression. *Neuro Endocrinol Lett*. 2008 Feb; 29(1):117-24.
10. Goebel A, Buhner S, Schedel R et al. Altered intestinal permeability in patients with primary fibromyalgia and in patients with complex regional pain syndrome. *Rheumatology (Oxford)*. 2008 Aug; 47(8):1223-7.
11. de Magistris L, Familiari V, Pascotto A et al. Alterations of the intestinal barrier in patients with autism spectrum disorders and in their first-degree relatives. *J Pediatr Gastroenterol Nutr*. 2010 Oct; 51(4):418-24.
12. Kirschner N, Poetzl C, von den Driesch P et al. Alteration of tight junction proteins is an early event in psoriasis: putative involvement of proinflammatory cytokines. *Am J Pathol*. 2009 Sep; 175(3):1095-106.
13. Hijazi Z, Molla AM, Al-Habashi H et al. Intestinal permeability is increased in bronchial asthma. *Arch Dis Child*. 2004 Mar; 89(3):227-9.
14. Kukkonen K, Kuitunen M, Haahtela T et al. High intestinal IgA associates with reduced risk of IgE-associated allergic diseases. *Pediatr Allergy Immunol*. 2010 Feb; 21(1 Pt 1):67-73.

SECTION V
Inflammation: The Stealth Monstrosity as Target for Seven-X Plan

CHAPTER 14

Inflammation: The Good, the Bad, and the Ugly

KEY POINTS

- Inflammation and infection are not the same thing, although inflammation occurs as a result of an infection.
- The signs of acute inflammation demonstrate that the body is trying to combat the danger and heal the damaged tissues.
- The process of inflammation occurs not just at the site of injury – it may also be seen in distant parts of body.

The word inflammation is derived from the Latin term *"inflammo,"* meaning "I set alight, I ignite."

Inflammation is part of the body's intelligence and judgment. It is a complex and interactive cascade of modification of the local and systemic environment involving inflammatory cells and pro-inflammatory chemicals in the blood, blood vessels, the site of tissue injury, and beyond.

PURPOSE OF INFLAMMATION

Inflammation is the body's natural immune reaction to combat any offending irritant or disease-producing bug that attacks our body. Inflammation performs the follows actions:

- Isolates the damaged area
- Protects against harmful agents and stimuli
- Demolishes or eliminates the harmful agent
- Clears the damaged cells attacked by the harmful agent

- Begins the repair process after the offending agent has been addressed, to allow for healing to bring the tissue back to its healthy baseline

The goal is to limit inflammation in a controlled fashion, commensurate to the severity of injury. The best benefits of inflammation are achieved when the body individualizes the response to the danger and adjusts accordingly.

Too little or too much inflammation is bad! Uncontrolled inflammation is bad!

WHEN DOES THE INFLAMMATION OCCUR?

When the body senses danger, it organizes the immune system forces to combat the offender and then to help repair in the aftermath. The harmful agent or danger may be physical, chemical, or a biological organism. Inflammation may be good or bad, depending upon the context.

WHAT CAUSES ACUTE INFLAMMATION?

- Acute inflammation occurs when a harmful or irritating agent affects any part of our body. It is frequently a self-limiting or relatively easily treatable phenomenon that resolves upon effective treatment of the cause. Chronic inflammation is the other end of the spectrum.
- Acute inflammation gets resolved as the healing process wins the day, converts into an abscess (a pocket of pus), or evolves into chronic inflammation.

WHAT CAUSES CHRONIC INFLAMMATION?

Chronic inflammation occurs as a result of an uncontrolled, poorly regulated, over-active, and self-sustaining torrent of events:

- Infections (especially chronic infections like tuberculosis) provide continued stimulus for inflammation

- Environmental offenders and toxins like pollens, smoking, traffic, industrial pollution, or a persistent foreign body irritate the system
- Inflammation is initiated because of something in the body, then autoimmune disease sets in and it becomes a self-perpetuating uncontrolled inflammation

ACUTE VERSUS CHRONIC INFLAMMATION

Acute inflammation starts quickly, rapidly progressing to its peak. Manifestations of acute inflammation may last a few days or as long as a few weeks. It requires the constant presence of the offending agent and resolves once the offender has been eliminated. Examples include acute respiratory infection and injury to the hand or foot.

Chronic inflammation lasts from months to years due to the inability of the body to effectively combat infection. It may also occur due to a self-sustaining inflammatory process seen in autoimmune diseases like rheumatoid arthritis and lupus. where the immune system actually attacks the body's own tissues, mistaking it as alien and harmful. Still another scenario would be a persistent low-grade inflammation, for example due to bad dental hygiene or stomach ulcers.

COMPONENTS OF INFLAMMATION

Leukocytes or white blood cells (WBCs) are critically involved in the initiation and sustaining of inflammation. These WBCs arrive at the site of injury or infection from their usual location in the blood, and then migrate across the blood vessel wall into the surrounding tissues.

Acute inflammation involves a variety of inflammatory cells like neutrophils, basophils, eosinophils, and mononuclear cells like macrophages, monocytes, and a variety of inflammatory chemicals.

Chronic inflammation involves different type of white cells that are involved in chronic inflammation, and these, coupled with oxidative stress (see Chapter 15) due to excess of reactive oxygen species and other pro-inflammatory biochemicals like interferons, causes damage which the body tries to heal by scarring. This process then continues unabated.

Plasma cascade systems involved in inflammation include the complement system, kinin system, coagulation system, and fibrinolysis system.

SIGNS AND SYMPTOMS OF INFLAMMATION

The names for classic features of inflammation are derived from five Latin terms:

- *Rubor* or redness: Redness occurs as a result of increased blood flow to the site of inflammation.
- *Calor* or heat/warmth.
- *Tumor* or edema/swelling: This occurs as more fluid and proteins, including antibodies, exude out of the blood vessels into the tissue surrounding the injury or infection.
- *Dolor* or pain.
- *Functio laesa* or decreased function/immobility.

The first four features were documented in *De Medicina* by a Roman medical writer named Aulus Cornelius Celsus. It is unclear who came up with the fifth feature.

The signs of inflammation, specifically acute inflammation, show that the body is trying to combat a danger and heal the damaged tissues.

All of the signs may not be present in every circumstance. Many of the signs of inflammation may not be visible if the site of inflammation is deep inside the body, such as with a lung infection that manifests with pneumonia.

PROCESS OF ACUTE INFLAMMATION WITH SPECIFIC REFERENCE TO GUT

The first defense is mounted by cells already present in the injured tissues. The gut, which has the highest amount of pathogens due to trillions of bacteria and toxins present, is the largest immune organ of all. The inflammatory cells of the gut include resident macrophages, dendritic cells, histiocytes, and mast cells.

Initially, there is dilation of the vessels that supply blood the site of injury. The blood capillaries become leaky, facilitating seepage of fluid out of the blood vessels into the surrounding tissue. Along with the fluid seepage also come the cells involved in inflammation, starting with neutrophils. A wide variety of WBCs are involved. Neutrophils form the "tip of the spear" and are the first ones to arrive at the site of inflammation.

The surface of these cells have Pattern Recognition Receptors (PRRs), which recognize pathogenic bugs and can differentiate between an invading organism and the body's own cells. Activation of PRRs by infection, trauma, irritant, or toxin initiates inflammation. WBCs engulf the pathogenic organisms and kill it, using armaments like oxygen free radicals.

Neutrophils also release many antimicrobial proteins and pro-inflammatory cytokines like tumor necrosis factor and interferon, which in turn stimulate increased synthesis and release of acute phase reactant proteins and spread the process of inflammation throughout the body.

PROCESS OF CHRONIC INFLAMMATION

The main white cells involved in chronic inflammation are monocytes, which engulf and kill the pathogens, as well as the older, damaged cells. Like other white cells, they are also the source of pro-inflammatory chemicals. Over time, lymphocytes also arrive at the scene.

Antibodies directed against the purported pathogen are formed and released. Sometimes, these antibodies have a "mis-recognition" and target the body's own tissues. Another process involves the antibody-antigen complex, stimulating the complement system and further kindling the release of intermediaries of inflammation.

The reactive oxygen species and pro-inflammatory mediators, in addition to killing the harmful pathogens, can also damage the body's own tissues. Chronic inflammation involves healing damaged tissues and forming new blood vessels at the site, along with regeneration of cells and scar tissue.

DISEASES RELATED TO CHRONIC INFLAMMATION

Chronic low-grade inflammation, due to something as simple as bad teeth and gums, can have widespread health consequences. These include an increased risk of the following:

- Heart disease
- Stroke
- Obesity
- Pregnancy complications
- Diabetes mellitus
- Nonalcoholic fatty liver disease
- Ageing prematurely
- Alzheimer's disease

Read about Dr. M's Recommendations for Controlling Inflammation and Potentiating Antioxidant Defenses Naturally in Chapter 45.

REFERENCES

1. Fullerton JN, O'Brien AJ, Gilroy DW. Pathways mediating resolution of inflammation: when enough is too much. *J Pathol.* 2013 Sep; 231(1):8-20.

2. Cardona SM, Garcia JA, Cardona AE. The fine balance of chemokines during disease: trafficking, inflammation, and homeostasis. *Methods Mol Biol*. 2013; 1013:1-16.

3. Moutsopoulos NM, Madianos PN. Low-grade inflammation in chronic infectious diseases: paradigm of periodontal infections. *Ann N Y Acad Sci*. 2006Nov; 1088:251-64.

4. Barth K, Remick DG, Genco CA. Disruption of immune regulation by microbial pathogens and resulting chronic inflammation. *J Cell Physiol*. 2013 Jul; 228(7):1413-22.

CHAPTER 15

Oxidative Stress

KEY POINTS

- Reactive oxygen species (ROS) damage or destroy cells indiscriminately – both normal cells and invading bacteria.
- Appropriate timing, amount, and location of ROS are critical for the body's healthy defense system. Inappropriate and uncontrolled ROS can lead to chronic diseases.

REACTIVE OXYGEN SPECIES (ROS)

Reactive oxygen species and reactive nitrogen species are frequently grouped together under the broad term *Reactive Oxygen Species* or ROS. Under healthy conditions, the production of ROS is offset by a well-organized system of antioxidants in the body. These antioxidants are molecules adept at "scavenging" ROS, which in turn prevents damage to the normal cells.

ROS are an integral component of our immune system that we are born with. They form the first line of defense against an injury or a noxious stimulus. They occur as a result of metabolic processes in the cells.

OXIDATIVE STRESS

In an unhealthy state, the ROS may be present in relative excess, or the body's own antioxidant system may be deficient. This shift of the balance in favor of oxidation is termed "oxidative stress."

Oxidative stress is the combined effect of all concurrent ROS insults. They may have detrimental effects on cellular and tissue structure and function, thus contributing to diseases like heart failure, Alzheimer's, and cancer, as well as the normal process of aging.

REACTIVE OXYGEN SPECIES ARE TWO-FACED

Because of perceived involvement in many modern diseases, ROS were thought to be a "necessary evil" associated with oxidation metabolism in the body. A superficial reading may suggest that they are a byproduct of an imperfect system. However, the fact that ROS have been conserved over the course of human evolution makes that unlikely.

> Reactive oxygen species play a dual, seemingly contradictory role, with positive and negative effects on health. The "two-faced" character of ROS has now been clearly established.

It has long been known that ROS can destroy cells, both normal as well as invading bacteria. While high levels of ROS cause damage to the normal cells, low to intermediate levels actually play an important role in maintaining critical health functions including communication within and between cells of the body.

CAUSES AND SOURCES OF ROS

- Cellular respiration involving mitochondria and other components of the cells
- Environmental pollutants
- Low-grade inflammation over a long period of time
- Radiation (ultraviolet light, X-rays)
- Malnutrition

Current evidence has revealed new roles for ROS in health and disease. A proper understanding and manipulation of ROS can provide therapeutic targets to enhance the healing.

KEY FUNCTIONS OF ROS

These highly energetic and potent molecules interact with basic but critical biological components, like proteins, lipids, carbohydrates and DNA. They play a wide variety of key roles in the body:

- Immune defense
- Development and control of blood vessels
- Regulation of various hormones
- Communications among different parts of our cells, as well as between the cells of our tissues, promoting a "healthy team" for a healthy metabolism.
- Wound disinfection and clearance of dead cells, while promoting regeneration of healthy tissue to replace the diseased one
- Tissue regeneration and healing

Different ROS species also affect different genes and thus "control the destiny" of any cell. In short, ROS are *critical* to our healthy well-being.

MECHANISM OF HARMFUL EFFECTS OF ROS

Repair of injured tissues involves a finely-controlled balance of the beneficial and harmful effects of reactive oxygen species. ROS need to be kept under tight control in order to maximize the beneficial effects and minimize the harm.

Harm results when a finely-tuned balance of ROS and the body's antioxidant system is disrupted. While produced in well-synchronized amounts in a healthy body, the level of ROS increases dramatically in times of sickness or strenuous exercise.

Change of such a magnitude has potential for errors in any complex system, and ROS are no exception. When not well-controlled, ROS can induce dysfunctional changes in biologically-critical molecules like proteins, cell membranes, and DNA.

> ROS damage cells, especially the cell membranes. Although the body's antioxidant systems try to fight such damage, over a period of time, there is an increased risk of chronic illness.

HARMFUL EFFECTS OF ROS

The precise effect depends upon the amount, duration, and site of ROS generation. Both very low and very high levels are bad for health. While a lower level of ROS may increase risk of infection, an unusually high amount of ROS can damage or kill the body's own cells.

Evidence suggests that oxidative stress is a co-factor in a wide variety of diseases and aging processes. These actions are also, in part, associated with inflammation.

> While a decrease in or lack of ROS increases the risk for chronic granulomatous disease and autoimmune disorders, an excess of ROS is responsible for increasing cardiovascular and neurodegenerative diseases.

WHY DO WE HAVE MORE CHRONIC DISEASES NOW?

Inflammation is an important part of the body's defense mechanisms, and ROS are produced during inflammation as part of the body's fighting capacity. Both inflammation and ROS work hand-in-hand to stave of bad stimuli like infections.

It is easier for the genes and the body to gradually adapt to bad changes during the evolutionary process, leading to healthy natural selection and survival. However, the abrupt changes of the human diet, lifestyle, and environment that have occurred over the last few decades may not allow enough time for modification of the genes and the process of natural selection to occur. This has resulted in a mismatch between the rapidly changing modern environment and the body's defense strategies.

SOME DISEASES ASSOCIATED WITH OXIDATIVE STRESS

Heightened oxidative stress has been incriminated in a wide spectrum of disorders involving multiple organ systems, including:

- Autoimmune disorders
- Heart disease
- High blood pressure
- Diabetes
- Obesity
- Premature aging
- Parkinson's disease
- Skin eczema
- Autism and ADHD (ADD)

REFERENCES

1. Nathan C, Cunningham-Bussel A. Beyond oxidative stress: an immunologist's guide to reactive oxygen species. *Nat Rev Immunol*. 2013 May;13(5):349-61.
2. Babizhayev MA. New concept in nutrition for the maintenance of the aging eye redox regulation and therapeutic treatment of cataract disease; synergism of natural antioxidant imidazole-containing amino acid-based compounds, chaperone, and

glutathione boosting agents: a systemic perspective on aging and longevity emerged from studies in humans. *Am J Ther.* 2010 Jul-Aug;17(4):373-89.

Section VI
Healing Nutrition Plays Central Role in Seven-X Plan

CHAPTER 16

Paleolithic Diet: Learning From Our Ancestors

KEY POINTS

- There was a conspicuous absence of grains in the Paleolithic diet.
- The Paleolithic diet may be better than the diabetic diet or the Mediterranean diet for patients with diabetes.
- The best health benefits of the Paleolithic diet are accomplished when we exclude things that our ancestors did not eat, rather than following what they did.

According to Drs. Konner and Eaton from Emory University, anthropological evidence suggests that ancestral human diets were characterized by lower concentrations of "refined carbohydrates and sodium, much higher levels of fiber and protein, and comparable levels of fat (primarily unsaturated fat) and cholesterol." Higher levels of physical activity also caused higher energy utilization.

COMPONENTS OF ANCIENT HUMAN DIET

The diet was essentially what was available. This included fruit and berries, plant shoots, leaves and flowers, meats including organ meats, fish, insects, and eggs. The relative proportion of different components of food in the Paleolithic diet is debatable. Nevertheless, the Paleolithic diet components currently provide only about 25 percent of modern calorie intake.

Here is one huge difference between the Paleolithic diet and what we eat: there was a conspicuous absence of grains in the ancient diet.

Studies by Dr. Kuipers and colleagues published in the *British Journal of Nutrition* have documented much higher levels of long-chain polyunsaturated fatty acids (PUFA) and lower levels of lenoleic acid in ancient diet.

HEALTH IMPLICATIONS OF PALEOLITHIC DIET

Evolutionary Discordance Hypothesis states that deviations from diet, exercise, and lifestyle patterns of our hunter-gatherer ancestors are responsible for many of the chronic medical ailments that characterize our Western society.

> Modern-day diseases like atherosclerosis, obesity, and metabolic syndrome were extremely rare among ancient populations. They are still rare among tribal people in remote areas unaffected by modern influences and continuing the Paleolithic lifestyle.

Dr. Jonsson and colleagues from Lund University have shown that the Paleolithic diet is superior to the diabetic diet in improving glucose control and cardiovascular risk factors in patients with diabetes.

The Paleolithic diet is superior to the commonly-practiced Mediterranean diet for improving glucose tolerance and producing more satisfaction and "fullness" per calorie consumed in patients with heart disease.

THE PALEOLITHIC DIET IS HEALTHY DESPITE ITS "NONHEALTHY" COMPONENTS

Perhaps we are looking at the wrong concept. Instead of looking at what was *included* in the Paleolithic diet, clues for the absence of modern day diseases might lie in what was *absent*.

HEALTH CONCERNS OF PALEOLITHIC DIET

FRUIT IN PALEOLITHIC DIET AND CONCERN ABOUT HIGH FRUCTOSE CONSUMPTION

Fruit was a large component of the Paleolithic diet for at least 50 million years, with some changes occurring about 5 million years ago. Fructose in fruits comprises as much as 40 percent of the carbohydrate content. While high fructose ingestion has been linked to rising obesity and metabolic syndrome in modern society, consumption of less than 60 grams of fructose per day appears to be safe.

In addition to studies of hunter-gatherers, diet of non-human primates may provide clues. For example, fruits comprise as much as 75 percent of a chimpanzee's diet.

So how can we explain the lower incidence of obesity and metabolic syndrome in our ancestors? Most of the fructose in the modern world is derived from non-natural sources, such as refined sugars and high-fructose corn syrup. There may be differences in metabolic processes and health outcomes when fruit as a whole is consumed along with other plant components.

HIGH STARCH CONTENT OF PALEOLITHIC DIET AND HEALTH CONCERNS

Starchy foods became part of the staple diet about 1-2 million years ago. Just like fructose, high starch content has been implicated in obesity and cardiovascular disease, although it may not be the sole causative factor.

Studies by Dr. Lindeberg and colleagues from Lund University show that people from the island of Kitava in Africa are still consuming a Paleolithic diet, including high starch but unaffected by modern influences. However, no cases of heart disease and stroke have been seen in the population.

HIGH MEAT CONTENT OF PALEOLITHIC DIET AND HEALTH CONCERNS

Meat was consumed in substantial amounts early during evolution. Studies on different hunter-gatherer populations reveal that the majority of them consumed meat, fish, and shellfish for 26-68 percent of their energy needs. Adult chimpanzees consume about 65 grams of meat per day.

> Although high meat consumption in modern society has been linked (although not proven as a cause) to high cholesterol, hypertension, and heart disease, such disorders were uncommon among hunter-gatherers.

High fish content of the Paleolithic diet may in part explain the beneficial effects of fish on cholesterol and the heart. Omega-3 fatty acids in fish appear to shift the blood-fat profile towards healthy proportions and prevent coronary artery disease. This may not be the entire answer, since seafood availability early in evolution was at best sporadic, and consistent access to seafood for ancient humans occurred only after they left Africa.

Another potential explanation may lie in the fact that wild meat has low fat and higher omega-3 fatty acid content, compared to farmed animal meat. The same is true for wild fish as compared to farmed fish. In fact, most of fish consumed these days is farmed fish.

HIGH INSECT AND LARVAE CONTENT OF PALEOLITHIC DIET AND HEALTH CONCERNS

The fact that insects and larvae were a significant proportion of the Paleolithic diet in most early humans is not disputed. They continue to be a significant part of the non-human primate diet and are a rich source of proteins and calories. There is, however, a paucity of data on implications for health.

HIGH CONSUMPTION OF NUTS EARLY IN EVOLUTION AND HEALTH CONCERNS

Nuts are a rich source of proteins, fats, and carbohydrates. Overall consumption of nuts has been associated with a lower risk of heart disease.

HIGH CONSUMPTION OF SEEDS EARLY IN EVOLUTION AND HEALTH CONCERNS

Wild seeds were part of the Paleolithic diet but were not derived from the same family as wheat and rice. A large variety of seeds were consumed. No single seed type was used on a daily basis. Seeds also formed a small component of Paleolithic energy needs.

In contrast to the past, the modern diet contains fewer varieties of grains. Wheat and rice form a substantial portion of energy needs on a daily basis. The modern grain consumption may allow a toxic component from a "bad" grain to bombard the gut on a daily basis and gain access to the body to assert harmful effects in an otherwise vulnerable person.

CONTRASTING PALEOLITHIC DIET AND CURRENT DIET

As much as 75 percent of the current diet is derived from foods like wheat and other grains, dairy products, refined fats especially trans-type, and refined sugar. Sodium intake is high. Such foods were practically absent from the Paleolithic diet.

HEALTHY CLUES FROM PALEOLITHIC DIET

Obviously, it would be difficult to pinpoint why our ancestors on the Paleolithic diet had a lower incidence of heart disease and metabolic syndrome.

There is a possibility that modern-day ailments are more related to the foods that were *absent* early in the course of evolution. Perhaps Dr. Knight of University of Adelaide said it best when explaining the explosion in rates of obesity: "Most people are simply not designed to eat pasta."

Read about Dr. M's Strategies for Healing Nutrition in Chapter 46.

REFERENCES

1. Lindeberg S. Paleolithic diets as a model for prevention and treatment of Western disease. *Am J Hum Biol*. 2012 Mar-Apr; 24(2):110-5.
2. Jönsson T, Granfeldt Y, Erlanson-Albertsson C et al. A Paleolithic diet is more satiating per calorie than a mediterranean-like diet in individuals with ischemic heart disease. *Nutr Metab (Lond)*. 2010 Nov 30; 7:85.

CHAPTER 17

Gluten: What, How, and Why?

KEY POINTS

- A "gluten-free" product must contain fewer than 20 parts per million of gluten.
- Gluten may be present in unexpected places, like candy and medications. Always read labels carefully.
- A strict gluten-free diet has nutritional deficits that can be overcome by careful dietary planning.

Most people with celiac disease improve on a gluten-free diet, but there is increasing study on the use of a gluten-free diet in other patients. Patients with non-celiac gluten sensitivity have seen some beneficial effects; some studies even show benefits in patients with non-gastrointestinal disorders, like autism.

Studies conducted by Packaged Facts estimate that the sales of gluten-free products were $4.2 billion in 2012 and will rise as high as $6.6 billion by 2017.

WHAT IS GLUTEN AND GLUTEN-FREE?

The term "gluten" is used for a diverse complex of water-soluble proteins derived from wheat, rye, barley, and triticale (a cross between wheat and rye). This complex includes potentially toxic proteins: gliadins and glutenins.

INGREDIENTS EXCLUDED FROM GLUTEN-FREE PRODUCTS

Based on FDA and NIH publications, gluten-free food or product does not contain any of the following:

- A "prohibited grain": any species of wheat, rye, barley, or a crossbred hybrid of these grains
- Any ingredient derived from a prohibited grain that has not been processed to remove gluten (such as wheat flour)
- Products of prohibited grain that have been processed to remove gluten (such as wheat starch) with any products containing over 20 parts per million (ppm) of gluten

CONTAMINATION OF GLUTEN-FREE FOODS

- Patients may be consuming small amounts of gluten from hidden sources, like additives, preservatives, and stabilizers made with wheat.
- Many corn and rice products are produced in factories that also manufacture wheat products. They can get contaminated with wheat gluten.
- Cross-contamination of gluten into inherently gluten-free foods may occur. While oat contamination is the most talked about, cross-contamination with other grains, seeds, and flour is also a possibility.

Thompson and colleagues examined 22 gluten-free grains, seeds, and flours for gluten. The results were reported in the *Journal of American Dietetic Association*. Gluten was detected in 41 percent of the products, varying from 8.5 ppm to 2950 ppm. In fact, 32 percent of these products contained greater than the allowed 20 ppm.

THE GLUTEN-FREE DIET

A gluten-free diet means avoiding foods that contain rye, barley, and wheat. The foods and food products made from these grains should also be avoided. Patients should avoid most grain, pasta, cereal, and many processed foods.

Patients can get complete nutrition by eating a well-balanced diet with a variety of foods; however, a dietary consultation to accomplish this goal may be important.

NUTRITION IMPLICATIONS OF GLUTEN FREE DIET

Unless properly undertaken, the gluten-free diet tends to be:

- High-fat
- Low-carbohydrate
- Low-fiber
- Low in elements/minerals (iron, zinc, calcium, phosphorus)
- Low in vitamins (B3, folic acid, Vitamin B12)

OVERCOMING NUTRITIONAL SHORTCOMINGS OF THE GLUTEN-FREE DIET

- Consume whole grains like brown rice, wild rice, whole corn, sorghum, teff, amaranth, quinoa, and buckwheat.
- Consume enriched or supplemented gluten-free products.
- Take vitamin-mineral supplements.
- Consume healthy amounts of vegetables and fruit.
- Eat legumes, seeds, and nuts, as allowed. Many nuts contain allergens and may need to be avoided as appropriate.
- Non-vegetarians should prefer fish, lean meats, and poultry over red meat. All fish do not have similar effects on health.
- Drink milk (if allowed) or milk substitutes, like gluten-free soy milk or almond milk, as tolerated.
- Consume calcium-rich foods or calcium-enriched gluten-free products.
- Choose products with lower fat content. You should say no to *trans-fat*.

- Most importantly, seek consultation with a dietician.

ALLOWED GLUTEN-FREE ALTERNATIVES

- Amaranth, buckwheat, bean flour, pea flour, potato, rice, soy, and quinoa
- Gluten-free bread and pasta
- Arrowroot, cassava, corn, flax, Indian rice grass, legumes, millet, nuts, job's tears, sago, seeds, sorghum, soy, tapioca, teff, wild rice, and yucca

COMMON FOODS DEVOID OF GLUTEN

"Plain" meat, fish, rice, fruits, and vegetables do not contain gluten; people with celiac disease can eat these foods.

LOOK OUT FOR THE FOLLOWING ON PRODUCTS NOT LABELED GLUTEN-FREE

- Wheat
- Rye
- Barley
- Malt
- Oats (do not consume if not labeled gluten-free)
- Brewer's yeast

EXERCISE EXTRA CARE IN THE FOLLOWING PLACES

- Restaurants
- Lunch at school or work
- Grocery store
- Parties
- Snack vending machines

GLUTEN MAY SOMETIMES BE PRESENT IN UNEXPECTED PLACES

- Medications

- Additive in products like lipstick and Play-Doh
- Meat, poultry, and egg products
- Candy, potato chips, sauces (especially soy sauce), cold cuts, sausage, gravy, imitation sea food, and soups

Most of these foods can be found gluten-free. When in doubt, check with the food manufacturer.

A FEW WORDS ON WHEAT STARCH

According to the *Academy of Nutrition and Dietetics*, "Studies have shown that both natural and wheat starch based [gluten-free] diets produce similar histological and clinical recovery in people with [celiac disease]."

Wheat starch may be included in gluten-free foods if it has been processed for gluten content down to less than 20 ppm. However, most gluten-free products do not include that, as many patients consuming gluten-free diet are inclined to avoid it.

GLUTEN AND OATS CONTROVERSY

Most people can safely eat small amounts of oats (up to 50 grams of dry oats per day), as long as the oats are not contaminated with gluten during mill processing.

According to a study published in the *New England Journal of Medicine*, gluten content of commercial oat products not labeled as gluten-free varies widely. Mean gluten content of four lots of Quaker Old-Fashioned Oats was found to vary from 338 ppm to 1807 ppm. Another brand, McCann's Street Cut Irish Oats, contained as few as three ppm and as many as 725 ppm of gluten, depending upon the lot.

In fact, the researcher concluded in her report, "None of the three brands of oats included in this assessment could be relied on to be gluten-free."

A WORD ABOUT OAT AVENIN

A few patients with celiac disease have avenin sensitivity. Avenin is a protein found in oats with properties similar to gluten. It may cause problems in patients with gluten sensitivity. Oat avenin contains glutinous proteins similar to wheat gliadin. As such, some celiac disease patients may have an adverse immune reaction to oat avenin.

Note: Parts of this chapter have been taken from or adapted from publications by U.S. National Institute of Diabetes and Digestive and Kidney Diseases and the U.S. Food and Drug Administration.

REFERENCES

1. Thompson T. Gluten contamination of commercial oat products in the United States. *N Engl J Med*. 2004 Nov 4; 351(19):2021-2.
2. Saturni L, Ferretti G, Bacchetti T. The gluten-free diet: safety and nutritional quality. *Nutrients*. 2010 Jan; 2(1):16-34.

CHAPTER 18

Increasing Wheat Consumption and Gluten Related Sickness

KEY POINTS

- There was a massive rise in production and consumption of wheat in the mid-20th century, in order to meet the rising needs during the war.
- New varieties of wheat were developed to increase production. However, some of these also have a much higher gluten content.
- Adverse reaction to a toxin depends in part on the amount of the toxin consumed.
- Celiac disease is a textbook example of gluten-related sickness.

SOURCES AND FATE OF INGESTED PROTEINS

Proteins are combinations and permutations of naturally-occurring amino acids. Sources of dietary proteins include animal muscle, milk, egg, and plants.

- Muscle proteins are derived from the ingested meat.
- Most of milk protein is comprised of caseins and whey proteins.
- Egg proteins are contained in both the egg white and yolk.
- Sources of plant proteins include cereals, lentils, and beans.

The intestines digest dietary proteins into smaller components so that they can be absorbed into the body. The digestion in the gut occurs via digestive enzymes that break the protein down into simple amino acids or combinations of amino acids known as peptides.

Larger peptides are further broken down into amino acids or smaller peptides. The absorbed breakdown products are then utilized by the body for energy needs and synthesis of other proteins.

Some of the breakdown products of gluten can bind to morphine-like opioid binding sites in the brain and are known as *exorphins*. Similar compounds generated in the body are called *endorphins*.

DISCRIMINANT ROLE OF GUT

The digestion and absorption process is complicated by the presence of many intestinal bacteria, proteins, and toxins in the gut. The immune system of the gut "samples" protein and bacteria to distinguish between harmful and harmless and deals with them accordingly.

A healthy gut does not provoke any reaction from our immune system when interacting with dietary proteins or harmless bacteria. If sampling reveals that the protein or bacteria is foreign and potentially harmful, a protective inflammation response is generated.

FATE OF PROTEINS IN IMMATURE/UNHEALTHY GUT

The gut and GI immune system may sometimes be inadequately developed. This can occur due to complex interactions of early age, unhealthy genes, or exposure to environmental injury that make the gut wall barrier highly permeable or leaky.

The breakdown of the selective intestinal barrier in the presence of immature immune system allows for sensitization to food proteins or allergens which might not have occurred in a healthy system. Food protein-related allergic reactions are seen in many cases of asthma, hives, and eczema. A leaky gut also allows for larger molecules to pass through the gut, allowing them access to the entire body, including the brain.

DIETARY PROTEINS OF INTEREST IN BRAIN DYSFUNCTION

Two dietary sources of proteins have been getting increasing attention for their widespread effects in the body, especially neurobehavioral dysfunction. These are the gluten from grains and casein from cow's milk proteins. We will discuss milk in subsequent chapters.

There is some evidence that public opinion about changing dietary habits may be far ahead of the scientific community, which is trying to figure out whether such claims are valid.

GLUTEN

Adverse response to gluten is not just seen in celiac disease. Rather, there is a wide spectrum of gluten-related disorders, including non-celiac gluten sensitivity. Patients suffer symptoms on exposure to gluten-related products and improve upon gluten exclusion. Likewise, celiac disease not only affects the gut; its effects can extend beyond the gut, including skin diseases and cancer.

WHEAT GLUTEN AS PART OF OUR DIET

Wheat is the most popular grain grown, followed closely by rice and corn. Most of the dietary wheat is ingested in a processed form, such as pasta, pizza, bread, and cakes.

Wheat was originally grown in the Fertile Crescent of southwestern Asia. This region was the birthplace of the first ancient civilizations; hence, it has been labeled the cradle of civilization. Older strains of wheat grown during the Middle Ages contained much fewer toxic proteins than that are presently available.

RAPID RISE IN WHEAT CONSUMPTION IN THE 20TH CENTURY

With the start of World War II and the rationing preceding it, many parts of the world experienced a big push to increase agricultural production to meet the nutritional needs of the population. Even the establishment of the Nutrition Society in Britain in 1941 had its roots in the underlying goal of increasing wheat production. Not surprisingly, the world wheat production by the end of the 20th century had increased by 500 percent.

> While technology has allowed development of newer wheat varieties, many of these have a higher gluten content.

RESULT OF RISING WHEAT CONSUMPTION

Our original genes were based on a hunter-gatherer diet. The movement from a Paleolithic diet to an agriculture-based diet several thousand years ago marked a dramatic evolutionary swing.

This move to an agriculture-based diet marked a critical defiance of the well-established earliest human immune system. The result was the abrupt assault on the gut defenses and the immune system, leading to the advent of gluten-related diseases. Wheat allergy and celiac disease has been with us since then. Baker's asthma, due to inhalation of wheat and cereal flour, has been with us since the ancient Roman Empire.

Increasing wheat production by utilizing newer varieties of wheat in the mid- to late 20th century finally broke the camel's back.

INCREASINGLY HIGH GLUTEN EXPOSURE IN DIET

Increasing the amount of potentially toxic compounds over a "short" period of evolution can make the human gene system and the body's defenses unable to adapt. Current consumption of gluten worldwide is the highest it has ever been.

> This high consumption may allow the body to be overwhelmed by the large amount of toxic exposure, even in subjects at lower risk to develop illness.

DISORDERS ASSOCIATED WITH GLUTEN

The rapidly increasing proportion of the population potentially affected by gluten makes one wonder how and why gluten is so toxic to so many in so many different ways.

- Celiac disease
- Non-celiac gluten sensitivity: Patients have diarrhea and frequently are diagnosed with irritable bowel syndrome (IBS)
- Dermatitis herpetiformis, a skin disease found in many patients with Celiac disease
- Gluten ataxia, a disease involving the cerebellum part of the brain
- Autoimmune diseases (Type-1 diabetes, Addison's disease, autoimmune hepatitis)

HOW DO DIFFERENT CLINICAL SYNDROMES OCCUR IN DIFFERENT PATIENTS?

The variation in immune reaction suggests that the response to harmful substances depends in part upon the patient's genetic vulnerability to certain disorders. But studies suggest that genetics can only explain part of the problem. Research on the other potential factors involved is in its infancy. Although evidence is limited, current data points to the following:

- The variety of skin, cancerous, and neurobehavioral symptoms may depend upon how our diet and environmental toxins affect our genes, gut, skin, brain, and other parts of our bodies.

- Some gluten breakdown products have an affinity for morphine-like opioid binding sites in the brain. These are called exorphins and they have the potential to affect brain.
- Not all gluten breakdown products absorbed are the same, creating another element of complexity in variability among patients. Different gluten peptides may bind selectively to different areas of brain, creating symptoms unique to that part of the brain.
- The total amount of gluten that a person consumes also plays a role. For example, some people may be able to handle small amounts without adverse consequences, while becoming symptomatic on further ingestion. That may be one of the reasons underlying the Food and Drug Administration's push to define gluten-free foods with much lower gluten content than before.

The final clinical outcome depends upon how the body's immune system reacts to the toxic breakdown products of gluten. For example, different reactions in different areas of the brain would lead to different behavioral changes. These complex interactions depend upon the body's immune architecture and its manifestations (depressed or excess), depending upon the other environmental factors interacting with the genes.

REFERENCES

1. Sapone A, Bai JC, Ciacci C et al. Spectrum of gluten-related disorders: consensus on new nomenclature and classification. *BMC Med*. 2012 Feb 7; 10:13.

CHAPTER 19

Cow's Milk: The Good, the Bad, the Ugly

KEY POINTS

- Milk from each species is different and designed to meet the needs of that particular species.
- Experience with animals across nature tells us that lactation, breastfeeding, and milk consumption are meant to be for a limited duration.
- Milk and dairy products are part of the *MyPlate* menu recommended by U.S. government agencies.

Before we start, let us just stipulate that, irrespective of the source, milk is full of nutritious components. Let us also stipulate that cow's milk overall has served as a good source of nutrition to humans over thousands of years.

Cow's milk has been an essential component of the everyday adult diet. It is a good source of proteins, vitamins, and minerals. In fact, dairy and dairy products are an important component of the *MyPlate* menu recommended by the Centers for Diseases Control.

EVOLUTIONARY UNDERSTANDING ABOUT MILK

According to Oftedal from the Smithsonian Environmental Research Center, as published in the journal *Animal*, the evolutionary origin of milk goes back to its secretion from the skin glands about 310 million years ago. In fact, the origin of nutritious milk may predate the origin of mammals.

The mammary glands likely arose from skin glands along with the hair follicles. Along the way, different components of milk, both nutritious and non-nutritious defensive components, came into being for delivery to the helpless baby.

Changes in digestive enzymes and bioactive metabolic compounds came about as a result of the evolution of new types of sugars.

During the late Triassic period (200-250 million years ago), milk replaced egg as the primary source of nutrition for newborns. However, the framework of milk, with its main components, occurred prior to the appearance of mammals. Thus the roots of the milk industry were established long before the dinosaur era.

Modern milk owes its origin to the continued changes in milk and mammary genes over the course of evolution, allowing for selection and conservation of beneficial genes based on different needs of the evolving species.

MILK AND THE LACTATION PROCESS

Milk is a biologic fluid that is a unique feature of mammals. Unlike the standardized formula feed, biologic milk is a dynamic fluid that changes to meet the needs of the baby as it grows.

Milk at the time of birth is not the same as the milk when the baby is one week old. Nature created milk as a maternal lactating secretion, a nutrient and defense complex for the newborn during its most vulnerable period of life. Subsequently, as the baby's own defenses come to fruition, the weaning process occurs.

SO WHAT HAS CHANGED?

CHANGES IN GENES

Our core genes have stayed relatively stable, with some mutations or epigenetic phenomenon along the way, over tens of thousands of years of evolution.

ROLE OF EPIGENETICS

The mere presence of a gene does not mean that it is functionally active. Genes could be present in the cells but silent.

- Epigenetics is the study of changes in the functioning of the genes as a result of environmental factors (such as diet or toxins).
- Changes in gene functioning may involve turning the gene "on" or "off." These functional changes can be genetically passed on to the next generation of the animal. An example of non-genetic influences affecting the functioning of genes is the cessation of milk secretion when the breasts are inflamed and/or infected, or as the breasts shrink.

Other cow-related factors with the potential to affect gene functioning include tight living conditions, use of hormones, and antibiotics.

WE HAVE CHANGED, AS HAS OUR ENVIRONMENT

Ancient humans lived as part of nature as 'hunter-gatherers.' We now have a fast-paced world, higher environmental pollution, and a relatively sedentary lifestyle.

It is not surprising that our genes are not functioning the same way as they did in ancient times, when human beings actually had to hunt for food rather than just driving to the supermarket.

THE COWS HAVE CHANGED

Even the cows don't drink the cow's milk we do. Cows drink milk from free-living cows, while we drink milk from caged animals. The cow's milk consumed by humans is not "natural" since it is:

- Modified due to specialized and selective breeding,
- Altered by unnatural living conditions,
- Altered by drugs and hormones administered to the cows to increase milk yield, and
- Altered by antibiotics given to cows for frequent infections.

INCREASING MILK PRODUCTION TO MEET 20TH- CENTURY DEMANDS

The average herd size in developed countries has been increasing dramatically in recent years, as has been the annual milk production per cow. Dairy cattle are now bred with the purpose of increasing milk production.

Cows in Israeli dairy farms produce 12,546 kg of milk per year, compared to cows in New Zealand, which yield 4,100 kg per year. The factors affecting the yield include production systems and cows' diet. For example, cows in New Zealand graze freely all year; in Israel, the cows are fed an energy-rich mixed diet in closed quarters.

> However, cow's milk itself cannot be the sole factor in causing problems in humans. A genetic vulnerability is critical, along with many other factors, including pollution.

FUNCTIONS OF MILK

Milk is not just a source of energy and building blocks for growth and development. It plays an important role in immune health, especially during the early vulnerable period of life. Milk proteins can act as enzymes, antibacterial agents, and hormones.

Many breakdown products of milk proteins have biological functions like the modification of the immune system, enzyme systems, and platelets.

ALL MILK IS NOT THE SAME

The composition of human milk is different depending upon the time of day, age of the baby, mother's diet, race, and ethnicity. Likewise, all cow's milk is not the same. Composition of cow's milk depends on breed, season, living conditions, and type of feed.

SPECIES-SPECIFIC MAMMALIAN MILK

Milk of each mammal is unique and intended to meet the needs of the newborn of each species. Thus, cow's milk has a much higher level of proteins designed to help with skeletal and muscular growth than human milk.

> Human milk is not just a source of energy for the baby. Humans have a highly developed nervous system, and the milk fed to human babies must be commensurate to the growth and development of this nervous system relative to the musculoskeletal system.

We should not just look at the macronutrient composition of milk, but also micronutrients and the relative proportions. Looking at cow's milk through this prism, it is clear and not surprising that cow's milk is simply not designed for humans. For example, cow's milk has blood components, albeit in small amounts, with potential to cause problems in at-risk individuals.

Non-nutritive bioactive factors in a mother's milk include growth factors to promote growth and development, maternal immune cells, antibodies, and other antimicrobial substances to fight against infections, erythropoietin to support blood formation, and prebiotic oligosaccharides to promote beneficial gut bacteria.

MERITS OF DRINKING COW'S MILK

Cow's milk is a near-complete source of nutrition for the human body. It is rich in calcium, phosphorus, and vitamin D. Among animal sources of nutrition, cow's milk is perhaps the most economical source of protein and many micronutrients. It serves as a valuable means for prevention and treatment of malnutrition in developing countries.

Besides the obvious nutritional benefit, there are other bioactive ingredients, as well. For example, some protein components in cow's milks lower blood pressure. Data suggests lower incidence of high blood pressure among people drinking milk.

NUTRITIONAL DEFICITS OF COW'S MILK

The use of cow's milk is constantly in lay press as well as peer-reviewed journals with respect to its association with iron deficiency anemia, lactose intolerance, diabetes, and many neurobehavioral disorders. The connection is controversial.

Perhaps one of the biggest nutritional deficits is low iron content. To make things worse, cow's milk prevents absorption of iron in the human baby. The iron deficit in those consuming cow's milk exclusively may be exacerbated by occult (hidden) bleeding from the gut, seen in as many as 40 percent of babies fed cow's milk.

WHY DO WE DRINK COW'S MILK?

Obviously cow's milk is a great source of nutrition, especially in developing countries. While we drink cow's milk based on culture and tradition, is it wise and healthy?

There is a good reason why milk of every animal is distinct and naturally designed to fulfill the needs of that particular species. Just look at a cow. Does the cow bear any similarity to the human in size, height, musculoskeletal structure, or intelligence?

Is it really plausible that it was God or nature's plan for one species to consume milk from another? If indeed it was her intention for us to drink cow's milk, would the milk from all species – or at least the cow and the human – not be similar? While it may be good for many people in certain circumstances, it may not be good for all.

COMPONENTS OF MILK

Human milk contains about 12 g of protein, 35 g of fat and 70 g of lactose per liter.

PROTEINS

Milk proteins are mainly comprised of caseins and whey.

Whey protein complex includes include alfa-lactoalbumin, lactoferrin, antibodies, lysozyme, and albumin.

The proportion of various proteins in the milk varies by species and breed. These proteins are digested in the gut into smaller components for absorption. For any species, the higher the protein content, the faster that offspring can double its weight.

While the protein content of the milk (colostrum) when the baby is born is as high as 2.3 percent, the mature human milk is just 1 percent protein.

The types of caseins are also different between the two species.

Most mammalian milk has three or four types of caseins. Caseins form only about 40 percent of the total human protein. In contrast to 1 percent protein in human milk, the cow's milk has 3.4 percent protein with as much as 84 percent of it being caseins.

Whey has been recognized as beneficial since ancient times. An ancient proverb states, "If everyone was raised on whey, doctors would be bankrupt." There are remarkable differences between cow and human milk with respect to the whey proteins. The level of alpha-lactoalbumin in human milk is twice as high as in cow's milk.

Human milk has high concentrations of lactoferrin, an important antibacterial and anti-inflammatory multi-functional protein, which also stimulates cell growth. Lactoferrin is present in cow's milk in only minimal amounts. The total antibody levels in human milk are much higher than cow's milk.

BENEFITS OF CASEIN DURING EARLY LIFE

Dr. Fiat asserts that a "strategic zone" containing immune-stimulating and opioid peptides occurs among the cow as well as human beta-caseins.

Studies By Dr. Tanabe and colleagues suggest that protein breakdown products (peptides) derived from the digestion of casein in the milk can strengthen the intestinal barrier, reinforcing the importance of breastfeeding for growth and immune defenses of the baby.

CARBOHYDRATES IN MILK

Carbohydrates in milk are mainly composed of lactose. Human milk has much higher lactose than cow's milk (6.6 percent versus 4.8 percent). In addition, human milk also provides 10 grams per liter of non-digestible oligosaccharides. These act as a prebiotic and promote the growth of beneficial protective gut bacteria in the infant.

FATS

Fat content of human milk is 3.9 percent, compared to 3.7 percent in cow's milk. While the total fat content is not too far apart, there are marked differences in the fatty acid and triglyceride composition.

Fatty acids

Human milk has a much higher concentration of important essential fatty acids compared to cow's milk.

Cow's milk has more short-chain and saturated fatty acids and very few long-chain polyunsaturated fatty acids compared to human milk. In fact, cow's milk has only about 0.2 percent of polyunsaturated fatty acids.

Saturated fatty acids (1.9 percent) are thought to contribute to heart disease, increased cholesterol, and obesity. However, not all saturated fatty acids are bad. Some of these saturated fatty acids, like butyric acid, may actually be beneficial for health as well.

- Breastfed infants have a higher concentration of docosahexaenoic acid (DHA) than formula-fed infants. Studies by Dr. Gale and colleagues indicate that children fed breast milk or DHA-fortified formula during infancy have a higher full-scale and verbal I.Q. scores by the age of four years, compared to those fed unfortified formula.
- A mother's consumption of cod liver oil, which contains important fatty acids, improves her child's I.Q., compared to moms provided with a corn-oil supplementation.

This suggests that mother's milk is better able than formula to provide key nutrients in a balanced fashion for optimal development of the brain.

The proteins in human milk are balanced and more tuned to human digestive and absorption processes. This meets the baby's unique protein requirements while protecting the baby's immature kidneys from an overload of protein wastes.

For example, human milk casein, when processed in the baby's gut, mimics a morphine-like substance called casomorphin that can affect the baby's mood and behavior. This early priming of behavior may have life-long impact of the personality profile.

A recent study by Dr. Andres and colleagues from the Arkansas Children's Nutrition Center puts the spotlight on differences between human milk, cow's milk-based formula, and soy-based formula milk. While there was no difference between cow-based or soy-based formula milk consumption, the breastfed babies fared better on cognitive function and performance tests at six and twelve months of age.

Similar study by Dr. Jing and colleagues showed that functioning of the brain as indicated by its electrical activity differed between those who are breastfed and with those fed milk-based or soy formula. There were no differences in brain activity between cow's milk- or formula-fed infants, highlighting the importance of human milk for humans.

Above reports suggest that one or more components of breast milk may be critical to cognitive development.

HUMAN MILK IS NOT PERFECT

Mom's milk meets the nutritional needs of babies for six months, except for vitamins D and K. Infants may benefit from an injection of vitamin K. Similarly, breastfed infants should get vitamin D supplementation.

Human milk is low in docosahexaenoic acid (DHA), so supplementation may be needed in exclusively breastfed babies.

Maternal diet varies, and it affects the composition of milk. As such, it is prudent for lactating moms to take multivitamin-mineral supplements.

HUMAN CONSUMPTION OF COW'S MILK

Cow's milk has become part of staple diet based on our culture and traditions. But has it become a problem in recent decades, at least more so in the developed countries?

While many of us may be able to handle cow's milk reasonably well, subjects at risk may be harmed. Subjects at risk include:

- Those with unhealthy genes,
- Those with a deficiency of digestive enzymes, which does not allow the gut to break down the relative high amounts of proteins like casein, and
- Those with leaky gut, which allows passage of larger, semi-digested breakdown products across the gut wall into the body.

> The potentially adverse impact of cow's milk may in part be a function of "unnatural" alterations in the cow's milk produced by a variety of methods used to increase the amount of milk produced.

POTENTIAL FOR ALLERGY

Human milk is less likely to cause allergic reaction in the baby, as it lacks many of the foreign proteins present in cow's milk. For example, milk from different animals all contain alpha-lactoalbumin but with slightly different structures. It is not surprising that lactoalbumin in human milk is best tolerated by human babies.

While some kids who are allergic to cow's milk may still be able to drink goat's milk, camel's milk has less cross-sensitivity with cow's milk and is a better alternative than goat's milk for children with cow's milk allergy.

MILK IS NOT THE PROBLEM, IT'S WHERE IT COMES FROM

In contrast to cow's milk that is homogenized and pasteurized, human milk is uniquely constructed to meet a human baby's needs. Mom's milk for the baby provides highly individualized nutrition for the particular baby, based on the stage of infancy along with bioactive immune-beneficial compounds.

Each human's milk can be different from the next, based on changing needs of the baby, while the cow's milk stays same.

The importance of proper nutrition in early life is highlighted by the fact that premature infants need dietary quality more than quantity for optimal growth and development. Studies suggest that dietary pattern during infancy and early childhood affects development of brain.

Since human milk is just produced for one baby, it is produced in smaller amounts, usually about 600-900 ml per day. In contrast, cow's milk is produced in large quantities for bulk consumption.

HOW CAN COW'S MILK CAUSE HARM TO CERTAIN PEOPLE?

When consuming another animal's product, potentially coded and critical genetic information can be passed on from the producer to the consumer – in this case, from cow to human. Such metabolic information may be useful or harmful; in some cases, it may be beneficial to the producer while being harmful to the consumer of the milk.

We know that casein in the milk is digested into a variety of smaller breakdown products or peptides with actual biological activity. These smaller peptides are capable of attaching to the morphine-like opioid binding areas in the brain, producing functional changes in the signaling and messaging networks.

This is not just a wild theory.

- Studies of milk have documented opioids occurring freely, as well as bound to other substances in the milk. This is one example of an external influence of one species (cow) on the other (human).
- Some of the synthetic casein byproducts act especially on mu-type opioid receptors and are widely used as an opioid tool for research purposes. Much of the data for the functional role for casein byproducts pertains to beta-casomorphins.

- The antibodies to cow's caseins are increased in patients with schizophrenia.
- Actions and interactions of casein byproducts in acting as "food hormone" in the body, especially during infancy and early childhood, may theoretically alter the brain function and even reset "normal" brain function.

According to Dr. Roncada and colleagues from Italy, there may be a latent biologic or metabolic activity that becomes unmasked when the proteins are broken down into smaller peptides.

One factor that determines the adverse effects of any toxic substance is the total amount of toxin. The human body is able to handle breast milk with low casein proteins for a short time during infancy. However, depending upon predilection, it may not be able to handle a constant bombardment of a toxic substance (like casein from cow's milk) day after day for the rest of the person's life. Such is even more likely if the exposure is in the absence of potentially protective metabolic substances in milk.

Consistent with this theory, studies from Dr. Nakamura's laboratory have demonstrated that consuming predigested casein increases work efficiency, stabilizes brain activity, and reduces anxiety.

WHY IS COW'S NOT HARMFUL TO EVERYONE? THINK EPIGENETICS.

It should be noted that milk is not the sole culprit for a disease when it occurs, but likely acts in conjunction with other insults whose onslaught forms a big insult and causes damage.

Other insults may include living in areas exposed to high traffic or war pollution, eating a high-gluten diet, and consuming meat from animals exposed to pesticides and contaminated with antibiotics.

POTENTIAL IMPACT OF CONTINUED MILK CONSUMPTION

Mother's milk is not just critical for the brain. Babies that are not breastfed are usually fed cow's milk-based formula. However, this strategy only increases the long-term risk of a variety of diseases, like diabetes, obesity, and allergies.

> Humans are the only species that consume milk past infancy. In some persons, the continued lifetime exposure to very high concentrations of casein of cow's proteins has the potential to cause continued and worsening damage in those vulnerable to such toxicity. And, of course, the ability to digest lactose declines past childhood and has its own potential for problems.

Breastfed and formula-fed babies have a different growth curve, fewer infections, and a reduced risk for many diseases, like celiac disease, diabetes, obesity, hypertension, allergies, and high cholesterol. Lack of breastfeeding has been implicated in the causation of inflammatory bowel disease and autism.

A recent systematic review by Pereira and colleagues concluded that the absence of breastfeeding is a modifiable risk factor for development of diabetes. Breastfeeding is of benefit to moms as well. It reduces the risk of breast cancer!

INFANTILE COLIC

Babies fed cow's milk tend to have more problems with infantile colic. Kids get relief from the colicky pain when they are fed pre-digested cow's milk, suggesting that the deficiency of digestive processes in the baby leads to colic.

Dr. Lacovou and colleagues from the Monash University in Clayton, Australia, conducted a meta-analysis of the health impact of dietary management of infantile colic and published their findings in the journal *Maternal and Child Health*. They concluded that switching from cow's milk formula to predigested protein-based or soy-based formula reduces infantile colic.

COW'S MILK ALLERGY

Cow's milk allergy is a well-known, widely prevalent, and growing problem in the West. It occurs in about 2 to 5 percent of kids. Allergic reaction is usually due to milk's casein and/or whey proteins. It should be noted that some of the cow's milk allergens like bovine alpha-1 casein may also be found in human milk, but usually do not cause problems. Treatment involves complete exclusion of milk from diet. Sensitivity to cow's milk may also occur without the involvement of allergy mechanisms.

Switching animal source of milk may help. Studies by Dr. Monti's laboratory indicate that donkey milk is well-tolerated by kids with a cow's milk allergy. Current evidence suggests that modification of intestinal bacteria using pre- and probiotics may be a possible therapeutic target for kids with cow's milk allergy.

LACTOSE INTOLERANCE: LACTASE DEFICIENCY OR LACTOSE SENSITIVITY?

Milk contains a large amount of lactose. Lactose intolerance is not the same as milk allergy. Most patients with lactose intolerance can tolerate about a glass of milk per day, especially when taken with a meal. Fermented milk is better tolerated since it contains less lactose.

It should be noted that most of us digest lactose very well in early childhood, and the ability declines as we grow older.

Perhaps Mother Nature is trying to tip us off!

The cause of lactose intolerance is deficiency of the lactase enzyme, which breaks down the lactose in milk. The prevalence of lactose intolerance is high worldwide, depending upon race and ethnicity and reaching as high as 90 percent in some populations.

The prevalence is low in Caucasians of Northern European descent and very high in Hispanics and African-Americans.

No wonder there has been an explosion of lactose-free products in the grocery store. Patients frequently suffer nausea, abdominal pain, and diarrhea.

Lactose intolerance is not as simple as it sounds. Controlled studies have actually shown that the severity of symptoms is not related to the severity of lactase deficiency.

Many patients continue to have symptoms after switching to a lactose-free diet, suggesting other factors may be at play. Could it be a "milk sensitivity" that is causing the GI symptoms?

Studies by Dr. Olivier and co-investigators indicate that sensitization to cow's milk, as manifested by increased antibodies to cow's milk proteins, may be involved.

EFFECT OF MILK ON GROWTH AND OTHER LONG-TERM CONSEQUENCES

According to Dr. Molgaard and colleagues from the Department of Human Nutrition, University of Copenhagen, milk stimulates linear growth during childhood by its effect on hormones and the immune system. Its effect on insulin-like growth factor and insulin may have positive or negative long-term consequences.

In fact, Dr. Thorsdottir and colleagues reviewed effects of the consumption of cow's milk in early infancy and deemed it as having "unfortunate effects on growth, especially weight acceleration and development of overweight in childhood."

ACNE

According to Dr. Melnik from the University of Osnabrück, Germany, the "rising incidence of acne in the Western society may be related to increased insulin- and IGF-1-stimulation of sebaceous glands mediated by milk consumption." Hormonal changes induced by cow's milk cause changes in sebaceous glands leading to acne.

CANCER

Recombinant bovine growth hormone (rBGH) increases cows' milk production by as much as 15 percent. This is allowed in the U.S. but banned in the European Union.

Cows given rBGH have increased concentrations of insulin-like growth factor (IGF-1) According to the American Cancer Society, while there may be a link between IGF-1 blood levels and cancer, the exact nature of this link remains unclear.

AUTISM

The opioid excess theory suggests that autism is a neuro-metabolic malfunction, wherein large amounts of biologically-active morphine-like opioid compounds from the breakdown of gluten and casein are absorbed through the leaky gut and enter the brain. They bind to the opioid binding sites in different regions of the brain affecting brain function.

Such a situation may occur in subjects who drink cow's milk but also have leaky gut with defective or deficient digestive enzymes. Continued consumption of cow's milk in such cases allows metabolically active chemicals to enter the brain in toxic amounts.

> Absorption of toxic compounds is likely to be higher during early formative years of life when the intestinal barrier is not mature. This fact alone can contribute to an increased harmful effect on the brain during its critical period of development.

It is noteworthy that a recent Israeli government report of social services documented a 500 percent increase of autism in Israel between 2004 and 2011. (The absolute numbers are quite low, however, compared to the West.) This may in part be related to awareness of autism, the stigma of autism diagnosis, and differences in health delivery programs.

FINALLY, A LINK BETWEEN GLUTEN AND IRRITABLE BOWEL SYNDROME (IBS)

For many years, patients were complaining that their IBS would get better upon excluding gluten from their diet. However, the medical community frequently poked fun at that notion, since these patients did fulfill criteria for diagnosis of celiac disease. We know from clinical studies that many of the patients with IBS have what we call "non-celiac gluten sensitivity."

Likewise, numerous parents report that their kids with various disorders (like eczema, colic, or acne) get better when milk is excluded from their diet. Perhaps similar mechanisms are involved.

HEALTH CONSIDERATIONS BEYOND CONSUMING COW'S MILK

Long-term milking of cows increases the risk of breast infections like mastitis requiring antibiotic for treatment. Low levels of antibiotics can also be detected in milk that we consume.

Such antibiotic exposure in the gut can alter the gut flora, affecting the whole body, especially the immune system. In addition, this contributes to the rise in drug resistant bacteria, which can afflict us just like any other animals.

IS MILK TOTALLY BAD?

Milk is not bad. Infants should drink milk, preferably their mother's milk, and then be weaned off. The problem is that it is difficult to clearly define who may be at risk or benefit from exclusion of cow's milk before a disorder occurs. Even then, literature on problems related to cow's milk is mostly circumstantial. At the other end, it is hard to ignore the fact that cow's milk has been a boon for preventing malnutrition, especially in the developing countries. Until more hard data is available, the debate will continue to be opinion-based and passionate. Do you own due diligence.

REFERENCES

1. Zhang Z, Adelman AS, Rai D et al. Amino Acid Profiles in Term and Preterm Human Milk through Lactation: A Systematic Review. *Nutrients.* 2013 Nov 26;5(12):4800-21

2. Bode L. Human milk oligosaccharides: every baby needs a sugar mama. *Glycobiology.* 2012 Sep; 22(9):1147-62.

3. Tekinşen KK, Eken HS. Aflatoxin M1 levels in UHT milk and kashar cheese consumed in Turkey. *Food Chem Toxicol.* 2008 Oct; 46(10):3287-9.

4. Maskatia ZK, Davis CM. Perinatal environmental influences on goat's and sheep's milk allergy without cow's milk allergy. *Ann Allergy Asthma Immunol.* 2013 Dec; 111(6):574-5.

5. Fleischer DM, Spergel JM, Assa'ad AH, Pongracic JA. Primary prevention of allergic disease through nutritional interventions. *J Allergy Clin Immunol Pract.* 2013 Jan; 1(1):29-36.

6. Kamal Alanani NM, Alsulaimani AA. Epidemiological pattern of newly diagnosed children with type 1 diabetes mellitus, taif, Saudi Arabia. *Scientific World Journal.* 2013 Oct 9; 2013: 421569.

7. Topal E, Eğritaş O, Arga M et al. Eosinophilic esophagitis and anaphylaxis due to cow's milk in an infant. *Turk J Pediatr.* 2013 Mar-Apr; 55(2):222-5.

8. Kagalwalla AF, Amsden K, Shah A et al. Cow's milk elimination: a novel dietary approach to treat eosinophilic esophagitis. *J Pediatr Gastroenterol Nutr.* 2012 Dec; 55(6):711-6.

9. Arvola T, Ruuska T, Keränen J, Hyöty H, Salminen S, Isolauri E. Rectal bleeding in infancy: clinical, allergological, and microbiological examination. *Pediatrics.* 2006 Apr; 117(4):e760-8.

10. Uijterschout L, Vloemans J, Vos R et al. Prevalence and Risk Factors of Iron Deficiency in Healthy Young Children in the Southwestern Region of the Netherlands. *J Pediatr Gastroenterol Nutr.* 2013 Oct 17.

11. Patelarou E, Girvalaki C, Brokalaki H et al. Current evidence on the associations of breastfeeding, infant formula, and cow's milk introduction with type 1 diabetes mellitus: a systematic review. *Nutr Rev.* 2012 Sep; 70(9):509-19.

12. Hsu CL, Lin CY, Chen CL, Wang CM, Wong MK. The effects of a gluten and casein-free diet in children with autism: a case report. *Chang Gung Med J.* 2009 Jul-Aug; 32(4):459-65.

13. Marcason W. What is the current status of research concerning use of a gluten-free, casein-free diet for children diagnosed with autism? *J Am Diet Assoc.* 2009 Mar; 109(3):572.

14. Hak E, de Vries TW, Hoekstra PJ, Jick SS. Association of childhood attention-deficit/hyperactivity disorder with atopic diseases and skin infections? A matched case-control study using the General Practice Research Database. *Ann Allergy Asthma Immunol.* 2013 Aug; 111(2):102-106.

15. Sozańska B, Pearce N, Dudek K, Cullinan P. Consumption of unpasteurized milk and its effects on atopy and asthma in children and adult inhabitants in rural Poland. *Allergy.* 2013; 68(5):644-50.

16. Sackesen C, Assa'ad A, Baena-Cagnani C et al. Cow's milk allergy as a global challenge. *Curr Opin Allergy Clin Immunol.* 2011 Jun; 11(3):243-8.

17. Krissansen GW. Emerging health properties of whey proteins and their clinical implications. *J Am Coll Nutr.* 2007 Dec; 26(6):713S-23S.

18. Dohan FC. Genetic hypothesis of idiopathic schizophrenia: its exorphin connection. *Schizophr Bull.* 1988; 14(4):489-94.

19. Reichelt KL, Knivsberg AM. The possibility and probability of a gut-to-brain connection in autism. *Ann Clin Psychiatry.* 2009 Oct-Dec; 21(4):205-11.

20. Turck D. Cow's milk and goat's milk. *World Rev Nutr Diet.* 2013; 108:56-62.

CHAPTER 20

FODMAP Diet: Role in IBS, Leaky Gut and Altered Gut Bacteria

KEY POINTS

- High FODMAP foods undergo rapid fermentation in the intestines. This creates metabolic breakdown products that cause increased intestinal permeability, altered intestinal bacteria, intestinal gases, and predisposition to small intestinal bowel bacterial overgrowth (SIBO).
- A low FODMAP diet helps improve symptoms in many patients with IBS.
- Cut-off levels of high FODMAP content versus low FODMAP content have not been scientifically standardized.
- FODMAP is the abbreviation used for a cluster of short-chain carbohydrates and sugar alcohols comprised of Fermentable Oligo- Di and Monosaccharides And Polyols.

POTENTIAL DISEASE ASSOCIATIONS

A high-FODMAP diet can affect factors involved in the causation of many diseases. Such factors include altered gut bacteria and leaky gut. There is strong evidence that high-FODMAP foods contribute to symptoms of irritable bowel syndrome (IBS).

Drs. Gibson and Shepherd from the Box Hill Hospital in Victoria, Australia, state that "rapid fermentation of FODMAPs in the distal small and proximal large intestine induces conditions in the bowel that lead to increased intestinal permeability, a predisposing factor to the development of Crohn's disease." Similar processes may be seen in disorders associated with leaky gut where GI problems are common.

Patients with functional bowel disorders and chronic pain disorders frequently suffer from IBS, as well. As such, high-FODMAP foods may contribute to IBS-like GI symptoms, irrespective of whether FODMAPs are actually involved in causing or sustaining the disease.

PROPERTIES OF FODMAP

- Poor absorption in small intestine
- Osmotically active small molecules (meaning they induce osmosis of water across a semi-permeable membrane)
- Rapid fermentation of undigested FODMAP foods by intestinal bacteria – the shorter the carbohydrate molecule, the faster the fermentation

High FODMAP foods in the intestines undergo rapid fermentation and create metabolic breakdown products that cause increased intestinal permeability, altered intestinal bacteria, intestinal gases, and predisposition to SIBO.

COMPONENTS OF FODMAP

FRUCTOSE

Examples of fructose sources include honey, variety of fruits (apples, pears, mango, watermelon), and high fructose corn syrup. Thirty percent of the population has problems absorbing fructose across the gut. Fructose restriction is needed only in those with fructose intolerance and can be tested by hydrogen breath tests.

LACTOSE

Lactose is present in milk and other dairy products like margarine, yogurt, and soft, unripened cheeses (ricotta, cottage). The prevalence of lactase deficiency varies from 5 to 90 percent in any population, depending upon ethnicity. Low FODMAP options include the use of lactose-free dairy products, rice milk, and sorbet.

FRUCTANS

Shorter molecules are called fructo-oligosaccharides (FOS) or oligofructose, whereas the longer ones are referred to as inulins. FODMAP-rich sources include chocolate, fennel, wheat, rye, and many vegetables like Jerusalem and globe artichokes, shallots, asparagus, beets, leeks, and onions.

The lack of intestinal enzymes limits intestinal absorptive capacity to less than 5 percent. Fructo-oligosaccharides and inulin are frequently added to foods for health benefits.

GALACTANS OR GALACTOOLIGOSACCHARIDES (GOS)

These are present in a variety of lentils, beans (baked beans, kidney beans), chickpeas, and vegetables like cabbage and onions. The capacity of the intestines to absorb is limited, due to a lack of necessary enzymes.

POLYOLS

These are naturally present in a variety of vegetables (avocado, mushrooms) and fruits (apples, pears, peaches, cherries, nectarines, plums, stone fruits). Absorption of polyols depends upon size of the molecule. Sweeteners like sorbitol are too large for absorption. Other examples of polyols include xylitol, mannitol, maltitol, erythritol, and arabitol, They may be present in the form of additives, humectants, and/or low-calorie sweeteners.

WHAT HAPPENS WHEN YOU INGEST HIGH FODMAP FOODS?

- Excess intake and delivery of undigested carbohydrates to the colon renders them subject to bacterial fermentation.
- The breakdown products of these FODMAP foods include increased acids (short-chain fatty acids), increased surfactant activity, increased gases (hydrogen, carbon dioxide, methane and hydrogen sulfide), and gut dilation. All these affect gut leakiness.
- Short chain fatty acids (SCFAs) excess has been shown to increase intestinal permeability in animal models. Although butyric acid strengthens the barrier, others can overwhelm the protective effect.
- The gas content of the gut plays an important role in GI symptoms like pain and bloating.

It should, however, be noted that cut-off levels of high versus low FODMAP content have not been scientifically standardized.

PROBLEMS OCCUR WHEN HIGH FODMAP FOODS ARE CONSUMED FAST

The process of diffusion of water into the gut lumen due to FODMAPs, if rapid, can be especially "explosive." This occurs when large amounts of undigested carbohydrates are exposed to disproportionately high and potentially harmful bacteria in the gut, as with small intestinal bacterial overgrowth.

TYPE OF FOOD VERSUS SPEED

Oligosaccharides (smaller chain length carbohydrates) and sugars are metabolized at a much faster rate than the longer chain length molecules like dietary soluble fiber. The speed of bacterial fermentation and generation of metabolic products varies according to substrate (lactulose, inulin, or resistant starch).

LOW FODMAP OPTIONS

FRUITS

Banana; berries like blueberries, raspberries, and strawberries; cantaloupe; grape; kiwi; lime or lemon; orange; and tangelo

VEGETABLES

Alfalfa, bell peppers, bok choy, carrots, celery, corn, eggplant, green beans, lettuce, scallions, spinach, squash, sweet potato, and tomato

DAIRY PRODUCTS AND ALTERNATIVES

Cheddar, Colby, Parmesan, and Swiss cheese; lactose-free milk and yogurt; almond milk; and rice milk

GRAINS AND GRAIN ALTERNATIVES

Wheat-free grains, oat, spelt, rice, quinoa, and sorghum

NUTS AND SEEDS

Almonds, peanuts, pecans, and sesame seeds

DEMERITS OF A LOW FODMAP DIET

A low FODMAP diet diminishes access to benefits of prebiotics like fiber. The gut is deprived of the following:

- Increased bowel fluid by osmotic effects
- Increased motility
- Increased production of short chain fatty acids that serve as food for colon cells
- Increase in beneficial strains of bacteria like bifidobacteria

TURNING HARMFUL EFFECTS OF FODMAPS INTO BENEFITS

- A lower proportion of rapidly fermentable carbohydrates, along with greater amount of slowly fermentable carbohydrates, has potential for ameliorating harmful effects of FODMAPs and shifting the balance towards benefits.

- For example, ingestion of raw potato starch and guar gum causes intestinal injury. The deleterious effects of these foods do not occur if they are consumed along with slowly fermentable wheat bran.
- Considering the demonstrated potential health benefits of prebiotics, the harm versus benefits may be individual-specific based on diet, types of gut bacteria, rapidity and amount of bacterial fermentation, and presence of other bodily dysfunction in the context of genetic vulnerability to sickness.

FODMAP DIET AND VEGETARIANS

Legumes and milk products are a major source of nutrition for vegetarians. Since the goal of FODMAP strategy is overall reduction, greater cuts need to be made in other categories in order to accomplish the desired goals.

Eat good carbs! A FODMAP elimination diet plan requires global and not individual product restriction. A consultation with a dietician would be prudent.

REFERENCES

1. Gibson PR, Shepherd SJ. Food choice as a key management strategy for functional gastrointestinal symptoms. *Am J Gastroenterol*. 2012 May; 107(5):657-66; quiz 667.
2. Barrett JS, Gibson PR. Fermentable oligosaccharides, disaccharides, monosaccharides and polyols (FODMAPs) and nonallergic food intolerance: FODMAPs or food chemicals? *Therap Adv Gastroenterol*. 2012 Jul; 5(4):261-8.

CHAPTER 21

Other Food Exclusions to Chew On

KEY POINTS

- The Six-Food-Elimination-Diet calls for exclusion of six foods, based on the relative incidences of allergies to different foods.
- Some persons are sensitive to the foods that contain chemicals like salicylates, amines, mono-sodium glutamate, sulfites, benzoates, antibiotics, and tartrazine.
- There are several other foods or substances in foods that a person may be intolerant to. Such sensitivities may not be detected by skin prick tests for allergies. Patients benefit from exclusion of such foods from their diet.

SIX-FOOD ELIMINATION DIET (SFED)

The Six-Food-Elimination-Diet (SFED) specifically excludes foods shared among most people with food allergies. These include milk, soy, egg, wheat, peanut/tree nuts, and seafood, including all fish. Interestingly, these six foods are also linked to damage to esophagus seen in the rising tide of eosinophilic esophagitis.

SIMPLE, PRACTICAL AND EASY TO FOLLOW

The best part about the SFED plan is its simplicity. Since food exclusion based on allergy testing achieves only limited success, this diet eliminates the need for prior testing and goes straight to a therapeutic trial. Eliminate six foods, that's it, and see what happens! Since these are the foods most frequently linked to food allergies, eliminating them also increases chance of success. SFED is very practical and easy to follow, resulting in high degree of compliance.

It has a low risk of creating nutritional deficiencies. A consultation with a dietician can make sure of that.

LOW RISK OF CROSS-CONTAMINATION

SFED also has a low risk of cross-contamination or "eating by mistake," compared to the gluten-free diet. It should be noted that some patients may need to be on SFED on top of a gluten-free diet. Federal laws require that foods be clearly labeled for the eight most common foods with potential to cause allergies. These include cow's milk protein, soy, egg, wheat, peanuts, tree nuts, seafood, and shellfish.

EVIDENCE FOR SUCCESS OF SFED

Clues come from its successful application come from its use in patients with eosinophilic esophagitis, the cause of which is not fully established. It is a chronic inflammation of the esophagus and is strongly associated with food allergies. Like many other chronic conditions, genes as well as environmental factors play a critical role in causing it.

Exclusion of intact protein and substituting it with predigested protein for ingestion heals this condition, establishing the link between food proteins and unrestrained chronic inflammation.

Well-designed clinical trials have documented the success of SFED plan in healing eosinophilic esophagitis. Based on this model, the SFED has the potential to benefit patients with other conditions characterized by chronic inflammation with strong link to food allergies.

MOST COMMON ALLERGENS BASED ON SFED DIET

Based on a study conducted by Dr. Gonsalves and colleagues, the most common food allergen based on reintroduction strategy is wheat (60 percent of the patients), whereas milk contributes to the disease in 50 percent of the cases. Clearly, many patients were allergic to more than one food. Interestingly, the skin prick testing was able to identify a specific allergen in only 13 percent of the cases in that study.

FOOD EXCLUSIONS BASED ON CHEMICAL SENSITIVITIES

Chemicals present in foods may become a part of food during cultivation or be added by the manufacturer. Any or some of them may be the cause of chemical sensitivity and intolerance in certain individuals.

The chemicals with high potential for causing chemical sensitivity include salicylates (found in herbs and spices, tea, and coffee), amines (chocolate, canned or smoked fish, sauces, stock, and vinegar), mono-sodium glutamate (strong cheeses, soy sauce), sulfites, benzoates, antibiotics, and tartrazine. Adverse effects of offending chemicals occur when these interact with intestinal nerve endings in people who are sensitive to them.

> Exclusion of foods based on chemical sensitivities may benefit people with frequent allergies and intolerances. However, foods to avoid, along with potential alternatives, are not fully standardized, and there may occasionally be conflict with other elimination diets.

Caution: In some cases, a product may appear among foods to avoid as well as in category of alternate option, depending on mechanism of action. Individual responses may also vary based on the amount of food ingested as well as foods ingested along with, genetic vulnerability, intestinal bacterial patterns, and exposure to the foods during childhood.

DISEASES ASSOCIATED WITH FOOD SENSITIVITIES

- Asthma
- Eczema

- Attention deficit hyperactivity disorder (ADHD)
- Irritable bowel syndrome
- Fibromyalgia

FOODS TO EXCLUDE AND ALTERNATE OPTIONS

- Avoid milk. Alternate options include rice milk, kefir, and plain lactose-free yogurt.
- Avoid eggs. Use alternate sources for protein needs.
- Non-vegetarians should avoid beef, pork, and all canned meats. Alternate options include organic lean chicken and turkey. Fish to avoid include shark, tuna, swordfish, and orange roughy. Alternate options include sardines, salmon, and shrimp. Note that organic vegetarian foods are less likely to cause chemical sensitivities than any non-vegetarian meats.

Grains and cereals to avoid include corn and gluten-containing foods like wheat, barley, rye, spelt, bulgar, farina, kamut, semolina, and triticale. Oats are best avoided. Beware of breaded foods. Read labels carefully; gluten may even be in a variety of products ranging from beer to imitation meats. Alternate options are the gluten-free foods like amaranth, arrowroot, buckwheat, maize, rice, soy, beans, quinoa, and tapioca.

Fruits to avoid include apples, strawberries, citrus fruits, mangoes, nectarines, lychee, plums, and pears. Avoid frozen, canned, or sweetened products. Alternate options include bananas, blueberries, raspberries, grapes, honeydew melon, cantaloupe, cranberries, grapes, resins, figs, and papaya.

Vegetables and condiments to avoid include potatoes, tomatoes, peas, peppers, paprika, chili pepper, cayenne, soy sauce, barbeque sauce, teriyaki, vinegar, mayonnaise, and cinnamon. Alternate options include vegetables (cauliflower, broccoli, green onions, lettuce, and carrots), low-sodium salt, basil, cumin, garlic, ginger, mint, parsley, cumin, rosemary, thyme, dill, mustard, and tarragon.

Avoid fats like butter, margarine, and shortenings. Better options include olive oil, clarified butter, or ghee.

Nuts and seeds to avoid include peanuts, walnuts, sesame, sunflower, pecans, and hazelnuts. You may try coconut, pine nuts, flax seeds, or cashews.

Both alcohol and its nonalcoholic components can be harmful. Wine is the worst culprit. Avoid dark beers and alcohols. Having said that, red wine is associated with better health outcomes, assuming you can tolerate it well and drink in moderation.

Minimize carbonated and caffeinated beverages and mineral water. Filtered or distilled water and decaffeinated herbal teas may be easier on the unhealthy gut.

Practice the SFED as outlined above. Reintroduce one at a time after a trial of at least eight weeks. Wheat and cow's milk are the worst of these offenders and should be reintroduced last.

MISCELLANEOUS EXCLUSIONS AND ALTERNATIVES

- Avoid raw vegetables. Try steamed, boiled, or lightly sautéed vegetables. Based on my experience, they are easier to digest and less likely to cause problems in patients with GI problems.
- Avoid deep-fried cooking. Alternate options include steamed or boiling dishes. Grilled and roasted are also acceptable.

REFERENCES

1. Gonsalves N, Yang GY, Doerfler B et al. Elimination diet effectively treats eosinophilic esophagitis in adults; food reintroduction identifies causative factors. *Gastroenterology*. 2012 Jun; 142(7):1451-9.
2. Chobtang J, de Boer IJ, Hoogenboom RL et al. The need and potential of biosensors to detect dioxins and dioxin-like polychlorinated biphenyls along the milk, eggs and meat food chain. *Sensors (Basel)*. 2011; 11(12):11692-716.

3. Gordon BR. Approaches to testing for food and chemical sensitivities. *Otolaryngol Clin North Am.* 2003 Oct; 36(5):917-40.

4. Rhind SM. Endocrine disruptors and other food-contaminating environmental pollutants as risk factors in animal reproduction. *Reprod Domest Anim.* 2008 Jul; 43 Suppl 2:15-22.

CHAPTER 22

The Sugar Monster

KEY POINTS

- Much of the obesity around us is due to high sugar consumption.
- Stevia offers a natural, no-calorie option as a sweetener.

Sugar intake has increased 40 to 50 times since the American Revolution and about five times since the 1950s. Annual American consumption of sugar has been rising in recent decades and is currently at 152 pounds per person per year. This also correlates with the rising consumption of carbonated beverages and the rise in obesity and metabolic syndrome, with all its complications.

Any excess consumption of added sugars is stored in the body. The harm afflicted by the rising use of sugar on the health of society can be seen all around us. Much of our obesity is due to sugar sweeteners and not fat consumption.

This fact was not lost on Dr. Atkins, who popularized the Atkins diet, which broadly restricts carbohydrate intake. Remember, complex carbohydrate intake is not bad; the main culprit is the simple carbohydrate – sugar and even fructose. Rather than having to explain the differences between types of carbs, Dr. Atkins just simplified it for the masses: No carbs!

Think of sugar as a slow poison, just like alcohol might be. Excess consumption is toxic!

SUGAR SUBSTITUTES

Although sugar substitutes are thought to have no effect on metabolism, recent reports suggest that they can affect glucose metabolism. They also affect the gut bacteria and, thus, the entire body. Studies in animals raised in a germ-free environment suggest that the bacteria preferentially consume nutritive sweeteners compared with sweeteners without calories.

CONTROVERSIAL SUGAR SUBSTITUTES

HIGH FRUCTOSE CORN SYRUP (HFCP)

HFCP is widely used as sweetener and has been implicated in the increasing tide of obesity, metabolic syndrome, and heart disease. According to Dr. Bray at Louisiana State University, fructose is hazardous to the health of some people. Fructose-associated damage is not solely related to its effect on obesity, since metabolic changes due to fructose may occur even in the absence of obesity.

Many experts have challenged the hypothesis blaming fructose as a cause of many of our health problems. Dr. Bantle, in a review article titled, "Is fructose the optimal low glycemic index sweetener?" states, "There is not yet any convincing evidence that dietary fructose does increase energy intake." The latter is consistent with reports by Dr. Soenen and colleagues from The Netherlands, who found no differences in satiety or energy intake after HFCP, sucrose, or milk.

According to Drs. Rippe and Angelopoulos from the University of Central Florida, "Whether there is a link between fructose, HFCS, or sucrose and increased risk of heart disease, metabolic syndrome, or fatty infiltration of the liver or muscle remains in dispute." In fact some studies suggest that use of artificial sweeteners is associated with increased weight gain.

As always, moderation is the key. Defining moderation can also be controversial. Just because there is a paucity of evidence to support harmful effects of fructose does not mean that you should load up on fructose in your diet. Naturally-occurring fructose in your daily consumption of fruits and vegetables should not be a major problem.

ASPARTAME (NUTRASWEET, EQUAL)

Aspartame is made of phenyl alanine, aspartic acid, and methanol. Aspartic acid is a predecessor for glutamate. Both aspartic acid and glutamate are involved in transmission of messages in the brain. Methanol is broken down into formaldehyde, which is toxic to the body. Subjects with phenylketone urea are especially at risk for aspartame toxicity.

Daily consumption of aspartame should be well below the 50 mg per kilogram of body weight per day, according to the Food and Drug Administration. Toxicity studies in animals have not found an increased risk of cancer or an effect on the brain function.

Although some epidemiologic data suggests an increased risk for some cancers in humans, according to Dr. Marinovich and colleagues, there is "no consistent association for cancers of the upper aero-digestive tract, digestive tract, breast, endometrium, ovary, prostate, and kidney."

> Some experts have implicated aspartame in increased headaches, sleeplessness, and seizure disorders. While evidence is lacking thus far, these problems could potentially occur due to the components and metabolic products of aspartame, causing changes in the levels of neurotransmitters in different areas of the brain.

Similarly, while implicated, there does not appear to be association of aspartame with vascular diseases and preterm deliveries.

SACCHARINE (SWEET 'N LOW)

Saccharine is 500 times sweeter than sugar. Although initial reports indicated an increased risk of cancer due to saccharine consumption, recent data has not confirmed these findings.

HEALTHY NATURAL SWEETENERS

STEVIA

Stevia is a natural sweetener. It is a purified extract from the plant *Stevia rebaudiana* (Bertoni) and is 300 times sweeter than sugar but without any added calories.

Studies suggest the stevia consumption is associated with lowering blood pressure in patients with high blood pressure. Stevia has also beneficial effect on glucose metabolism and thus may help patients with diabetes.

HONEY

Honey is sweet and does contain calories! Upon ingestion, it also affects the gut bacteria.

Honey is well known to have a healing effect on a cough or a common cold. Medical-grade honey is used for wound healing. Studies show that honey reduces glucose levels and is better tolerated than most common sugars or sweeteners.

Not all honeys are the same.

According to Dr. Erejuwa and colleagues and as published in the journal *Molecules*, "Honey, administered alone or in combination with conventional therapy, might be a novel antioxidant in the management of chronic diseases commonly associated with oxidative stress." The list of such diseases includes diabetes, hypertension, heart disease, cancer, and Alzheimer's.

MISCELLANEOUS NATURAL SWEETENERS

- Maple syrup is not just sweet but full of antioxidants.

- Molasses is sweet and also contains the highest content of antioxidants of the sweetening options, even higher than maple syrup and honey.
- Sucanat is basically dried whole cane juice and includes molasses, which is not present in refined sugar. Because of its composition, it does cause fluctuations in blood glucose.
- Monk Fruit in the Raw is natural sweetener derived from monk fruit.
- Coconut sugar contains both glucose and fructose but has low glycemic index, plus a truckload of essential minerals.
- Agave has been rising in popularity in recent years. It is derived from a plant which is also the source of tequila.

There is nothing special about agave, since it is manufactured just like any other sugar. A tablespoon of agave has 60 calories, in contrast to refined sugar, which has 40 calories. However, agave is 1.5 times sweeter than sugar, so you require less of it for the same degree of sweetness. Commercial agave is 55 to 90 percent fructose, and the rest is glucose.

Agave does have lower glycemic index than sugar. Although labeled as "diabetes friendly," diabetics should limit agave intake. In fact, healthy diet should limit intake of simple sugars in any form and that includes agave.

REFERENCES

1. Pepino MY, Bourne C. Non-nutritive sweeteners, energy balance, and glucose homeostasis. *Curr Opin Clin Nutr Metab Care*. 2011 Jul; 14(4):391-5.

2. Ulbricht C, Isaac R, Milkin T et al. An evidence-based systematic review of stevia by the Natural Standard Research Collaboration. *Cardiovasc Hematol Agents Med Chem*. 2010 Apr; 8(2):113-27.

3. Magnuson BA, Burdock GA, Doull J et al. Aspartame: a safety evaluation based on current use levels, regulations, and

toxicological and epidemiological studies. *Crit Rev Toxicol.* 2007; 37(8):629-727.

CHAPTER 23

Is Vegetarianism Healthy or Unhealthy? You Decide

KEY POINTS

- A variety of plant foods, eaten in different meals throughout the day, can adequately meet all essential protein needs in healthy adults.
- The American Dietetic Association has concluded that macronutrient intake by pregnant vegetarian females is similar to that of non-vegetarians.
- Well-planned vegetarian diets, including a vegan diet, may be undertaken during any and all stages of the lifecycle, including childhood, pregnancy, and lactation.

Pythagoras is considered the founder of vegetarianism. The proponents from modern history include Benjamin Franklin. Until then, vegetarianism was promoted based on moral and metaphysical grounds. Former President Bill Clinton, Dr. Neal Bernard, and Hollywood stars Alec Baldwin, Pamela Anderson, and Anne Hathaway are a few of the many famous Americans who are vegans.

CLASSES OF VEGETARIANISM

- A lacto-vegetarian diet excludes eggs and all kinds of meat, fish, and poultry.
- Lacto-ovo-vegetarians do eat eggs.

- The vegan diet is the most restrictive. Subjects do not ingest eggs, dairy, and other animal products. Some vegans also avoid honey and animal products such as leather and wool.
- Macrobiotic diet followers consume mostly grains, legumes, and vegetables, while fruits, nuts, and seeds are avoided. Organic meat is allowed during transition at least, and some of these people do not exclude fish from the diet.
- A raw foods diet, also known as the "living food diet," consists mainly of uncooked and unprocessed foods, including fruits, vegetables, nuts, seeds, grains, and beans. Some followers may consume unpasteurized dairy products and even raw meat and fish.
- A fruitarian diet involves fruits, nuts, and seeds. Subjects avoid vegetables, grains, beans, and animal products. (Avocados and tomatoes are included in the diet.)
- Semi-vegetarians do consume some fish, chicken, or even meat. These self-described vegetarians may be identified in research studies as semi-vegetarians. Individual assessment is required to accurately evaluate the nutritional quality of the diet of a vegetarian or a self-described vegetarian.

In our overfed society, vegetarianism is a healthy option unless it results in a nutritional deficiency. Availability of numerous fortified food products in the market reflects an improvement of a vegetarian diet of the past.

HEALTH ADVANTAGES OF A VEGETARIAN DIET

- Reduced cholesterol levels
- Reduced risk of heart disease
- Reduced risk of high blood pressure (hypertension)
- Reduced risk of cancer. A recent expert review led by Dr. Huang concluded that vegetarians have 18 percent less incidence of cancers
- Improved glucose control

- Reduced risk of gallbladder stones
- Improvement of arthritis
- Reduced risk of obesity

According to Dr. McEvoy from the Queen's University Belfast, "Plant-based diets contain a host of food and nutrients known to have independent health benefits."

> Dr. Key and colleagues from the Cancer Epidemiology Unit in Oxford, United Kingdom combined data from five different studies and found that, compared to non-vegetarians, "mortality from ischemic heart disease was 20 percent lower in occasional meat eaters, 34 percent lower in people who ate fish but not meat, 34 percent lower in lacto-ovo-vegetarians, and 26 percent lower in vegans."

POTENTIAL NUTRIENT DEFICIENCIES

Depending upon the type of vegetarianism practiced, deficiency of vitamins (B_{12}, D), zinc, long chain omega-3 fatty acids, calcium, iodine, and riboflavin may occur.

Dr. Jenkins and colleagues from the St Michael's Hospital in Toronto, Canada, compared the cholesterol-lowering potential of a diet with that of a cholesterol-lowering statin drug. The authors found that a near-vegan diet rich in fiber, nuts, and soy protein reduces serum LDL-cholesterol levels as much as a low-saturated fat diet and a statin for lowering serum LDL-cholesterol levels.

SPECIAL DIETARY CONSIDERATIONS

PROTEINS

Nitrogen is an integral part of protein. It is used as a measure of protein intake and output, in broken down form. Most nitrogen balance studies do not show significant difference in protein, based on the source of dietary protein. Even vegetarian athletes can meet their protein needs well.

IRON

The Institute of Medicine, a nonprofit organization formed by Congress, recommends almost twice the iron intake by vegetarians as compared to non-vegetarians.

OLDER ADULTS

Dietary intake of vegetarian older adults is similar to non-vegetarians. There may be reduced iron absorption, and fortified supplements may be used. Similarly, Vitamin D production declines with age, and supplements are helpful.

ATHLETES

A well-planned vegetarian diet provide adequate nutritional intake to athletes without requiring supplements. Creatine supplementation may benefit athletes involved in high-intensity exercise.

KIDNEY FAILURE

The vegetarian diet is high in phosphorus. As such, increased use of phosphate binder drugs may be needed. Plant proteins contain higher amounts of non-essential amino acids and thus generate more urea and pose a difficult challenge in severe renal failure. A carefully-designed vegan diet can be effectively used to treat mild chronic renal failure. It may in fact be the diet of choice when a patient is unable to tolerate a conventional low-protein diet. Ingestion of low-potassium fruits, vegetables, and grains is needed to compensate for the relatively higher potassium content of plant foods like legumes and nuts.

REFERENCES

1. Craig WJ and Mangels AR: American Dietetic Association: Position of the American Dietetic Association: vegetarian diets. *J Am Diet Assoc* 2009 Jul; 109(7):1266-82.

2. Drake R, Reddy S and Davies J: Nutrient intake during pregnancy and pregnancy outcome of lacto-ovo-vegetarians, fish-eaters and non-vegetarians. *Veg Nutr* 1998; 2:45–52.

3. Key TJ, Fraser GE, Thorogood M et al.: Mortality in vegetarians and nonvegetarians: Detailed findings from a collaborative analysis of 5 prospective studies. *Am J Clin Nutr* 1999; 70 (suppl): 516S–524S.

4. Giem P, Beeson WL and G.E. Fraser. The incidence of dementia and intake of animal products: Preliminary findings from the Adventist Health Study. *Neuroepidemiology 1993;* 12:28–36.

5. Tipton KD and Witard OC. Protein requirements and recommendations for athletes: Relevance of ivory tower arguments for practical recommendations. *Clin Sports Med* 2007; 26:17-36.

CHAPTER 24

Organic Foods: Are They Better?

There has been a great deal of hype about the recent Stanford study that found no substantial difference in essential nutrients between organic and conventional foods. Let's put the issues in the study (as published in the journal *Annals of Internal Medicine* and reported in the *New York Times*) in the context of the confusion it has caused among people trying to make difficult choices.

Seventeen studies in humans and 223 studies of nutrient and contaminant levels in foods were included in the analysis. Bacterial contamination of retail chicken and pork was common but did not vary by farming techniques. However, bacteria resistant to three or more antibiotics were found more commonly in conventional than in organic meats.

While there is not much difference in essential nutrients, organic foods have lower levels of pesticides, fewer highly antibiotic-resistant, food-borne, disease-causing bacteria and many more cancer-fighting phenols than conventional foods.

GOING BEYOND THE HEADLINES

Unfortunately, most of the headlines have focused on the part of the study showing no difference in nutrients and not the remaining results. This has led a lot of people to jump to conclusions that we might as well have conventional foods in lieu of the more expensive organic foods.

The proponents of this argument, in my opinion, are only half-correct. They miss the point that the reason why many people prefer organic foods over conventional foods is because of potential pathogens and toxins in conventional foods. This is a result of the growing and processing of these foods, which then winds up in the food we eat on an everyday basis.

LIMITATIONS OF THE STUDY TO PUT RESULTS IN THE CONTEXT

Even the authors of this study conceded that studies were heterogeneous and limited in number and publication bias may be present. Given these substantial limitations, one should be careful in drawing any far-reaching conclusions about organic foods. One conclusion from the study, however, was a lot more definitive: "consumption of organic foods may reduce exposure to pesticide and antibiotic-resistant bacteria."

REFERENCES

1. Smith-Spangler C, Brandeau ML, Hunter GE et al. Are organic foods safer or healthier than conventional alternatives?: a systematic review. *Ann Intern Med*. 2012 Sep4; 157(5):348-66.

CHAPTER 25

Cancer-Fighting Diet

KEY POINTS

- A diet high in fruits and vegetables lowers the risk of cancer.
- The Mediterranean diet offers significant protective benefits.
- Garlic and onions help prevent cancer.
- Fiber protects against cancer.
- Excessive cooking and frying increases the risk of cancer.

Food factors can affect the development of several cancers. Potential factors that can modify the risk of colon cancer include fat, red meat, fiber, fruits, vegetables, and alcohol.

VEGETARIAN VERSUS NON-VEGETARIAN

Results of the studies provide conflicting results. Dr. Huang and colleagues recently conducted an expert systematic review of the scientific studies. They included seven published studies comprising 124,706 subjects in their analysis. Their results were reported in the journal *Annals of Nutrition & Metabolism*. The investigators concluded that vegetarians have an 18 percent lower cancer incidence and 29 percent lower death rate due to heart disease than the non-vegetarians.

RED, PROCESSED MEAT

Meat has been implicated in the pathogenesis of cancer. Examination of the relationship between recent and long-term meat consumption and the risk of colon cancer suggests that high intake of red, processed meat carries a greater risk of colon cancer. Lean meat carries a lesser risk.

EFFECT OF COOKING

Cooking meat and fish under usual conditions results in compounds that induce cancer. A population-based study of colon cancer found that intake of red meat increases the risk for colon cancer. Associations were strongest for pan-fried red meat, as was the association with well- or very well-done red meat.

WHOLE VERSUS REFINED GRAINS

While refined grain does not appear to increase the risk of cancer, increased intake of whole grains protects against colon cancer, probably because of additional fiber in the diet and other elements that may be lost in refining.

WESTERN VERSUS "PRUDENT" DIET

A population-based study examined the dietary intake of 1,993 cases and 2,410 controls. The "Western" dietary pattern was associated with an increased risk of colon cancer in both men and women. Subjects in the "prudent" dietary lifestyle had high intake of fiber and folate, and this group showed lower risk of colorectal cancer.

Another study of patients with colon polyps and cancer reported that intake of fried, preserved, and grilled meat, animal fats, and sugar increase the risk of colon polyps, as does obesity.

MEDITERRANEAN DIET

Subjects on the Mediterranean diet have a lower risk of heart disease and cancer. According to Dr. Giacosa at the University of Genoa in Italy, "The mechanism of cancer prevention is likely due to the favorable effect of a balanced ratio of omega-6 and omega-3 essential fatty acids and high amounts of fiber, antioxidants and polyphenols found in fruit, vegetables, olive oil, and wine."

GERSON REGIMEN

This is a dietary approach to cancer management that includes low-sodium, high-potassium lactovegetarian diets and fruit juices. Data indicates that this is not effective in treating cancer.

MACROBIOTIC DIET

This consists of a low-fat, high-complex carbohydrate vegetarian diet. Some data suggests that it may improve quality of life in patients with pancreatic cancer. Many of the dietary components indicate therapeutic potential. Despite many anecdotal reports, there is lack of good scientific data to support its use in the treatment of cancer. Adoption of such a diet should not delay seeking medical care by a cancer specialist.

KELLY-GONZALEZ REGIMEN

The program involves dietary restrictions and the use of digestive aids and a detoxification regimen, including coffee enemas. A two-year, non-blinded pilot study reported that such an aggressive nutritional regimen, paired with high doses of pancreatic enzymes, results in increased survival in patients with advanced pancreatic cancer. Larger randomized controlled trials are needed before any recommendations can be made.

SELECTED VEGETABLE AND HERB MIX

This is a proprietary boiled and freeze-dried formula blend (SV) of multiple vegetables and herbs, including soy, mushrooms, beans, red dates, scallion, garlic, lentils, leek, hawthorn fruit, onion, ginseng, angelica, dandelion, senegal, licorice, ginger, olives, sesame, and parsley. There is a lack of data to support its use in treating digestive cancers.

VEGETABLES AND FRUITS

ALLIUM VEGETABLES

Allium vegetables like garlic, onions, leeks, shallots, and chives have been reputed across various cultures to have beneficial health effects.

- Most case-control studies have demonstrated a reduced risk of cancer as a result of Allium vegetable consumption. The evidence for a protective effect is strong for stomach and colon cancer, while the data on breast, lung, and other cancers is mixed. Of all the allium vegetables, the protective effect is the strongest with scallions, garlic, and Chinese chives.
- Results from the Prostate, Lung, Colorectal, and Ovarian Cancer Screening Trial show that diets rich in fruit, deep-yellow and dark-green vegetables, onions, and garlic are modestly associated with reduced risk of colon polyps. Best protective effects were seen for subjects consuming high intakes of deep-yellow vegetables, onions, and garlic.

CRUCIFEROUS VEGETABLES

Cabbage, broccoli, and Brussels sprouts are rich in anti-cancer compounds that protect against liver, colon, and breast cancer in animals. Data indicates protective effects in humans as well.

ROLE OF FIBER

- An expert systematic review from Queens University in Belfast, U.K. concluded that dietary fiber protects against cancer of the esophagus. The investigators speculated that the mechanisms may "include gastroesophageal reflux and/or weight control."
- Similarly, Dr. Thompson from the University of Arizona recently concluded in a review that a low-fat, high-fiber diet is "weakly protective" against breast cancer.
- Some studies indicate a protective effect of fiber against colon polyps and cancer.

FRUIT VERSUS VEGETABLE FIBER

Examination of data from a food-frequency questionnaire used in a population-based prospective mammography screening study of women in Sweden found that fiber consumption was inversely associated with colon cancer risk during an average 9.6 years of follow up. The risk was the highest for those consuming the least amounts of fruit and vegetables. High consumption of cereal fiber did not have any beneficial effect.

SELECT FOODS

BERRIES

Berries contain antioxidant, anti-inflammatory components that protect against cancer and neurodegenerative processes.

- Cranberry extracts affect several cancer-associated mechanisms in breast, colon, prostate, and other cancer cells in laboratory. Blueberry juice results in significant reductions in the formation of abnormal cells in the colon leading to colon cancer in animals.
- The extracts of blackberry, blueberry, raspberry, cranberry, and strawberry inhibit growth of cancer cells in human oral, breast, colon, and prostate tumors.
- Black raspberry and strawberry extracts have the most anticancer effects against colon cancer.

GARLIC

It inhibits growth of cancer cells and induces programmed cell death.

- One study from China attributed a tenfold difference in the death rate from stomach cancer in two Chinese provinces to the differences in garlic consumption. Garlic intake was 20 g/day in the low-risk region, while the high-risk group consumed less than one g/day.

- The majority (but not all) of cohort studies have found reduction in risk for colon cancer associated with higher consumption of garlic.
- Dr. Kim and colleagues have reported that there is limited evidence of a relationship between garlic consumption and reduced risk of colon, esophagus, larynx, oral, ovary, prostate, or renal cell cancers, while there was no beneficial effect against stomach, breast, lung, or uterus cancer.

While high dietary garlic is linked to reduced cancer risk, garlic supplements do not appear to have the same effect.

GINGER

Mice given free access to extract of ginger in water are found to have a decrease in breast cancer. Beneficial results have been seen for colon cancer, as well, in laboratory experiments.

OLIVES

Olive ingestion protects against colon tumors in rats. The effect may in part be due to maslinic acid present in wax-like coating of olives, which inhibits growth of colon-cancer cells.

ONIONS

- Diets supplemented with onion or tomato has a preventative effect against the formation of colon polyps in animals.
- A report from China showed that people from low-risk areas for stomach cancer consume high amounts of Welsh onions, onions, and Chinese chives.

SAGE

It is used as a spice and has been associated with decreased risk of lung cancer as part of the Mediterranean diet.

TOMATOES

Tomato and garlic, individually as well as combined, reduce colon polyps in rats. One study examined the inhibitory potential of garlic and tomato, individually and in combination against colon polyp in rats. The protective effect was greater when the combination of garlic and tomato was used, compared to each individually, suggesting a possible synergistic action of garlic and tomato.

REFERENCES

1. Giacosa A, Barale R, Bavaresco L et al. Cancer prevention in Europe: the Mediterranean diet as a protective choice. *Eur J Cancer Prev.* 2013 Jan; 22(1):90-5.
2. Huang T, Yang B, Zheng J et al. Cardiovascular disease mortality and cancer incidence in vegetarians: a meta-analysis and systematic review. *Ann Nutr Metab.* 2012; 60(4):233-40.
3. Pauwels EK. The protective effect of the Mediterranean diet: focus on cancer and cardiovascular risk. *Med Princ Pract.* 2011; 20(2):103-11.
4. Coleman HG, Murray LJ, Hicks B et al. Dietary fiber and the risk of precancerous lesions and cancer of the esophagus: a systematic review and meta-analysis. *Nutr Rev.* 2013 Jul; 71(7):474-82.
5. Schmid A. The role of meat fat in the human diet. *Crit Rev Food Sci Nutr.* 2011 Jan; 51(1):50-66.
6. Gonzalez NJ, Isaacs LL. Evaluation of pancreatic proteolytic enzyme treatment of adenocarcinoma of the pancreas, with nutrition and detoxification support. *Nutr Cancer.* 1999; 33(2):117-24.
7. Millen AE, Subar AF, Graubard BI et al. PLCO Cancer Screening Trial Project Team. Fruit and vegetable intake and prevalence of colorectal adenoma in a cancer screening trial. *Am J Clin Nutr.* 2007 Dec; 86(6):1754-64.
8. Michels KB, Giovannucci E., Joshipura KJ et al. Prospective study of fruit and vegetable consumption and incidence of colon and rectal cancers. *J Natl Cancer Inst.* 2000 Nov 1; 92(21):1740-52.

Section VII
Gut Psychology and Eating Dysfunction

CHAPTER 26

Anorexia Nervosa

KEY POINTS

- The use of most modern drugs for pharmacotherapy of anorexia nervosa raises more questions than answers.
- There is lack of good pharmaceutical agents to treat this challenging condition. Most efforts are directed at treating complications.
- Behavioral therapy aims to empower the patient to learn to refrain from potentially harmful eating behaviors.
- Cognitive behavioral as well as family therapy are effective.
- Hypnotherapeutic techniques can help uncover the origin of the disrupted cognition and emotional conflicts and empower patients to develop feelings of control over their thoughts and actions.

Most illness, irrespective of the label, reflects a disruption of the intricately-interacting links in the life network of an individual, and eating disorders are no exception. These include anorexia nervosa and bulimia nervosa.

While psychological issues have long been focused on, there are biological underpinnings to eating disorders as well. Hunger-satiety signals play an important role in the pathogenesis of eating disorders. Abnormalities may be seen in brain-gut axis, compounded by abnormalities in hormonal balance. Specific gene mutations have recently been identified in patients with eating disorders.

Antibodies against brain tissue and hormones have been documented. According to Dr. Smitka and colleagues, the presence of such autoantibodies supports the hypothesis that intestinal bacteria and their components provoke the body's immune system into formation of such antibodies in healthy individuals.

Anorexia nervosa (AN) is a multifactorial convoluted complex of learned behaviors which grows out of patient's own defense system. Complex interactions of body weight, body shape, dietary issues, and fantasy impact proneness.

- Patients are overly sensitive about their body weight and have an altered perception of body size.
- Simple and natural developmental processes like weight gain around the time of first menstrual cycle lead to loss of self-confidence and self-esteem.
- Patients suffer from feelings of inadequacy, hopelessness, shortcomings, poor self-confidence, and inadequate coping mechanisms.
- There is a close relationship between emotions and different bodily experiences.

ANOREXIA NERVOSA VERSUS BULIMIA

Anorexia nervosa is characterized by failure or refusal to maintain a minimum healthy body weight, fear of weight gain and being "fat," distorted and dysfunctional body image, and lack of regular menstrual cycles.

Bulimia nervosa involves recurrent binge eating followed by inappropriate and tactless counterbalancing behavior, including self-inducing vomiting, use of laxatives and diuretics or other such medications, fasting, and relatively too much exercise.

ADOLESCENT VERSUS ADULT ANOREXIA NERVOSA

Anorexia nervosa manifests differently in children and adolescents than in adults.

- Diagnostic strategies and multidisciplinary management approach should be tailored to the unique developmental, medical, nutritional, and psychological needs of children and adolescents.
- Although a variety of therapies are used in treating adolescents, evidence suggests that the Maudsley model of family therapy may be the best strategy for treating anorexia nervosa in adolescents.

PATHOGENIC FACTORS UNDERLYING FEEDING DISORDERS

Patients with eating disorders need to be investigated as to the underlying psychodynamics behind the symptoms.

- Eating disorders may co-exist with post-traumatic stress disorder (PTSD).
- Patients often have a history of physical or sexual trauma and/or current trauma symptoms.
- Stress is frequently involved.
- A person's personality, along with their environment, modifies the manner of coping with stress differently for anorexia and bulimia.

DIAGNOSIS OF ANOREXIA NERVOSA

- It can be difficult to detect in the early stages.
- Patients hide their condition and do not want medical help.
- Medical treatment occurs usually when the patient's condition becomes serious or even life-threatening.
- Severely ill patients have difficulty understanding the problem. This tends to resolve once re-feeding starts.

TREATMENT STRATEGY FOR ANOREXIA NERVOSA

- Promise of a long-term treatment from the patient and the family
- Focus is to achieve healthy weight and to accept that as normal
- Creative ways to develop and implement individualized therapeutic strategy
- Weight gain
- Address interactive psychosocial factors

A focused approach addressing the various diverse but overlapping areas of psychopathology is likely to achieve better and sustained response to therapy than a non-specific strategy.

TREATMENT OPTIONS

Management of anorexia nervosa is very expensive and involves complex and intensive inpatient and outpatient approaches.

The most common components of treatment include:

- Re-nutrition
- Psychotherapy
- Family therapy
- Additional psycho-education strategies, especially cognitive and interpersonal psychotherapy, for sustained response.

ROLE OF MODERN THERAPIES

- Studies show that the core symptoms of anorexia nervosa are resistant to currently available psychotropic medications.
- Antidepressants benefit patients with depressive symptoms and may help prevent relapse.
- Even electroconvulsive therapy (ECT) has been used for some patients.

PSYCHOTHERAPIES

Behavioral modification

- Elimination of all disordered eating behavior may be unrealistic. The main goal is to get the patient to learn to refrain from potentially harmful eating behaviors and maintain healthy and controlled eating patterns.
- Eating behaviors are learned behaviors and as such have the potential to be unlearned. A patient must relearn normal eating habits. The aim is to restore normal eating behaviors. However, the success is gradual at best.
- Behavioral approaches alone or combined with cognitive behavior therapy may be used.
- Indirect suggestions are more effective since they serve to enhance rather than challenge the patient's need to have control.
- Rehearsal, age progression, or assertiveness training may be used, as appropriate.
- A lenient attitude is likely to be more acceptable to patients than one that involves punishment.

Behavioral modification may be comprised of:

- Gaining insight into the eating behavior and reasons for persisting
- Diet and nutrition counseling
- Dispelling myths about food and eating
- Lifestyle modifications
- Shopping-style modifications, like avoiding certain stores and purchasing trigger foods
- Establishing new habits to replace the vacuum created by eliminating the older ones, like reading books at a bookstore instead of spending most time alone at home
- Modification of eating behavior, like not watching television at the same time as eating

Cognitive behavioral therapy (CBT)

Cognitive behavioral therapy may be helpful in improving outcomes and preventing relapse in weight-restored anorexia nervosa. This leads to significant reduction in symptoms of eating disorders, depression, and overall psychological issues.

- Outpatient cognitive-behavioral therapy for the treatment of anorexia nervosa is effective. Good EAT scores have been observed in as many as 70 percent of the patients at the end of treatment and in 60 percent after one year. (The Eating Attitudes Test is a screening tool to examine if person might have an eating disorder requiring professional attention help. It is not a tool to make an actual diagnosis.)
- Combined cognitive-behavioral, medication, and nutritional therapy results in improvement in body mass index as well as psychological function.
- Nurses are a valuable resource in CBT management. They can help patients address and overcome the beliefs that form the core of their disorder, such as too much focus on body weight or figure.
- CBT reduces the risk of relapse in patients with anorexia nervosa after weight restoration, although its efficacy in the underweight patients remains to be established.

According to Dr. Murphy and colleagues from Oxford University, CBT is the leading therapeutic strategy, and a new "enhanced" version of the treatment is more effective and provides additional advantages for treating all eating disorders.

Biofeedback relaxation system

One study examined the effect of multi-pronged therapies for eating disorders, including a biofeedback relaxation system. The results showed that electrodermal response biofeedback improves eating disorders, especially AN.

A variety of strategies are used. Overall, it is helpful as a part and not necessarily as an exclusive treatment for AN.

Family therapy

A five-year follow-up on patients who had participated in a previous trial of family therapy for anorexia and bulimia nervosa found that while much of the improvements after five years can be attributed to the natural outcome of the illness, significant benefits attributable to previous psychological treatments were still evident, favoring family therapy for patients with early onset and short history of anorexia nervosa and favoring individual supportive therapy for patients with late-onset AN.

Conjoint family meetings should be avoided, at least in earlier stages when parental criticism is quite evident.

A recent Cochrane database meta-analysis review concluded that family therapy may be more effective than usual treatment; however, it is not superior to other forms of psychological interventions.

Hypnosis

Hypnosis has the potential to help establish a reality-based body image in the patients.

- Hypnotherapy can help uncover the origin of the disrupted thinking processes and emotional conflicts at the core of the patient's problem.
- Hypnosis may empower patients to develop feelings of control and mastery over their thoughts and actions.
- Different patients may respond differently because of interaction between the individual characteristics and the hypnosis.
- Hypnosis is a useful addition to other psychotherapeutic techniques as a way to reach the goal of conflict resolution, creating coping mechanisms, and managing anxiety.

Hypnosis, singly or in combination with other therapies, helps achieve relaxation, guided imagery, ego strengthening, cognitive reorientation, and reframing. Success of hypnosis is indirectly related to the number of visits for hypnotherapeutic interventions, indicating that likelihood of success after four sessions is low.

A caveat about hypnosis: While hypnosis plays an important role in improving self-confidence and self-esteem, patients with anorexia nervosa have an extreme need for control and as such they tend to be poor subjects for hypnosis.

Art-based therapies

A therapeutic approach combing art therapy, guided role playing, and verbal therapy has a greater potential for success than these therapies if undertaken individually.

- Anorexia nervosa can be seen even in mentally-challenged subjects and presents difficulties in diagnosis and management. Music may be used to explore the patient's inner self.
- Arts-based therapies are being increasingly used in combination with other therapies, especially as part of inpatient programs.

Spirituality

Dr. Richards from Brigham Young University led a randomized, controlled trial comparing the effectiveness of a spirituality group with cognitive and emotional support groups in subjects receiving inpatient eating disorder treatment for anorexia nervosa. Patients in the spirituality group scored higher on spiritual well-being and lower on psychological disturbance and eating disorder symptoms at the conclusion of treatment compared to patients in the other groups. Thus spiritual therapy during inpatient treatment may help calm the psychological and relationship distress, social role conflict, and other symptoms.

Traditional Chinese Medicine

Acupuncture

A randomized crossover trial from Dr. Fogarty's laboratory examined the efficacy of acupuncture as an adjunct treatment for treatment of eating disorders. Treatment resulted in an improvement in quality of life, along with improvement in anxiety and perfectionism.

TREATMENT SETTING

Patients with concurrent medical issues are likely to benefit from inpatient treatment. Multi-modal treatment strategy is also more feasible for inpatients and potentially less stressful on the family.

Outpatient specialist services may provide more benefit over inpatient psychiatric treatment in the treatment facility. A multi-center randomized, controlled trial compared inpatient psychiatric treatment, specialist outpatient treatment, and general outpatient treatment for cost-effectiveness at baseline, one, and two years. The authors concluded that the provision of specialist outpatient services for adolescents with anorexia nervosa is the most cost-effective.

MISCELLANEOUS

A case of a 38-year-old woman with anorexia nervosa (AN) who successfully used alternative (Zen) therapy instead of conventional treatment has been described.

PREVENTION OF ANOREXIA NERVOSA

The interventions to prevent eating disorders have not been promising and, in fact, may have led to a cascade of increasing and worsening manifestations.

REFERENCES

1. Hebebrand J. Pharmacotherapy of anorexia nervosa: more questions than answers. *J Am Acad Child Adolesc Psychiatry.* 2011 Sep; 50(9):854-6.
2. Robin AL, Gilroy M, Dennis AB. Treatment of eating disorders in children and adolescents. *Clin Psychol Rev.* 1998 Jun; 18(4):421-46.
3. Keel PK, Haedt A. Evidence-based psychosocial treatments for eating problems and eating disorders. *J Clin Child Adolesc Psychol.* 2008 Jan; 37(1):39-61.
4. Casper RC. How useful are pharmacological treatments in eating disorders? *Psychopharmacol Bull.* 2002 Spring; 36(2):88-104.

CHAPTER 27

Bulimia Nervosa

KEY POINTS

- Bulimia nervosa occurs in up to one percent of young women, starting in teenage years.
- Prognosis and outcome of bulimia nervosa is better than for anorexia nervosa.
- Cognitive behavioral therapy offers the best chance of success and is superior to pharmacological treatment.
- Combined psychological plus pharmacological treatment may not be superior to psychological treatment alone.

Bulimia nervosa (BN) is characterized by recurrent episodes of impulsive, uncontrolled, and rapid binge eating, along with compensatory behaviors such as self-induced vomiting and intake of laxatives and diuretics.

Typically, it occurs at least twice weekly for at least three months and is associated with persistent over-concern for body shape and weight. Patients who do not binge but indulge in self-induced vomiting are not considered to be bulimia nervosa. Often, the patient's weight is actually normal.

Age of onset is in the teens, typically between the ages of 14 and 16 years, while a full-fledged disorder may be seen between the ages of 17 and 24 years of age. Ten percent of the patients are males.

CAUSATION

Bulimia nervosa is a multifactorial disorder involving genetics, family dynamics, and psychosocial and cultural factors. Familial disturbances, distorted cognitions, and learned behaviors may be involved. Developmental arrest has been implicated.

As is the case for anorexia nervosa, abnormalities of hunger-satiety signals along with gene mutations may be seen. Abnormal antibodies against brain tissue and/or hormones have been documented implicating the intestinal bacteria in causation.

There is a high incidence of sexual abuse during childhood among patients. Bulimia nervosa is more common in the West, due likely to the higher emphasis on a slender figure.

Disease associations include depression, bipolar disorder, obsessive-compulsive disorder, and substance abuse, including alcoholism, cocaine addiction, and amphetamines addiction.

DIAGNOSIS

The diagnosis is primarily clinical. In contrast to anorexia nervosa, bulimia nervosa can be difficult to diagnose if the patient is not open and forthright about his or her history. Standardized self-reporting tests help aid the diagnosis.

TREATMENT

GENERAL MEASURES

- Nutritional counseling
- Food diaries
- Advance planning for meals

PSYCHOLOGICAL TREATMENTS

Multiple expert reviews have shown that psychotherapy (including cognitive behavioral therapy) and anti-depressants are effective for treatment of bulimia, especially when used in combination. The most effective strategy involves an interdisciplinary team including a physician, dietitian, and psychologist or psychiatrist.

Cognitive behavioral therapy (CBT)

The goal of CBT is to unlearn the distorted thinking process, normalize eating habits, and eliminate compensatory behaviors.

Multiple controlled trials have confirmed the effectiveness of CBT as compared to no therapy, nondirective therapy, psychodynamic therapy, stress therapy, and pharmacological treatments.

- A meta-analysis of randomized placebo-controlled drug and psychosocial studies found that CBT provides superior relief of binge eating, purging, and eating behaviors. As many as half of the patients are not binge eating at one year after treatment. On the other hand, up to one-third of patients show no response.
- An Internet-based self-help therapeutic approach utilizing CBT is a viable option, as compared to waiting list controls (patients waiting for treatment who can serve as controls). This approach is especially useful for less severe cases. Group treatment prefaced by a short individual therapy may be a cost-effective alternative to purely individual treatment utilizing CBT.
- Self-guided CBT provides a faster relief and is less costly than family therapy.
- A large number of bulimic patients also suffer from a substance use disorder. CBT can be adapted as integrated treatment for such patients, since it is effective for both disorders independently.

Cognitive orientation therapy

The therapy is targeted at behavioral modification based on underlying themes or processes presumed to contribute to illness, rather than the eating behavior itself. It does not involve telling the patient that his or her eating behavior is abnormal.

Cognitive analytic therapy (CAT)

CAT aims to figure out the evolution of the patient's problems in light of patient's personal history and determine how things can be improved. The therapist then helps patient organize their own strengths and weaknesses to develop a plan to bring about changes in behavior. There is a lack of data supporting its use in bulimia.

Motivational enhancement therapy

A randomized comparison of motivational enhancement therapy over four sessions found it to be equally effective as CBT specifically for bulimia. This form of therapy is more frequently used for anorexia nervosa rather than bulimia.

Interpersonal psychotherapy (IPT)

Individuals with eating disorders have a low sensitivity for interpersonal stressful situations. IPT targeted for bulimia nervosa facilitates the patient making specific changes for healing. This form of therapy does not focus specifically on eating habits or attitudes toward weight and shape and does not involve any specific behavioral or cognitive procedures.

IPT provides a beneficial short-term intervention especially helpful in patients with associated depression. It is considered inferior to CBT.

Dialectical behavioral therapy

This is a modified form of behavioral therapy that focuses on emotional dysfunction underlying the abnormal eating behavior. Dr. Safer and colleagues from the Stanford University in California studied 31 women who were randomized to 20 weeks of dialectical behavior therapy or a waiting-list comparison. There was a significant decrease in binge/purge behavior with dialectical behavior therapy, compared to controls.

Hypno-behavioral therapy

Hypno-behavioral therapy is effective. It results in a significant decrease in bulimic behavior as compared to controls. It is a therapeutic strategy combining behavioral techniques, such as self-monitoring to change abnormal eating patterns, and hypnosis with the goal of emphasizing and inspiring behavioral modification.

Family therapy

Family-based therapy focusing on BN is helpful in adolescents. Such therapy does not target the causes of BN. Rather, it utilizes parental assistance in monitoring the eating and purging behaviors in order to facilitate their kid's quitting such behavioral malfunction.

Family therapy is more effective than individual therapy in patients whose illness is not chronic and onset was before the age of 19 years. It accomplishes abstinence in 40 percent of cases at end of treatment. The Maudsley form of family therapy is more effective than supportive psychotherapy.

Family therapy is similar in efficacy to CBT-guided self-care. CBT-guided self-care has the slight advantage of faster relief and lower cost.

Guided imagery therapy

Dr. Esplen and colleagues from the Mount Sinai Hospital in Toronto, Canada, examined the effect of individual guided imagery therapy designed to enhance self-comforting in a randomized controlled trial of 50 subjects with bulimia nervosa over 6 weeks. The treatment group demonstrated a mean reduction of binges by 74 percent and of vomiting by 73 percent along with improvement of psychological parameters as well as attitudes about eating, dieting, and body weight.

All psychotherapies are not equal

Dr. Hay and colleagues conducted a systematic expert review of randomized controlled trials of psychological therapies for treatment of eating disorders including bulimia. Results indicated that CBT – especially bulimia nervosa-targeted CBT (CBT-BN) – is effective for bulimia nervosa. Other psychotherapies, especially interpersonal psychotherapy, are also effective. Self-help protocols using structured CBT treatment manuals may be helpful. Psychotherapy alone is not likely to be very effective.

LIGHT THERAPY

The role of light therapy is controversial. Braun et. al. recruited 34 bulimic subjects to a randomized controlled trial of light therapy for three weeks. The treatment group displayed a significant reduction in binge frequency.

Another double-blind, placebo-controlled study of light therapy daily for one week found that light therapy resulted in improvement of mood during the light period but did not affect binge eating behavior.

YOGA

Individualized yoga treatment may have the potential for efficacy as an adjunct treatment of BN. Dr. Carei and colleagues from the Seattle Children's Hospital conducted a randomized controlled trial of yoga in patients with BN. Individualized yoga treatment decreased Eating Disorder Examination scores at 12 weeks, and food preoccupation subsided immediately after yoga sessions in patients with eating disorders.

SPIRITUAL THERAPY

Religious beliefs affect attitudes and motivation in eating disorders. A randomized control group design study found that attention to spiritual growth and well-being of patients may help improve psychological manifestations as well as eating behavior in patients with eating disorders.

BIOLOGIC ENERGY THERAPIES

Results of studies have been mixed. Application of high-frequency repetitive transcranial magnetic stimulation reduces cue-induced food cravings in people with BN and may reduce binge eating.

DRUG TREATMENT

Medications are an option in patients' refractory to CBT and may include antidepressant drugs. The presence of depression is not a prerequisite for success with the use of antidepressants. Antiepileptic drugs like topiramate (Topamax) and selective serotonin antagonists like ondanestron (Zofran) have shown promise. Severe cases may need hospitalization.

Although a combination of drugs and psychological therapies is used, evidence for combining them is weak as compared to the use of drugs alone.

PROGNOSIS AND OUTCOME

Bulimia nervosa is characterized by remissions and relapses. The remission rate at 10 years is 50 percent. Bulimia carries a better prognosis as compared to anorexia nervosa, and it is not associated with risk of premature death.

Complications include fluid and electrolyte abnormalities, esophagitis, gastrointestinal bleeding, constipation, and dental damage. Menstrual abnormalities, infertility, and bone loss may occur.

Use of a "treatment contract" with the patients is controversial. Managed care strategies are not particularly helpful, since they tend to focus on shorter-term treatments, which may not work with such chronic illnesses.

REFERENCES

1. Hay PP, Bacaltchuk J, Stefano S et al. Psychological treatments for bulimia nervosa and binging. *Cochrane Database Rev* 2009 Oct 7; (4):CD000562.
2. Trace SE, Baker JH, Peñas-Lledó E, Bulik CM. The genetics of eating disorders. *Annu Rev Clin Psychol.* 2013; 9:589-620.
3. McElroy SL, Guerdjikova AI, Mori N, O'Melia AM. Current pharmacotherapy options for bulimia nervosa and binge eating disorder. *Expert Opin Pharmacother.* 2012 Oct; 13(14):2015-26.
4. Hoste RR, Labuschagne Z, Le Grange D. Adolescent bulimia nervosa. *Curr Psychiatry Rep.* 2012 Aug; 14(4):391-7.

Section VIII
Annoying GI Problems

CHAPTER 28

Belching

KEY POINTS

- Belching is a normal phenomenon and is an extension of "normal" aerophagia.
- A belch after a hearty meal is considered a compliment for the chef in some Eastern cultures.

Dictionaries describe belching or eructation as "the voiding of gas or a small quantity of acidic fluid from the stomach through the mouth." Aerophagia means swallowing of air. It frequently occurs while eating, drinking, chewing gum, and smoking and increases exponentially during anxiety. Belching in anxious persons is an extension of "normal" aerophagia and belching. While breathing in, the patients suck air into the food pipe in addition to the windpipe.

HOW DOES BELCHING OCCUR?

The air in the stomach is normally passed downstream into the intestines. Belching occurs when the stomach air, instead of going down, regurgitates up into the esophagus and is expelled through the mouth. As in acid reflux disease or GERD, this process requires that the valve between the esophagus and stomach, also known as lower esophageal sphincter (LES), relax to allow the spewing of air upward into the esophagus and then out through the mouth, making a sound.

BELCHING AFTER A MEAL MAY BE NORMAL

Belching after a meal, especially a big meal, may be normal. It occurs as a result of air being swallowed while eating. In addition, a lot of swallowed air accumulates in the stomach in between meals. The food, once it reaches the stomach, dislodges the air already present there. Belching after eating is further facilitated by relaxation of lower esophageal valve due to alcohol, carbonated drinks, and foods like onions, mint, tomatoes, and chocolate.

CULTURAL VARIATION AND ACCEPTANCE

Cultural acceptance of belching varies. While considered uncouth in Western society, a belch after a hearty meal is considered a compliment for the chef in some Eastern cultures.

Chronic belching is generally not due to any organic disease. Rather, it is a learned process, albeit subconsciously. In most cases, air is swallowed into the esophagus as described above but is promptly expelled out as a belch even before it has had a chance to reach the stomach. This develops into a habit in anxious persons. As such, excessive belching has been described by some as a behavioral disorder.

CLINICAL FEATURES

Many patients believe that belching is an indicator of disease of the digestive system. Frequently, they ascribe their digestive symptoms actually caused by other disorders to belching.

DIAGNOSTIC TESTING

Diagnostic tests are generally only performed in patients with additional symptoms that may point towards a disease.

TREATMENT

Treatment can be challenging in some cases. This primarily involves reassurance that chronic belching is a benign condition and would not have long-term health consequences.

MODIFICATION OF EATING HABITS

- Eat slowly
- Consume small meals
- Avoid foods that promote belching like mints, onions, large fatty meals, and chocolate
- Minimize carbonated beverages
- Quit drinking alcohol
- Quit smoking

ADJUNCT MEASURES

- Try stress reduction and relaxation
- Patients with severe symptoms may require professional help for anxiety and stress management

REFERENCES

1. Bredenoord AJ. Management of belching, hiccups, and aerophagia. *Clin Gastroenterol Hepatol.* 2013 Jan; 11(1):6-12.
2. Bredenoord AJ. Belching, aerophagia, and rumination. *J Pediatr Gastroenterol Nutr.* 2011 Dec; 53 Suppl 2:S19-21.

CHAPTER 29

Bloating and Indigestion

KEY POINTS

- Multiple factors are involved in the causation of bloating and indigestion.
- Dietary and lifestyle adjustments help relieve symptoms in many patients.
- Among alternative therapies, the Chinese herbal formulation STW5 and acupuncture have been shown to be of benefit.

Patients with bloating and indigestion do not have just one complaint. Usually it is a conglomeration of upper abdominal discomfort, with bloating and distention after eating associated with early fullness. There may be some burning sensation in stomach. This is labeled as functional dyspepsia when no cause can be found on testing, including an upper GI scope.

The 30-odd feet of our gastrointestinal highway has both country roads as well as freeways. This transport system needs to keep moving smoothly and easily. If it slows down in any region, the whole system is backed up, causing misery not just to the gut but the entire body, affecting quality of life. There is discomfort, and the belly can becomes bigger after a meal.

WHAT CAUSES BLOATING AND INDIGESTION

It is a myth that most people with bloating have more gas. This was proven by studies comparing gas amounts in patients with and without bloating. The same thing can be confirmed by comparison of the X-ray studies. Studies do suggest that patients may have slower movements of the small intestine, creating a logjam of traffic of intestinal contents. Fatty meals are especially to blame for the slowness.

The gut of many patients tends to be hypersensitive, so that it is more aware of the gas being present as compared to those who do not have bloating. The bloating sensation may occur with or without the belly getting distended. Patients that also have distended bellies frequently have dysfunction coordination of breathing and abdominal muscles.

FACTORS AFFECTING BLOATING AND INDIGESTION

GENDER

Females are more susceptible to bloating and indigestion because of the long colon being trapped in a smaller abdominal cavity. This results in multiple, smaller loops and sharp angles, causing pockets of food and air to get trapped.

HORMONES

Bloating tends to occur more when females start menstruating or at menopause. This indicates that the female hormones estrogen and progesterone play a role, although the mechanisms are not clear. Birth control pills also exacerbate bloating. Males seem to be protected somewhat from bloating because of higher levels of testosterone, which tends to tighten up the abdomen.

DIET

Eating too much, too fast on the run does not allow the stomach time to process and deliver the food to the small intestine in a timely fashion, resulting in a backlog that can cause stomach discomfort.

Fermentation of undigested or unabsorbed food results in increased gas. Reducing consumption of foods that reach colon without being digested and absorbed would result in lesser gas production. Patients tend to get relief when switching to low-FODMAP foods. Different foods can then be introduced into the diet one by one to see which ones matter the most! See Chapter 20 for more details about FODMAP diet.

Likewise, a diet that predisposes a person to constipation is likely to allow more time for bacteria to act on undigested food. Listen to your gut. The stools are the messenger. If your stools are pale, you need some more green vegetables in your diet!

ILL-FITTING DENTURES

Poorly-fitted dentures allow food of large sizes to be consumed, which can then not be efficiently emptied from the stomach into the small intestine. This also results in poor digestion of such big pieces, allowing a larger amount of undigested food to reach the colon and be acted upon by trillions of bacteria.

ANXIETY AND STRESS

Eating quickly lends to swallowing more air. Eating slowly, in a relaxed manner allows food to be consumed in much smaller particles, reducing the stress on the stomach and the time it takes to break it down to one- to two-millimeter particles before delivering it to the intestine. Slower emptying of the stomach contributes to bloating.

Increased stress, especially while eating, also creates a hormonal imbalance that allows blood to be shunted away from the gut and results in impaired digestive processes. Such a hormonal imbalance, while hastening the colon, actually slows the stomach, diminishing the downward momentum for the passage of food and air out from the stomach into the intestine. This accentuates the bloating problem.

FOOD INTOLERANCE

Bacterial fermentation of undigested food is a major source of gas in the gut. Digestive abilities and absorptive capacity for nutrients varies among people, leading to different components of food waste reaching the colon. Similarly, as we have learned earlier, everyone's bacterial fingerprint in the gut is different. Interaction of different foods with different patterns of bacteria can produce different responses of gas production – both type of gas and quantity – in different persons.

LIFESTYLE ISSUES

Unhealthy lifestyle choices, like smoking, insufficient water drinking, and lack of adequate exercise, promote bloating. People often use carbonated beverages for their fluids, which have gas and can actually worsen the situation. Some people chew gum and suck on hard candy to compensate for stress and anxiety. Again, these are counterproductive since more air gets swallowed, worsening bloating.

DRUGS

There are many medicines that slow down the gut and can promote fullness and bloating. These include aluminum-containing antacids, most drugs used for anxiety, stress and psychological dysfunction, narcotics painkillers, and many drugs that treat heart disease and high blood pressure. The package inserts for these drugs provide specific information.

BACTERIA

Everyone's intestinal bacteria are different. Gas production in the gut is likely to be higher with an overgrowth of bad bacteria or even just the overall number of bacteria is too high at the wrong place, as seen in small intestinal bacterial overgrowth. The bacterial balance can be transformed by taking appropriate measures, including dietary adjustments and probiotics. See Chapter 9 for more details.

MISCELLANEOUS FACTORS

The problem may be set off by an episode of infection, especially infectious diarrhea. Multiple other factors have been implicated and include a slow or lazy stomach (see Chapter 35 on gastroparesis), abnormal electrical rhythms of the stomach, *Helicobacter pylori* infection of the stomach, and reduced conformity or compliance of the stomach to the food being consumed. When food reaches the stomach, the stomach wall opens up to accommodate the incoming food, just like a balloon opens up to accommodate air. It is adapting to the food and conforming to the amount that gets in there, without stretching or causing problems.

Many patients with indigestion report a history of physical or sexual abuse. Psychological factors including anxiety, depression, and personality issues have also been reported.

DIET AND LIFESTYLE ADJUSTMENTS

Since multiple causative factors are involved, the treatment also calls for multiple adjustments.

- Eat slowly and in a relaxed fashion.
- Cut food into small pieces on the plate and chew at least 20 times.
- Avoid large, fatty meals.
- Make sure dentures fit well.
- Increase water intake.
- Increase soluble fiber in diet with chickpeas, broccoli, or cauliflower.
- Switch to low-FODMAP foods.
- Avoid constipation. Read Chapter 38 for more details.
- Avoid carbonated beverages.
- Exercise regularly.
- Quit smoking and drinking alcohol.

HERBAL THERAPIES FOR BLOATING AND INDIGESTION

AMALAKI

Amalaki is an Ayurvedic herbal remedy derived from pericarp of the dried fruit of Emblica officinalis. Dr. Chawla and colleagues compared the treatment of dyspepsia using Amalaki or gel antacids for four weeks. Patients included those with ulcers and non-ulcer dyspepsia. Compared to the baseline, symptoms improved in both treatments groups.

ARTICHOKE LEAF EXTRACT

A study by Dr. Holtmann and co-investigators studied the efficacy of artichoke leaf extract (two doses of 320 mg plant extract, three times a day, for six weeks) in the treatment of patients with functional dyspepsia in a double-blind, randomized, placebo-controlled trial. The artichoke leaf extract demonstrated superior efficacy in alleviating symptoms and improved the disease-specific quality of life in patients with functional dyspepsia.

ASPARAGUS RACEMOSUS (SHATAVARI)

Shatavari is used in Ayurveda for indigestion. It hastens the stomach emptying in healthy volunteers and reduces gastric acidity.

BANANA POWDER (PLANTAIN BANANA)

One study showed that banana powder treatment for eight weeks results in marked improvement (partial or complete relief) in patients with non-ulcer dyspepsia, compared to controls.

BRAHMI

Fresh juice from the whole plant of *Bocapa monniera Wettst*, commonly known as Brahmi, is used in Ayurveda for indigestion. Although used for centuries for dyspepsia, studies for its use are lacking.

CHILI POWDER (CAPSAICIN)

Dr. Bortolotti and colleagues examined the effect of red pepper (2.5 g per day) on the treatment of functional dyspepsia in a double-blind, placebo-controlled trial. The overall symptom score, as well as the stomach pain, fullness, and nausea scores, improved significantly in the red pepper group as compared to the placebo. Thus, while chili pepper may cause symptoms in susceptible subjects in the short term, it can relieve functional dyspepsia by causing desensitization of the pain nerve endings.

CURCUMIN (TURMERIC)

It reduces gastric acidity, promotes gallbladder contractions, and relaxes spasms of the intestines. A randomized controlled trial found that 87 percent of patients with dyspepsia responded to turmeric capsules, compared to 53 percent to placebo.

GINGER ROOT

Ginger hastens gastric emptying. However, its effect on dyspeptic symptoms is controversial.

LEMON BALM (MELISSA OFFICINALIS)

It is contained in many herbal combinations like STW 5 that are useful in dyspepsia. Studies on its use as a sole remedy are lacking.

LIQUORICE (LICORICE)

Most of the studies regarding beneficial effects involve licorice as a component of an herbal combination. Combinations like CAVED-S and STW 5 containing licorice have been shown to be effective in treating dyspepsia.

MASTIC

Mastic is a concrete resinous exudate obtained from the stem of the tree *Pistacia lentiscus*. Dr. Dabos, in a randomized controlled trial, found that mastic gum treatment results in significant improvement of symptoms of dyspepsia. Seventy-seven percent of the study group had improved, compared to 40 percent of the placebo group.

PEPPERMINT OIL

Peppermint oil has been used for dyspepsia and spasms/colic in various cultures for centuries. It may be used singly or in combination with other herbs. Peppermint oil enhances the early phase of stomach gastric emptying.

Dr. May's group conducted studies of the efficacy and tolerability of a combination of peppermint oil and caraway oil in patients with functional dyspepsia. They found the treatment was superior to the placebo with respect to pain intensity, sensation of pressure, and a full, heavy feeling, as well as the overall improvement.

TERMINALIA

Terminalia arjuna is a deciduous tree, and its bark is used in herbal medicine. It is commonly advocated in Ayurveda to improve indigestion. It is known to hasten stomach emptying in animals, but human studies are lacking.

HERBAL COMBINATIONS

The use of herbal combinations has the potential to affect a disease process at multiple levels in its pathogenesis.

Hange-koboku-to (Banxia-houpo-tang; HKT)

Hange-koboku-to accelerates stomach emptying in patients with dyspepsia, as well as healthy controls. This improvement in gastric emptying is accompanied by improvement in bloating.

Liu-Jun-Zi-Tang (TJ-43)

Liu-Jun-Zi-Tang, also known as Rikkunshi-to and TJ-43, is a compound Chinese herbal formulation of multiple plants. It increases gastric emptying and promotes relaxation of the stomach upon eating. Compared to placebo, TJ-43 improves GI symptoms of stomach fullness, heartburn, belching, and nausea.

Shenxiahewining

Shenxiahewining is a Chinese herbal medicine. In the Chen study of 100 patients with non-ulcer dyspepsia, improvement was seen in 92 percent of the treatment group, compared to only 20 percent of the control group.

STW 5

STW 5 is a fixed combination of nine herbs and is perhaps the best-studied herbal formulation. It modifies stomach emptying and reduces gastric acidity. Multiple meta-analyses of double-blind, randomized, clinical trials on the efficacy of STW 5 in patients with functional dyspepsia have demonstrated a highly significant therapeutic benefit. Tolerability of the drug is excellent.

Based on efficacy and safety, STW 5 is a valid therapeutic option for patients seeking natural herbal therapy for indigestion and bloating.

ACUPUNCTURE AND OTHER ELECTROMAGNETIC TREATMENTS

- Electroacupuncture at acupoint ST-36 improves stomach emptying in gastroparesis. It increases the number of the stomach's normal electrical waves in healthy volunteers.
- Clinical studies have shown that electro-acupuncture improves symptoms of functional dyspepsia in patients with normal and slowed stomach emptying. Acupuncture also helps in dyspeptic symptoms during pregnancy.

Acupuncture administered by an expert may be a reasonable option for patients with symptoms refractory to standard management.

PROBIOTICS FOR BLOATING AND INDIGESTION

An open label trial (where doctors and patient know the drug the patient is getting) found that *Lactobacillus acidophilus* improves symptoms of bloating, abdominal pain and pressure, and flatulence in patients with dysbiosis/maldigestion.

A randomized controlled trial conducted by Dr. Ringel-Kulka from the University of North Carolina documented that probiotic treatment with *Lactobacillus acidophilus NCFM* and *Bifidobacterium lactis* Bi-07 improves bloating.

Dr. Kalman and colleagues conducted a randomized double-blind placebo-controlled trial to compare the probiotic dietary supplement Digestive Advantage Gas Defense Formula to placebo, regarding effects on functional gas-related symptoms of pain, distention, and flatulence after eating. The probiotic group demonstrated significant improvements in abdominal pain and the total Gastrointestinal Symptom Rating Scale score.

Conflicting results on studies with probiotics are likely due to the different strains of bacteria used in different studies.

PSYCHOLOGICAL THERAPIES FOR BLOATING AND INDIGESTION

Multiple studies have documented the positive effects of psychological therapies for functional dyspepsia. Therapeutic modalities of benefit include the following:

- Hypnotherapy accelerates gastric emptying in dyspeptic and healthy subjects.
- Cognitive behavioral therapy is better than education alone for treatment of functional bowel disorders.
- Biofeedback has the potential to allow patients to manipulate the abnormal electrical and mechanical rhythms of the stomach

through imagery while watching the stomach's rhythm activity on the screen.

- Breathing exercises can increase drinking capacity and improve quality of life in patients with functional dyspepsia.

REFERENCES

1. Ringel-Kulka T, Palsson OS, Maier D et al. Probiotic bacteria Lactobacillus acidophilus NCFM and Bifidobacterium lactis Bi-07 versus placebo for the symptoms of bloating in patients with functional bowel disorders: a double-blind study. *J Clin Gastroenterol*. 2011Jul; 45(6):518-25.
2. Hasler WL, Wilson LA, Parkman HP et al. Bloating in gastroparesis: severity, impact, and associated factors. *Am J Gastroenterol*. 2011Aug; 106(8):1492-502.
3. Houghton LA. Bloating in constipation: relevance of intraluminal gas handling. *Best Pract Res Clin Gastroenterol*. 2011 Feb; 25(1):141-50.

CHAPTER 30

Morning Sickness Due to Nausea and Vomiting of Pregnancy

KEY POINTS

- Dietary modification and avoidance of triggers plays an important role in prevention.
- Studies on the role of hypnotherapy have shown encouraging results.
- Most data indicates ginger is effective and superior to vitamin B6.
- The data on the efficacy of complimentary therapies should be taken in the context that there is a lack of good data on the use of commonly used anti-nausea medicines and acid blockers.

Pregnant women frequently suffer from nausea and vomiting during pregnancy. Hyperemesis gravidarum represents the most severe form. Paradoxically, women who suffer from nausea and vomiting during pregnancy have a reduced risk of miscarriage.

TRIGGERS TO AVOID

The symptoms can be instigated by a variety of factors, and they are frequently different in different women.

- Empty stomach
- Large meals
- Crowded places, including small crowded rooms
- Smells of food and perfumes
- Bright lights
- Smoking

- Noise
- Heat
- Motion due to driving or flying
- Medications that may irritate stomach, like iron and NSAIDs

TREATMENT

GENERAL MEASURES

Usual management is supportive, including adequate hydration. Avoid triggers. Minimize contact with family members. Patients with a severe form usually respond to bowel rest and intravenous hydration.

NUTRITION

- Small, frequent, low-fat, high-carbohydrate meals
- Cold food without aroma
- Protein-predominant meals
- Frequent snacks in small amounts, like nuts and crackers
- Spicy or salty food, for some patients
- Cold, clear drinks like ginger ale or mint tea
- Electrolyte-replacement drinks and oral nutritional supplements, in small amounts

MEDICATIONS

Drugs used include anti-emetics (like Zofran) and acid-blocking drugs like histamine-2 blockers (like Zantac and Pepcid) and PPIs (like Prilosec, Prevacid, and Nexium), although there is lack of good data on the efficacy of these drugs. While tube feeding helps some women, intravenous nutrition via the veins may also be undertaken. Enteral and/or intravenous nutrition support may be needed in refractory cases.

NATURAL AND ALTERNATE TREATMENT OPTIONS

ACUPRESSURE/ACUPUNCTURE

Randomized controlled trials have shown that acupressure and vitamin B6 relieve nausea and vomiting in pregnancy to a similar degree. No pregnancy-related adverse events have been reported with P6 acupuncture or acupressure.

GINGER

Evidence suggests efficacy of powdered ginger (1-1.5 g per day in three to four divided doses). Ginger lollipops may be used. Another option is to chew on a thin slice of fresh ginger root two to four times a day as needed.

PYRIDOXINE OR VITAMIN B6

Randomized controlled trials suggest effectiveness of pyridoxine for management of nausea and vomiting during pregnancy. The recommended dose is 75 mg per day.

HYPNOSIS

Hypnotherapy has been successfully used for treatment of nausea and vomiting of pregnancy.

PSYCHOTHERAPY

Psychotherapy may be beneficial, especially as an adjunctive therapy in patients with severe stress or anxiety.

REFERENCES

1. Lee NM, Saha S. Nausea and vomiting of pregnancy. *Gastroenterol Clin North* Am. 2011 Jun; 40(2):309-34.
2. Ding M, Leach M, Bradley H. The effectiveness and safety of ginger for pregnancy-induced nausea and vomiting: a systematic review. *Women Birth*. 2013 Mar; 26(1):e26-30.
3. Mohammadbeigi R, Shahgeibi S, Soufizadeh N et al. Comparing the effects of ginger and metoclopramide on the

treatment of pregnancy nausea. *Pak J Biol Sci.* 2011 Aug 15; 14(16):817-20.

CHAPTER 31

Doc, I Have Hiatal Hernia

KEY POINTS

- The mere presence of hiatal hernia does not mean that it is a problem.
- Symptoms, if present, are usually related to acid reflux or GERD.

Hiatal hernia is a common finding on upper GI X-rays and endoscopy. It implies a pulling up of the stomach into the chest cavity. The most common type (comprising 95 percent of all hiatal hernia) is called sliding hernia, in which only the upper part of the stomach is pulled up. The uncommon kind is para-esophageal hiatal hernia, which is prone to complications.

CLINICAL FEATURES

Symptoms are basically the same as those of GERD. Fifty to 90 percent of patients with hiatal hernia complain of acid reflux or GERD.

- Heartburn
- Chest or abdominal pain
- Difficulty swallowing
- Hoarseness
- Chronic cough
- Frequent upper respiratory infections
- GI bleeding

DIAGNOSIS

Hiatal hernia may be diagnosed on imaging studies (upper GI X-ray) or endoscopy (upper GI scope).

The diagnosis is very common, and the mere fact that a person has it does not mean that it is the cause of patient's problems.

TREATMENT

Treatment is only undertaken if there are associated symptoms of GERD. Patients are managed like any other patient with GERD, using lifestyle measures and acid-blocking medications. See Chapter 34 for details. Surgery may sometimes be needed, especially in cases of para-esophageal hiatal hernia.

ENDOSCOPIC TREATMENTS

A variety of procedures may be undertaken, including applying sutures, fasteners, or staples at the gastroesophageal junction to tighten it up to prevent reflux of stomach acid into esophagus.

REFERENCES

1. Kahrilas PJ, Kim HC, Pandolfino JE. Approaches to the diagnosis and grading of hiatal hernia. *Best Pract Res Clin Gastroenterol*. 2008; 22(4):601-16.
2. McColl KE, Clarke A, Seenan J. Acid pocket, hiatus hernia and acid reflux. *Gut*. 2010 Apr; 59(4):430-1.

CHAPTER 32

Intestinal Gas

KEY POINTS

- Everyone has and passes gas. Gas is ubiquitous and that includes our digestive system. Everyone has it!
- Symptoms may occur due to gas trapped at sharp angles in the bowel or due to increased sensitivity of the gut, as seen in irritable bowel syndrome.

NORMAL AMOUNT OF GAS AND GAS EXPULSIONS (FLATUS)

An average adult produces one to three pints of intestinal gas every day, and the number of flatus expulsions may vary from 14 to 23 per day. The food you eat and the intestinal bacteria play a pivotal role in the amount and aroma of your flatulence.

DO OLDER FOLKS PRODUCE MORE GAS?

Many elderly people complain of increased frequency of flatus. However, they usually pass smaller amounts of gas with greater frequency, since their ability to hold gas may be impaired.

COMPOSITION OF INTESTINAL GAS

About 99 percent of gas is composed of nitrogen, hydrogen, and methane. The composition of intestinal gas also varies depending upon the part of the gut it is derived from and the types of intestinal bacteria acting upon the undigested food.

STOMACH GAS

In the stomach, gas is usually high in oxygen and nitrogen and represents the swallowed air. In an upright position, most of swallowed air is expelled through the mouth and does not appear in flatus. However, in a lying position, some of the swallowed air may go downstream.

FLATUS GAS

Much of the colonic gas (and gas expelled in flatus) is produced in the colon as a result of fermentation of unabsorbed carbohydrates by intestinal bacteria. Flatus is low in oxygen with a relatively higher level of methane. Most of the carbon dioxide, on the other hand, gets absorbed in the small intestine.

CAUSES OF EXCESS GAS

Numerous factors may play a role in production or awareness of excess gas. These include the following:

BLOCKAGE OR OBSTRUCTION OF THE INTESTINES

This may occur due to adhesions or scarring after surgeries or tumors.

SLOW MOVEMENTS OF THE GUT OR LAZY GUT

Factors include diseases like diabetes and scleroderma, as well as many medications especially psychiatric, neurological, and heart medicines. Sometimes the gut is just slow, and no cause can be identified.

IRRITABLE BOWEL SYNDROME

Patients with IBS usually do not have excess gas but have increased sensitivity and awareness of the gas being present.

MALABSORPTION OF FOOD

The more the undigested food in the gut, the more fermentation by the bacteria. This may occur when our ability to digest or absorb food is impaired. This may be seen in lactose intolerance, fructose intolerance, chronic pancreatitis, and celiac disease.

INFECTIONS

The small intestine has a low amount of bacteria and does not have much effect on the food that arrives there to be digested. In patients with small intestinal bacterial overgrowth, the number of bacteria increases many-fold and can ferment the yet-undigested food that arrives from the stomach. Increased gas may also be seen in patients with giardia infection.

PSYCHOLOGICAL FACTORS

Patients with severe anxiety tend to swallow a lot of air and, as such, may complain of gas.

DIETARY FACTORS

If we consume things that we cannot efficiently digest or absorb, the bowel bacteria will act upon them to ferment. Examples include sugars like fructose in fruits and vegetables that many of us cannot digest and sorbitol, which is used as low calorie sweetener. Sorbitol cannot be absorbed by our gut, and its fermentation by the bacteria can produce gas.

COMPLAINT OF GAS PROBLEM VERSUS AMOUNT OF INTESTINAL GAS

The volume of intestinal gas created is usually around 150-250 ml per day. It may rarely be as high as 1000 ml/day. The volume of gas produced is generally similar in people who complain of increased gas and those who don't.

FLATUS AROMA/ODOR

Most of the intestinal gas is odorless. The foul odor arises from trace amounts of sulfur-containing gases arising as a result of bacterial fermentation.

HOW DOES INTESTINAL GAS PRODUCE SYMPTOMS?

The symptoms of "gas" may arise because of increased gas or gas trapped in loops of the bowel (especially at sharp curves or angles) or increased sensitivity or awareness of gas. Irritable bowel syndrome, functional dyspepsia, and "intestinal gas" are associated with increased awareness. Food-related excess gas may occur in lactose intolerance and intolerance to sugars like fructose or sorbitol.

WHAT TO DO ABOUT GAS?

Diagnostic tests are based on associated symptoms that may suggest an underlying disease. A measurement of gas is not part of the testing strategy.

Treatment involves the underlying factors (outlined above) that may be contributing to excess gas. For example, better glucose control for cases of diabetes and antibiotics like rifaximin (Xifaxan) for small intestinal bacterial overgrowth.

Other widely-used options that are used by some patients include:

- Simethicone, which absorbs gas bubbles and is found in numerous over-the-counter formulations, including Gas-X, Maalox-Antigas, and Mylanta Gas
- Activated charcoal
- Beano
- Pepto-Bismol
- Charcoal cushions

Dietary manipulation is the only practical and beneficial strategy option in most cases. The less undigested food in the gut, the less gas is produced. In a nutshell, try a low-FODMAP diet. Details on FODMAP diet and alternatives are described in Chapter 20.

REFERENCES

1. Bolin T. Wind -- problems with intestinal gas. *Aust Fam Physician*. 2013; May; 42(5):280-3.
2. Azpiroz F. Intestinal gas dynamics: mechanisms and clinical relevance. *Gut* 2005 Jul; 54(7):893-5.

CHAPTER 33

Hemorrhoids and Anal Fissures

KEY POINTS

- Hemorrhoids are normal cushions made up of blood vessels and are present at birth.
- Local injection botulinum toxin is useful for treating anal fissure.

HEMORRHOIDS

Hemorrhoids are normal cushions made up of a network of blood vessels. They are underneath the lining of the anorectal wall and are called external or internal depending upon location. They are normally hidden inside the body. Hemorrhoids assist in normal continence. About five percent of the US population seeks medical attention for hemorrhoids at some point in their life.

CAUSES OF HEMORRHOIDAL DISEASE OR "HEMORRHOIDS"

While most hemorrhoids are asymptomatic, hemorrhoidal disease or "hemorrhoids" occur more commonly in the elderly. Other risk factors include chronic diarrhea, pregnancy, chronic constipation, and weight lifting. The factors contributing to hemorrhoidal disease may be multifactorial, including loss of connective tissue anchoring the hemorrhoidal cushion to the anal sphincters.

CLINICAL FEATURES

Patients have painless bleeding associated with bowel movements, especially bright red blood on the side of the stool or on the toilet paper. Blood may occasionally drip into the toilet. Bleeding can occasionally be severe, especially in patients on blood thinners. Bleeding associated with painful bowel movements suggests the possibility of an anal fissure. Pain may be present if a clot develops in hemorrhoids.

Perianal itching is usually related to other causes, such as suboptimal perianal hygiene, although hemorrhoids may contribute to it by permitting leakage of rectal contents, as well as by difficulty in cleaning skin tags. Aggressive cleaning, especially in cases of diarrhea, may also contribute to itching.

MEDICAL MANAGEMENT

- Avoid constipation. Read Chapter 38 for more details.
- Your diet should be rich in fruits and fiber. Fiber intake should be about 25 to 35 g per day.
- Fiber supplementation in the form of wafers, powders, or pills is effective in reducing acute episodes.
- Take bulk-forming laxatives like psyllium (Metamucil), methylcellulose (Citrucel), polycarbophil (FiberCon), and wheat dextrin (Benefiber). Start with a small amount and gradually increase it, along with increasing water in order to avoid adverse effects.
- Increase fluid intake. The bulking effect of fiber with the fluid may prevent perianal irritation by reducing seepage.
- Maintain clean, healthy perianal hygiene. Avoid irritating hemorrhoids. Use baby wipes to clean instead of toilet paper.
- Soak buttocks, preferably with cheeks spread, for 10-15 minutes twice a day to soothe the irritated hemorrhoids. One way to accomplish this is by lying in a bathtub of warm water. Do not add anything else to the bathwater like soap or bubble bath.
- Warm Sitz baths are effective for itching. Sitz baths should be performed three times a day. They help by reducing inflammation and relaxing the internal anal sphincter.
- Topical analgesic creams and suppositories for healing hemorrhoidal problems are available over the counter and may help. Creams and ointments containing hydrocortisone should

not be used for more than a week without the approval of the physician.

ROLE OF PHLEBOTONICS

This class of drugs is comprised of plant extracts as well as synthetic compounds. They act on blood vessels and are used for diseases related to blood vessels. A systematic review conducted by Dr. Perera and colleagues from the United Kingdom concluded that these drugs help in treating hemorrhoidal disease as well as post-procedural complications. Phlebotonics reduce bleeding, itching, discharge, and leakage.

> Examples of natural phlebotonics include bioflavonoids like quercetin, hesperidin, troxerutin, buckwheat extract, and ginko biloba and saponosides like horse chestnut seed extract. Synthetic drugs include naftazone, aminaftone, and chromocarbe. Miscellaneous phlebotonics include iquinosa and flunarizine.

MINIMALLY-INVASIVE PROCEDURES

These include rubber band ligation, cautery, laser, and cryosurgery. Patients who are non-responsive to simple measures are candidates. The choice of the procedure depends upon local expertise.

Rubber band ligation is one of the better options for most cases. It involves tying a rubber band around the hemorrhoid. The hemorrhoid then shrinks, separates, and falls off in a few days.

SURGERY

Surgical therapy involves excision of excess hemorrhoidal tissue. It is indicated in difficult cases, like large hemorrhoids with severe bleeding and those refractory to standard treatment. Mixed hemorrhoidal disease (involving external and internal hemorrhoids) also requires surgery. Serious complications due to surgery may however occur occasionally. These include bleeding, infection, fecal impaction, and urinary retention.

TREATMENT OF HEMORRHOID PLUS FISSURE

In patients with concomitant anal fissure, once the fissure is treated, the constipation should improve. The hemorrhoidal symptoms may then resolve without surgery.

ANAL FISSURE

An anal fissure is a tear in the lining of the anal wall.

CAUSATION

It occurs because of trauma due to large, hard stools or in association with inflammatory bowel disease (Crohn's disease and ulcerative colitis), tuberculosis, leukemia, or other conditions. Poor blood supply to the area may contribute to poor healing and creation of a chronic fissure.

CLINICAL FEATURES

The tear causes the surrounding muscles to go into spasms. Patients present with throbbing pain (most frequently occurring during or made worse following a bowel movement), bleeding, seepage, and difficulty with having a bowel movement. There may be anal itching. A finger rectal exam is painful and should be avoided.

DIAGNOSIS

This is made by inspection of the anal region by separating the buttocks. Patients who have bleeding need a lower GI scope to exclude other causes of bleeding.

TREATMENT

A multipronged approach is needed.

- Sitz baths with warm water two to three times a day
- Bulking fiber supplements (Metamucil, Citrucel, Benefiber)

- Stool softeners
- Pain control with pain-killer analgesics
- Local application of nitroglycerin ointment
- Local injection of botulinum toxin (BOTOX) injection

Calcium channel blockers diltiazem (Cardizem) or nifedipine (Adalat CC, Procardia) have also been used with success. However, there is the potential for side effects.

ROLE OF SURGERY

Surgery is undertaken for patients who fail to respond to medical therapy. Complications of surgery include minor fecal incontinence.

Note: An optimal treatment of anal fissures is still elusive.

REFERENCES

1. Lohsiriwat V. Hemorrhoids: from basic pathophysiology to clinical management. *World J Gastroenterol.* 2012 May 7; 18(17):2009-17.
2. Nelson RL, Thomas K, Morgan J, Jones A. Non surgical therapy for anal fissure. *Cochrane Database Syst Rev.* 2012 Feb 15; 2:CD003431.

SECTION IX
Chronic GI Problems Requiring Tailored Seven-X Plan

CHAPTER 34

Chronic Heartburn or Gastro-Esophageal Reflux Disease

KEY POINTS

- An upper GI scope is an insensitive diagnostic test for GERD since half of the patients do not have any grossly visibly damage.
- The heart should be excluded as a cause for atypical chest pain before consideration of more benign conditions like GERD.
- Lifestyle modifications help ameliorate esophageal symptoms in many cases.
- Acid blockers, while effective, also carry the risk of long-term consequences.
- Psychological therapies may benefit patients with GERD and non-cardiac chest pain.

Gastroesophageal reflux (GER) is a normal phenomenon occurring in healthy individuals, especially after meals. It is considered GERD when the reflux occurs to the degree that it produces esophageal and non-GI symptoms or causes damage to the esophagus or other organs.

HISTORICAL PERSPECTIVE

Until the late eighteenth and early nineteenth century, most symptoms of possible gastroesophageal reflux disease (GERD) and peptic ulcer disease (PUD) were lumped into various diagnoses, depending upon the culture or civilization. Some of the ancient treatments have stood the test of time and are still preferred over modern medicine by millions of people.

HOW COMMON IS GERD?

Prevalence estimates vary depending upon the definition used. While uncommon in Asian countries, GERD is thought to be primarily a disease of the West. However, its prevalence is increasing even in the Eastern countries, probably because of the adoption of Western diet and lifestyle. The prevalence of heartburn is eight percent in Italy and 10 percent in Japan.

Heartburn occurs in 15 to 44 percent of Americans at least once a month, weekly in 20 percent, while about 7 percent of Americans have heartburn every day. Only five percent of patients with heartburn seek medical attention, but this is rapidly changing because of the recognition of its potential seriousness and the availability of effective medications for treatment. GERD occurs more frequently in men and is uncommon in African-Americans.

The prevalence of heartburn increases with age. It increases dramatically after turning 40. Complications of GERD are more frequent in white males and increase with age.

CAUSATION

In contrast to physiologic reflux episodes, which are normal, especially after meals, pathologic reflux is associated with nocturnal symptoms and even complications. While the physiologic reflux episodes are short-lived, pathologic reflux may be prolonged.

The stomach's regurgitation causes damage to the tight junctions between the cells of the esophageal mucosa. This leads to widening of intercellular spaces and increased permeability in the lining of esophagus. This allows for increased acid penetration. The increased leakiness allows contact of acid with the underlying nerves, resulting in symptoms. At this point, the damage is only microscopic and may explain about 50 percent of GERD patients who have non-erosive reflux disease. In many patients, there is further disruption of junctions leading to cell damage, inflammation, and grossly visible ulceration.

FACTORS AFFECTING REFLUX OF GASTRIC CONTENTS INTO ESOPHAGUS

Reflux occurs due to numerous causes. The relative contribution of the causes varies between different individuals.

LOWER ESOPHAGEAL SPHINCTER

The most important factor is the one-way valve function of the lower esophageal sphincter (LES), which is at the junction of the esophagus and stomach. The LES is normally closed at rest and opens to facilitate the passage of food from the esophagus into the stomach when we swallow food.

About 71 percent of reflux symptoms occur within four hours of a meal. In fact, these transient relaxations are the major cause for GERD in many patients. The LES can also be weak, and such patients tend to get more serious complications.

ESOPHAGEAL FACTORS

These include gravity, peristaltic function of the esophagus, and the neutralization of the acid by alkaline salivary juices. Both the salivary secretions as well as peristalsis of the esophagus are decreased during sleep, and the protection by gravity is lost since we are lying down. This results in prolonging the contact of regurgitated material with the esophagus.

Esophageal factors providing resistance to acid-induced damage include tight junctions, buffering action of blood flow, mucous, bicarbonate, and epidermal growth factors.

STOMACH FACTORS

Delayed stomach emptying is present in many patients with GERD. Other factors include hiatal hernia, obstruction to outflow of food from stomach into small intestine, pregnancy, and patients with weight loss surgery.

HELICOBACTER PYLORI INFECTION

The role of *H. pylori* is controversial. Evidence suggests that chronic infection leads to chronic gastritis, which can then lead to decreased acidity. As such, *H. pylori* may be protective against GERD in many cases.

OTHER DISEASES

These include diabetes mellitus, scleroderma, and CREST syndrome.

CLINICAL FEATURES OF GERD

Patients typically complain of heartburn and a retrosternal burning sensation radiating to the neck. It frequently occurs after meals and may wake the patient at night. Some patients find it difficult to sleep unless they are in a recliner. The symptoms improve with antacids. Patients also may complain of effortless return of stomach contents to the throat.

ATYPICAL FEATURES

These fall along a wide spectrum and include the following:

- Angina-like chest pain, which can be difficult to distinguish from angina of the heart – remember, angina chest pain of the heart can kill, so always seek medical help.
- Water brash
- Asthma
- Globus sensation (a lump in the throat)
- Difficulty swallowing and choking while eating
- Aspiration of stomach contents into the lungs, causing bronchitis and pneumonia

- Hoarseness due to laryngitis
- Frequent upper respiratory infections
- Bad breath
- Chronic cough
- Chronic throat clearing

While GERD has been implicated in numerous extra-esophageal problems, a cause-and-effect relationship has been difficult to establish in many instances.

GERD IN CHILDREN

GERD is under-recognized in the pediatric population, especially during infancy. It occurs due to an underdeveloped lower esophageal sphincter that usually resolves by one to two years of age. The symptoms are nonspecific and include excessive fussiness, abnormal crying, aversion to food, inability to sleep, and even growth failure.

DIAGNOSIS

Patients with typical symptoms do not need to have any diagnostic evaluation and may be treated on clinical grounds. Exceptions include patients with alarm symptoms like weight loss, bleeding, and difficult or painful swallowing. Tests include upper GI scope, upper GI X-ray, and 24-hour pH check of acid in esophagus. A routine upper GI scope is less likely to be of benefit if done just to make diagnosis of GERD, since half of the patients will not show any grossly visible damage.

COMPLICATIONS OF GERD

Complications include inflammation and narrowing of the esophagus, bleeding, and cancer. Narrowing or stricture of the esophagus can be dilated during an upper GI scope. Bleeding can be severe. Food can become impacted if there is a significant blockage of the esophagus, requiring an emergency upper GI scope to dislodge the impacted food.

MEDICAL TREATMENT OF GERD

GERD is frequently a clinical diagnosis, and empiric treatment is used in patients without evidence of alarm symptoms.

LIFESTYLE MEASURES

Lifestyle modifications may provide symptomatic relief in up to 25 percent of the cases. These include:

- Elevate the head of the bed by using four- to six-inch blocks.
- Eat supper at least three hours before bedtime.
- Go out for a short, relaxed stroll after supper.
- Eat small, frequent meals. Avoid large, fatty meals, especially at dinner. Do not eat bedtime snacks.
- Dietary modifications should also be individualized, based on the patient's symptom triggers.
- Avoid foods that precipitate reflux like chocolate or that irritate esophagus like tomatoes and oranges
- Chewing gum helps increase the alkaline salivary juices to neutralize acid.
- Avoid carbonated or caffeinated beverages.
- Quit smoking. Smoking increases stomach acidity and adversely affects healing capacity. Smoking also increases the risk for esophageal cancer.
- Minimize or quit drinking alcohol. Alcohol has direct toxic effects on the lining of the esophagus, in addition to promoting reflux.
- Avoid tight clothes, especially at home.
- Attempt weight reduction if overweight.

OVER-THE-COUNTER RELIEF

Acid neutralization by antacids and alginic acid provide relief in many cases of intermittent heartburn. Many of these come as combination formulations like Gaviscon-2. The use of antacids for chronic heartburn on a regular basis may not be cost-effective and may cause significant side effects.

ACID BLOCKERS

Acid suppression is the cornerstone of treatment and can be carried out using H2 receptor antagonists (H2RAs), which provide relief in about 50 percent of cases, or proton pump inhibitors (PPIs), which provide relief in 85 to 95 percent of the cases. H2RAs include cimetidine (Tagamet), ranitidine (Zantac), nizatidine (Axid), and famotidine (Pepcid).

PPIs block the final step in the pathway to acid secretion and are more potent than H2RAs for acid suppression, as well as for relief of heartburn. These include omeprazole (Prilosec), lansoprazole (Prevacid), rabeprazole (Aciphex), pantoprazole (Protonix), and esomeprazole (Nexium). The drugs are best given 30 to 45 minutes before breakfast, which is sufficient for most patients with GERD.

ACID BLOCKERS ARE NOT RISK-FREE

In addition to the easily-recognized side effects and potential for drug interactions, it is being increasingly understood that the potent PPI type of drugs can have serious long-term consequences. These include:

- Malabsorption of nutrients
- Vitamin B-12 deficiency
- Increased risk of respiratory infections
- Increased risk of GI infections like *C. difficile* colitis
- Increased risk of fractures
- Osteoporosis

ROLE OF SURGERY

Surgery is an effective treatment for GERD and can be done via tiny incisions. While many surgeons consider all GERD an indicator for surgery, most gastroenterologists refer patients for surgery selectively.

The effectiveness of surgery depends upon the expertise of the surgeon. Patients who do not respond well to PPI drugs are less likely to respond well to surgery.

DEVICE TREATMENTS VIA UPPER GI SCOPE

Multiple devices have been approved over the years. Many of them subsequently fell out of favor because of complication. The purpose of many devices is to make the valve at the lower esophageal sphincter (LES) tighter so as not to allow reflux. This can be accomplished by devices that apply sewing or stapling at the LES. Still another device applies radiofrequency waves at the site, which then causes the LES to become narrow due to scarring by these waves.

Most of the trials done using devices exclude serious cases of GERD. In my opinion, the current technology is still in its infancy and should be considered only in the context of clinical trials.

ALTERNATIVE MEDICINE TREATMENTS

PLANT-BASED THERAPIES

Peppermint oil

Peppermint promotes gastric emptying and thus may be an antidote to GE reflux. Peppermint aromatherapy has major effects on decreasing pain and depression levels, suggesting another possible mechanism for non-cardiac chest pain and heartburn.

Patients with GERD have long been warned to avoid peppermint oil. However, this recommendation appears to be based predominantly on theoretical grounds and lacks data from randomized controlled studies to support it. This recommendation also flies in the face of the centuries-old use of peppermint after meals, with perceived beneficial effects against indigestion.

Hange-koboku-to (Banxia-Houpo-Tang, HKT)

Hange-koboku-to accelerates stomach emptying and is likely to play a beneficial role in combating GERD.

Liu-Jun-Zi-Tang (TJ-43)

Liu-Jun-Zi-Tang, also known as Rikkunshi-to and TJ-43, is a multi-herbal Chinese formulation. Compared to placebo, TJ-43 (2.5 g, three times a day) improves gastric emptying and heartburn.

STW 5

It protects against damage to the esophagus in animal models of esophagitis. This occurs without reducing the acidity, suggesting that its effects are mediated by enhancing the anti-inflammatory and repair mechanisms.

Tangweikang

Tangweikang is a Chinese herbal preparation used to treat diabetes. It hastens stomach emptying in gastroparesis and may be useful as an anti-GERD agent.

Terminalia

Terminalia chebula is commonly advocated in Ayurveda to improve GI movements. It has been shown to hasten gastric emptying in rats. As such, it has the potential to be helpful in treating GERD as a prokinetic agent.

Turmeric (Curcuma)

It blocks acid secretion in the stomach and, as such, may help in GERD.

Warm chamomile or lemon balm teas are also reputed to tame agitated stomachs. A variety of other herbs that have been used with success over the centuries include ginger, bitters, gentian root, goldenseal, aromatics, and ginseng.

ACUPUNCTURE

Multiple studies have documented that acupuncture speeds up stomach emptying. It is also an acid blocker. Studies done in patients with GERD have also demonstrated efficacy.

PROBIOTICS

Certain probiotics enhance stomach emptying. For example, the gastric emptying rate is significantly faster in the newborns receiving *L. reuteri* than in newborns receiving formula with placebo.

The probiotic combination formulation Ecologic Relief (*Bifidobacterium bifidum W23, B. lactis W52, B. longum W108, Lactobacillus casei W79, L. plantarum W62,* and *L. rhamnosus W7*) reduces reflux episodes in pregnant women.

Data suggests that some probiotics may benefit GERD patients.

CHIROPRACTIC TECHNIQUE

While there are no controlled trials, anecdotal reports suggest a benefit in treating GERD.

PSYCHOLOGICAL THERAPIES

Psychological factors are involved in GERD, non-cardiac chest pain, and functional heartburn. They offer a potential target for psychological interventions in the treatment of esophageal disorders.

- Relaxation exercises ameliorate reflux symptoms by reducing esophageal acid exposure.
- Use of psychological therapies for non-cardiac chest pain appears promising. A randomized, controlled trial of cognitive-behavioral therapy for treatment of persistent non-cardiac chest pain demonstrated significant reductions in chest pain,

limitations of daily life, autonomic symptoms, and psychological morbidity, compared to the control group.

- One study compared a psychological treatment package (including treatments like education, relaxation, breathing training, and graded exposure to exercise) to waiting-list controls for treatment of non-cardiac chest pain. Treatment significantly reduced chest pain episodes from 6.5 to 2.5 per week, accompanied by improvements in anxiety and depression scores, disability rating, and exercise tolerance.

Overall, the role of psychological therapies for GERD and non-cardiac chest pain appears promising.

HOMEOPATHY

Homeopathy is based on the principle of dilutions. It defies biological plausibility and continues to baffle scientists; the debate on its effectiveness is ongoing. There is a lack of data confirming or refuting the effect of homeopathy in esophageal disorders.

MINERALS

Most of the data in this category pertain to the use of zinc. Zinc reduces stomach acid. It protects the stomach wall against damage. The efficacy of zinc in treating GERD is supported by evidence of its local tissue healing properties, as well as its ability to reduce gastric acid.

REFERENCES

1. Lightdale JR, Gremse DA. Gastroesophageal reflux: management guidance for the pediatrician. *Pediatrics*. 2013 May; 131(5):e1684-95.
2. Bredenoord AJ, Pandolfino JE, Smout AJ. Gastro-oesophageal reflux disease. *Lancet*. 2013 Jun 1; 381(9881):1933-42.
3. Hom C, Vaezi MF. Extraesophageal manifestations of gastroesophageal reflux disease. *Gastroenterol Clin North Am*. 2013 Mar; 42(1):71-91.

4. de Milliano I, Tabbers MM, van der Post JA, Benninga MA. Is a multispecies probiotic mixture effective in constipation during pregnancy? 'A pilot study'. *Nutr J*. 2012 Oct 4; 11:80.
5. Abdel-Aziz H, Zaki HF, Neuhuber W et al. Effect of an herbal preparation, STW 5, in an acute model of reflux oesophagitis in rats. *J Pharmacol Sci*. 2010 Jun; 113(2):134-42.
6. Indrio F, Riezzo G, Raimondi F et al. The effects of probiotics on feeding tolerance, bowel habits, and gastrointestinal motility in preterm newborns. *J Pediatr*. 2008 Jun; 152(6):801-6.
7. McDonald-Haile J, Bradley LA, Bailey MA et al. Relaxation training reduces symptom reports and acid exposure in patients with gastroesophageal reflux disease. *Gastroenterology* 1994 Jul; 107(1):61-9.

CHAPTER 35

Gastroparesis

KEY POINTS

- Gastroparesis may be occult. Patients sometimes have non-specific symptoms like bad pain, diarrhea, poor appetite, and weight loss, especially in the absence of risk factors like diabetes or surgery that may not look like gastroparesis but may be related to it. The diagnosis is a consideration in any patient with refractory upper gut symptoms.
- Drug treatment of gastroparesis has been suboptimal.
- Dietary manipulation is of paramount importance.
- Gastric electrical stimulation may help some patients with gastroparesis.
- Therapies based on Chinese medicine (like STW 5 and acupuncture) are effective.
- Mind-body therapies have a beneficial effect in treating gastroparesis.

Gastroparesis is the slow emptying of stomach contents. Some experts suggest using the term *gastropathy*, which would consist of all disordered emptying (either too slow or too fast).

PREVALENCE OF GASTROPARESIS

Although widespread, the prevalence and the age and sex distribution of gastroparesis is unknown. There are over 50,000 patients with severe gastroparesis symptoms in the United States. As many as 40 percent of diabetic patients have delayed gastric emptying; however, not all patients with delayed gastric emptying have symptoms. In fact, there is a poor correlation between the degree of slowness of emptying and the symptoms associated with it.

CAUSES OF GASTROPARESIS

Cause cannot be identified in a majority of cases. About half of the cases are preceded by an episode of infectious illness. Gastroparesis is fairly common after stomach surgery.

Delayed or disordered stomach emptying may be seen in systemic diseases like scleroderma, diabetes, thyroid dysfunction, multiple sclerosis, Parkinsonism, anorexia nervosa and bulimia, chronic liver or renal failure, pancreatitis, bone marrow transplantation, cancer, or abnormal stomach pacemaker activity due to nervous system damage. Many medications can slow the stomach as well, although they are usually the sole cause.

CLINICAL FEATURES

Patients present with nausea, vomiting, abdominal bloating and distension, feeling full shortly after initiating a meal, and sometimes weight loss. Initial evaluation assessment focuses just not on the GI systems but also on other body-wide disorders that may contribute to disordered emptying.

DIAGNOSIS

Upper GI endoscopy and/or upper GI barium X-rays are useful to exclude any structural abnormality. A four-hour stomach emptying scan is the standard. The patient consumes standard food laced with radionuclide material. The percent of the meal remaining in the stomach determines the diagnosis, as well as the severity of gastroparesis.

Electrogastrography (EGG) examines the electrical activity of stomach just as EKG does for the heart. It helps detect abnormalities of electrical rhythm in the stomach.

TREATMENT

Modification of lifestyle, including eating small, frequent meals and eating low-fat meals, is the first step. Medical therapy is effective in as many as 60 percent of the patients.

LIFESTYLE STRATEGIES

- Five to six small meals per day
- Low-fat diet
- Low-fiber diet
- Avoiding fried foods
- Stopping smoking
- Stopping drinking
- Avoiding carbonated beverages
- Weight control, if overweight

DRUG TREATMENT OF GASTROPARESIS

Metoclopramide (Reglan) is useful, but its utility is limited by its high incidence of nervous system side effects.

Domperidone is similar to metoclopramide, except that it does not penetrate the blood-brain barrier well and as such is devoid of troublesome movement-related side effects. However, it is available only in compound pharmacies in the United States and is very expensive. It is available in pharmacies in other countries, including Canada.

Erythromycin is effective in improving gastric emptying but loses its effects within a few weeks. Cisapride is an effective agent but is not available for widespread use in the US. Bethanecol has been used; however, its side effects preclude its widespread use.

Botulinum toxin (BOTOX) injection into the pyloric sphincter at the junction of the stomach and duodenum (the first part of small bowel) has been used in cases where a spasm of the pylorus is suspected to be the cause, as in diabetes mellitus.

SURGERY

Results from surgery as treatment of gastroparesis are disappointing.

GASTRIC PACEMAKER

Similar to a pacemaker for the heart, gastric electrical stimulation (GES) has been approved by the FDA for drug-refractory gastroparesis. Results from the studies have been mixed. GES appears to improve stomach emptying and nutritional status and reduce healthcare costs. Complications may occur. The most common complication of using a GES device is infection.

ALTERNATIVE MEDICINE THERAPIES

PLANT-BASED NATURAL THERAPIES

Asparagus (Shatavari)

Shatavari is used in Ayurveda to treat dyspepsia. It reduces gastric emptying time in normal, healthy volunteers.

Ginger

Administration of three ginger capsules (a total of 1,200 mg one hour before a meal) accelerates stomach emptying and stimulates stomach contractions in healthy volunteers.

Peppermint oil

Peppermint increases the early phase of stomach emptying. The effect of peppermint oil and caraway on stomach emptying is equivalent to that of the drug cisapride.

HKT

Hange-koboku-to (Banxia-houpo-tang; HKT) accelerates gastric emptying in patients with dyspepsia and in healthy controls.

STW 5

STW 5 is a fixed combination of nine herbs. It modifies the electrical rhythm waves in the stomach and stimulates stomach motility. It has different effects in different parts of stomach. It improves symptoms in patients with gastroparesis without affecting gastric emptying. A double-blind trial documented that the effects of STW 5 and STW 5-II given for four weeks are equivalent to those of cisapride for the treatment of the dysmotility type of functional dyspepsia.

TJ-13

Liu-Jun-Zi-Tang (TJ-43) is also known as Rikkunshi-to. Compared to placebo, TJ-43 (2.5 g three times a day) improves gastric emptying, as well as gastrointestinal symptoms of stomach fullness, heartburn, belching, and nausea.

Tangweikang (TWK)

Tangweikang is a Chinese herbal preparation used in diabetes. It hastens gastric emptying in diabetic gastroparesis.

ACUPUNCTURE

Electro-acupuncture hastens stomach emptying in several animals. It increases the normal stomach electrical waves in healthy volunteers.

Multiple studies have documented the efficacy of acupuncture in treating gastroparesis. A single-blind controlled trial found that electro-acupuncture results in improving symptoms of diabetic gastroparesis associated with faster solid stomach emptying. Effects were sustained for at least two weeks after the end of the trial. Acupuncture even improves gastric emptying in critically ill patients.

Based on the literature, acupuncture administered by an expert may be a reasonable option for patients with refractory gastroparesis resistant to standard management.

PROBIOTICS

Limited evidence exists regarding the role of probiotics in gastroparesis. The gastric emptying rate is significantly faster in the newborns receiving the probiotic L. reuteri in their formula than those receiving formula supplemented with placebo. In fact, L. reuteri-supplemented babies have a motility pattern resembling that of newborns fed with breast milk.

MIND-BODY THERAPIES

Psychological alterations may be involved both as a cause and effect of gastroparesis. Evidence suggests a potential target for psychological interventions in the treatment of gastroparesis. For example, gut-oriented hypnosis accelerates gastric emptying. Listening to enjoyable music increases the amplitude of electrical waves in the stomach of healthy humans.

Watching EGG activity on the screen, patients can see their body's contraction waves, then learn relaxation techniques to modulate gastric electrical waves. Breathing exercises with biofeedback increases drinking capacity.

HOMEOPATHY

Homeopathy, while extremely popular outside of the U.S., continues to defy biological plausibility and baffle scientists. The debate on its effectiveness continues. There is a lack of data examining the effect of homeopathy in treating gastroparesis.

REFERENCES

1. Abell TL, Malinowski S, Minocha A. Nutrition aspects of gastroparesis and therapies for drug-refractory patients. *Nutr Clin Pract*. 2006 Feb; 21(1):23-33.
2. Abell TL, Minocha A. Gastroparesis and the gastric pacemaker: a revolutionary treatment for an old disease. *J Miss State Med Assoc*. 2002; 43(12):369-75.
3. Inamori M, Akiyama T, Akimoto K et al. Early effects of peppermint oil on gastric emptying: a crossover study using a

continuous real-time 13C breath test (BreathID system). *J Gastroenterol*. 2007 Jul; 42(7):539-42.

4. Rösch W, Vinson B, Sassin I. A randomised clinical trial comparing the efficacy of a herbal preparation STW 5 with the prokinetic drug cisapride in patients with dysmotility type of functional dyspepsia. *Z Gastroenterol*. 2002 Jun; 40(6):401-8.

5. Sun BM, Luo M, Wu SB et al. Acupuncture versus metoclopramide in treatment of postoperative gastroparesis syndrome in abdominal surgical patients: a randomized controlled trial. *Zhong Xi Yi Jie He Xue Bao*. 2010 Jul; 8(7):641-4.

CHAPTER 36

Ulcers

KEY POINTS

- Most patients with ulcer-like symptoms do not have ulcers.
- Treatment of an ulcer involves therapy to heal the ulcer and to prevent its recurrence.
- Smoking and alcohol drinking increase gastric acidity and reduce the stomach's defense mechanisms.
- Chili pepper, while it may cause indigestion, has been shown to protect against stomach ulcers in animals.
- Limited data suggests that psychological interventions may be helpful in treating select patients.

PREVALENCE

Peptic ulcer disease accounts for billions of dollars each year in treatments in the United States. Peptic ulcer disease may occur in the stomach or duodenum, which is the first part of the small bowel adjoining the stomach. While some ulcers resolve on their own, others may progress and create complications, sometimes even requiring surgery.

CAUSATION OF ULCERS

Despite the recent surge in knowledge implicating *H. pylori* in the causation of the majority of stomach and duodenal ulcers, the old dictum "no acid, no ulcer" still applies.

The causative factors include increased stomach acid, smoking, and medications, especially NSAIDs. The ulcer occurs when the strength of injurious factors overwhelms the body's defenses.

Limited evidence suggests that stress plays a role in the causation of ulcers, although it is controversial. Ulcers are more common during wars and among war survivors.

Most ulcers can be accounted for by *H. pylori* infection and NSAID use.

Healing of ulcers is slower in elderly subjects, alcoholics, smokers, and patients in stressful life situations.

CLINICAL FEATURES

An ulcer in the duodenum typically causes stomach pain two to three hours after a meal. Pain improves with food. Patients tend to eat more and may become overweight. An ulcer in the stomach, on the other hand, causes pain soon after eating; as such, patients are afraid to eat and lose weight. Symptoms of complicated ulcer disease include upper GI bleeding and vomiting due to stomach obstruction. On rare occasions, the ulcer might burrow a hole through the stomach wall, causing a surgical emergency.

DIAGNOSIS

An ulcer is typically diagnosed by an upper GI X-ray and/or scope. Only 15 to 25 percent of the patients with ulcer-suggesting symptoms are actually found to have ulcers upon upper GI scope. A scope test is preferred, because it is more sensitive for small ulcers and also allows for the taking of biopsies.

H. PYLORI TESTING

All patients with an ulcer should undergo testing for *H. pylori*. During the upper GI scope, biopsies can be taken and examined under a microscope. A blood test, breath test, or stool test for *H. pylori* are other options, depending on the clinical situation.

HISTORY OF ULCER TREATMENT

The ancient description of the use of powdered coral, chalk, and seashells for relief of dyspepsia suggests that this problem occurred long before the modern descriptions of GERD and ulcers. Hunter in 1784 advocated the use of milk as a natural antacid.

Illogical treatments of the past include antimony, arsenic, mercury, alcohol rectal enemas, and complete bowel rest. Application of leeches to the abdomen was in vogue in the eighteenth century. Other treatments used in the past include synthetic resins, cabbage, pectin, pituitary extract, insulin, and histamine.

Surgeons like Dr. Billroth made the first advance in modern treatment by performing surgery for ulcers in the 1880s. Nevertheless, radiation treatment and rest in the hospital was routine in the first half of the 20th century.

MODERN TREATMENT OF ULCERS

The treatment of peptic ulcer disease is twofold:

- To heal the ulcer.
- To prevent the recurrence of ulcer.

HEALING THE ULCER

Changes to diet are not routinely recommended. Stop or minimize NSAID drug usage and smoking.

Antacids are effective, but the side effects make their routine use less attractive. Histamine-2 receptor antagonists (H2RAs) like cimetidine (Tagamet), ranitidine (Zantac), famotidine (Pepcid), and nizatidine (Axid) heal about 70 to 80 percent of ulcers within four weeks and 85 to 95 percent after eight weeks of therapy.

Sucralfate (Carafate) does not have any significant impact on stomach acid secretion, in contrast to acid blockers. Sucralfate heals ulcers mainly by its local effects on the stomach and duodenum wall and is equal in efficacy to H2RAs.

The PPI class of drugs, including omeprazole (Prilosec), lansoprazole (Prevacid), pantoprazole (Protonix), rabeprazole (Aciphex), and esomeprazole (Nexium), results in an 80 to 100 percent healing rate for duodenal ulcers within four weeks. The superiority of PPI drugs over H2RAs for healing of stomach ulcers is modest, however.

PREVENTION OF RECURRENCE OF *H. PYLORI* (HP)-RELATED ULCERS

Patients testing positive for Hp should use a 10- to 14-day treatment of at least 3-4 drugs. Multiple combinations of drugs are in vogue. Dose-packs like PrevPak combine all three commonly-used drugs and make it easier to follow instructions.

PREVENTION OF RECURRENCE OF NSAID-INDUCED ULCERS

NSAID-type pain/arthritis medications increase the possibility of ulcers. Thus, patients with NSAID-induced ulcers should stop using the drug, if medically allowed by their physician. Another option is giving the minimum needed dose of NSAID. If that is not feasible, patients can be treated with a PPI drug (see examples above) along with the NSAID to reduce the risk of ulcers. Combination dose-packs containing an NSAID and a prophylactic PPI medication are available (PREVACID-NapraPac 500).

Another option is to use COX-2 inhibitors, which have less (but not zero) risk for ulcers. They have lately fallen out of favor because of increased risk for heart problems.

MAINTENANCE TREATMENT OF ULCERS

Maintenance therapy is indicated in high-risk patients in whom *H. pylori* infection could not be eradicated or in those who have ulcers unrelated to *H. pylori* or NSAID drugs. Such patients are investigated for other causes of ulcers, like tumors and infection.

Histamine blockers or H2RA drugs (like Zantac) are effective in reducing the recurrence of ulcers. PPI drugs (like Prilosec) may also be used for maintenance, especially if H2RA drugs fail or if there are giant and/or persistent ulcers.

ALTERNATIVE MEDICINE TREATMENT OF ULCERS

PLANT-BASED THERAPIES

Several studies have shown the potential benefit of natural plant-based treatments.

Amalaki

Amalaki is an Ayurvedic herbal remedy. Dr. Chawla and colleagues from India compared the use of Amalaki or antacids. Patients included those with an ulcer and non-ulcer dyspepsia. Compared to the baseline, symptoms improved in both treatments groups.

Chili powder (capsaicin)

Chili powder given by mouth protects against aspirin-induced ulcers in healthy human subjects. On the other hand, capsaicin can increase heartburn after a meal. Interestingly, epidemiologic surveys in Singapore have shown that stomach ulcers are three times more common in people of Chinese descent than in those of Indian descent, who tend to consume more chili peppers.

Mastic

Mastic is a concrete resinous exudate obtained from the tree *Pistacia*. It decreases stomach acid. A double-blind trial of mastic for the treatment of duodenal ulcers showed that 70 percent of patients on mastic treatment had healed when a follow-up upper GI scope was done, compared to 22 percent of patients on placebo.

Turmeric (curcumin)

One study found that turmeric treatment using *Curcuma longa* for four weeks resulted in healing of 48 percent of cases of peptic ulcer. Seventy-six percent of patients had healed their ulcers by the end of 12 weeks.

Pepticare

It is an Ayurvedic herbal-mineral formulation. It reduces stomach acid and protects against experimentally-induced ulcers in rats. There are no comparable human studies.

PROBIOTICS

Probiotics may have a role in ulcer disease, especially in reducing the risk of side effects related to treatment of H. pylori. There is no good evidence to support their routine use in ulcer treatment at the present time.

PSYCHOLOGICAL THERAPIES

The role of war and stress in ulcer causation suggests the potential for psychological interventions in the treatment of ulcers, especially ulcers not responding to routine medical care.

Dr. Colgan and colleagues conducted a controlled trial of hypnosis to prevent relapse of duodenal ulcers after ulcer treatment with an acid blocker (ranitidine). After stopping ranitidine, patients either received hypnotherapy or did not receive hypnotherapy for 10 weeks. A follow-up upper GI scope at one year showed that, while all of the patients in the no-hypnotherapy group showed relapse, only about half (53 percent) of the hypnotherapy group had developed ulcers.

ZINC

Multiple studies have documented the benefit of zinc for treating ulcers. A multi-center, double-blind comparison of zinc acexamate and the acid blocker famotidine for four weeks showed that zinc acexamate is as effective as famotidine for symptom relief as well as healing of duodenal ulcer.

REFERENCES

1. ASGE Standards of Practice Committee, Banerjee S, Cash BD, Dominitz JA, Baron TH et al. The role of endoscopy in the management of patients with peptic ulcer disease. *Gastrointest Endosc.* 2010 Apr; 71(4):663-8.
2. Asher GN, Spelman K. Clinical utility of curcumin extract. *Altern Ther Health Med.* 2013 Mar-Apr; 19(2):20-2.
3. Milosavljevic T, Kostić-Milosavljević M, Jovanović I, Krstić M. Complications of peptic ulcer disease. *Dig Dis.* 2011;29(5):491-3.
4. Overmier JB, Murison R. Restoring psychology's role in peptic ulcer. *Appl Psychol Health Well Being.* 2013 Mar; 5(1):5-27.
5. Georgopoulos SD, Papastergiou V, Karatapanis S. Current options for the treatment of Helicobacter pylori. *Expert Opin Pharmacother.* 2013 Feb; 14(2):211-23.
6. Jhun HJ, Ju YS, Kim JB, Kim JK. Present status and self-reported diseases of the Korean atomic bomb survivors: a mail questionnaire survey. *Med Confl Surviv.* 2005 Jul-Sep; 21(3):230-6.
7. Colgan SM, Faragher EB, Whorwell PJ: Controlled trial of hypnotherapy in relapse prevention of duodenal ulceration. *Lancet.*1988 Jun 11; 1(8598):1299-300.

CHAPTER 37

Irritable Bowel Syndrome

KEY POINTS

- Irritable bowel syndrome is a clinical diagnosis based on specific diagnostic criteria. Both abdominal pain and bowel problems must be present for diagnosis.
- A biopsychosocial model, involving multiple exacerbating and perpetuating factors, has been suggested as involved in causation of this poorly understood condition.

Irritable bowel syndrome (IBS) is a "functional disorder" characterized by abnormal intestinal movement patterns or intestinal sensations, increased sensitivity to pain, and dysfunction of the brain-gut connections and functions. It results in abdominal pain associated with abnormal pattern of bowel movements. While knowledge continues to evolve, very little is understood about IBS, and many practitioners openly admit that it is a disorder about which we have few clues and the management of which is mostly "trial and error."

WHY IS IBS SO COMMON IN MODERN SOCIETY?

There have been numerous and complex changes in the human environment, including diet and other lifestyle conditions. These started with the introduction of agriculture, animal husbandry and have continued through the growth of city living, industrialization, and the use of processed food. Dietary changes include alterations in glycemic load, fat composition, proportion and variety of macronutrients, micronutrient density, sodium-potassium ratio, and amount of fiber. At the same time, we have evolved from a hunter-gatherer society to the modern era, where we drive to the gym to walk on the treadmill!

PREVALENCE

The estimated prevalence of IBS varies widely, depending on the study criteria used and the population studied. The overall prevalence of IBS is similar between Western and Eastern cultures. Approximately 10 to 20 percent of the worldwide population suffers from IBS. The prevalence is greater among women than men in the Western society. However, studies from India suggest IBS is more common among men. Patients usually present for the first time between the ages of 15 and 50.

Prevalence estimates of IBS among African-Americans and Hispanics are less established. Studies by Dr. Minocha's group of investigators suggest that the prevalence is similar among African-Americans and Caucasian-Americans.

USE OF HEALTHCARE RESOURCES

Patients seeking healthcare attention are just the tip of the iceberg of IBS sufferers. Twelve percent of the patients seen in primary care practice carry the diagnosis of IBS. Physician surveys suggest that as many as 41 percent of the outpatient GI diagnoses are functional GI disorders, of which IBS is the most common.

Patients with IBS seeking medical attention tend to have concurrent non-GI complaints. There is also a greater likelihood of prior hysterectomy and appendectomy amongst these patients. The cost to the healthcare system related to IBS is high. IBS accounts for 2.4 to 3.5 million physician visits annually in the United States, resulting in 2.2 million prescriptions.

The average annual healthcare cost of a patient with IBS is $4,044, compared to $2,719 for the patients without this diagnosis. Patients with IBS miss three times as many work days as those without IBS. The disorder is associated with $1.6 billion in direct and $19.2 billion in indirect costs annually to the healthcare system.

CLINICAL FEATURES

IBS is diagnosed with symptom-based criteria, none of which is ideal. The most popular is the ROME criteria, which keeps evolving. Currently, the ROME III criteria defines IBS as a group of functional bowel disorders in which the patient complains of abdominal pain or discomfort for at least six months (which need not be consecutive) and the symptoms have occurred for at least three days during the prior three months. The pain must be associated with at least two of the following three features:

- Improvement of pain with defecation
- Onset of pain with change in frequency of stool
- Onset of the pain associated with change in appearance of stool

The diagnosis of IBS also is supported by abnormal stool frequency, abnormal stool form, difficult defecation, urgency or incomplete evacuation, mucus in stools, and a sensation of bloating or abdominal distention. These criteria assume that there is no biochemical or structural explanation for the complaints. Work on the ROME IV criteria is in process.

The IBS symptoms wax and wane over extended periods.

HOW DOES IBS OCCUR?

IBS VERSUS NON-IBS PATIENTS

Abdominal pain and altered bowel habits can occur in everyone in response to abnormal stimuli like infection, dietary indiscretion (like alcohol intake), foreign travel, strenuous physical activity, or psychological stress. Thus, the differences between the IBS patients and healthy controls are largely quantitative and not qualitative with respect to causative factors. Patients with IBS have an exaggerated reaction to external stimulus like infection. While healthy patients may resolve their diarrhea within a few days, it may persist for months or years in cases of IBS.

ABNORMAL INTESTINAL MOVEMENT PATTERNS

Altered movement patterns in different parts of the gut are noted in patients with IBS; however, these findings are not consistent. IBS is characterized primarily by increased gut movements in response to psychological and physiological provocations that affect the bowel on an everyday basis.

VISCERAL HYPERSENSITIVITY

The gut is hypersensitive or hyper-vigilant to any provocation. This leads to a lower pain threshold. A stimulus that may be of little or no consequence to a healthy non-IBS subject may cause significant pain in those with IBS. As an example, as a balloon is inflated in the rectum, IBS patients experience pain much more quickly than controls.

ABNORMAL GI IMMUNE SYSTEM

Alterations in the intestinal immune, inflammatory profile and function have been implicated in some studies. An increased number of mast cells are present in the small intestine and colon. Many patients attribute the onset of their symptoms to a GI infection or gastroenteritis.

It appears that psychological distress also may play a role in determining which patients develop persistent symptoms after a bout of intestinal infection (post-infectious IBS).

GLUTEN SENSITIVITY

The gluten-free diet is increasingly popular, and IBS is one arena where science has lagged behind public perception of the diet. The mechanisms are not entirely clear.

IMPAIRED DIGESTION AND ABSORPTION

While long dismissed as a potential factor, the benefit derived from a low-FODMAP diet points to carbohydrate malabsorption as a factor in causing symptoms, but it is not critical enough to have an effect on the overall nutritional status. Undigested FODMAP carbohydrates are attacked by bacteria upon arrival in the large intestine, resulting in bacterial fermentation, increased acid production, intestinal inflammation, leaky gut, and increased gas.

DISORGANIZED/CHAOTIC FUNCTIONING OF NERVOUS SYSTEM

Autonomic dysfunction is noted in about 25 percent of IBS patients. The message system between the gut and brain play an important role in gastrointestinal health and disease. Chronic inflammation increases the intestinal sensitivity, as demonstrated by lower threshold pain. Stress, anxiety, or recall of past psychological trauma can heighten the perception of painful events.

ROLE OF STRESS

Stress may precipitate or worsen the symptoms. While not necessarily associated with the disease per se, there is a 40 to 80 percent prevalence of psychiatric diagnosis among patients with IBS. Increased stressful life events, chronic social stress, or anxiety disorder, and history of past sexual or physical abuse are associated with a poor clinical outcome. Those who seek healthcare generally report greater levels of psychological distress than those who do not.

DIAGNOSIS

Diagnosis is usually based on clinical criteria as well as the exclusion of any blood or structural abnormalities that may present with similar signs and symptoms.

A more aggressive investigative strategy is required when alarm features, such as weight loss, persistent diarrhea, bleeding, abnormal physical examination, laboratory test results like low hemoglobin, and a family history of colon cancer, are present.

Depending on the symptom presentation and the possibility of alternative diagnosis, patients should undergo routine studies, including a complete blood count, stools for occult blood, ova and parasites, and thyroid function tests. Patients with diarrhea-predominant IBS should be tested for celiac disease.

Colonoscopy (examination of the entire colon and rectum) is usually performed in patients above the age of 50, whereas sigmoidoscopy (examination of just the rectum and lower part of the colon) is often considered sufficient in younger subjects. Some experts recommend a colonoscopy in most subjects, regardless of age, since normal colonoscopy removes the fear of cancer—a stressor seen in many patients. In addition, it provides an opportunity to take biopsies for evaluation of microscopic evidence of colitis and to exclude inflammatory bowel disease, especially Crohn's disease, which might explain the patient's symptoms.

The extent and nature of the work-up requires some degree of common sense and is directed by the symptoms and clinical presentation.

MANAGEMENT

A trusting physician/patient relationship with compassionate support is of paramount importance. Learning about the disease is important. Patient education and reassurance helps patients cope with the symptoms. The underlying concept for treatment is to balance two factors, the stool pattern (e.g. diarrhea, constipation) or other symptoms (e.g. bloating), and the severity of symptoms, as determined by the pain.

DIET

Although a generalization regarding food sensitivities cannot be made across all IBS patients, certain foods may exacerbate symptoms in some patients. Diet diaries may help identify if things like large, fatty meals, beans, alcohol, caffeine, or lactose are offenders.

Lactose intolerance is widespread, affecting 80-90 percent of patients with IBS, within some ethnicities. Patients with diarrhea-predominant IBS should avoid lactose-free products.

Food allergies and intolerances depend upon individual sensitivities and need to be taken into account. Read details in Chapter 21.

Foods associated with increased gas (such as beans, onions, celery, carrots, raisins, bananas, apricots, prunes, and Brussels sprouts) should be avoided if "gas" is a significant problem.

Non-celiac gluten enteropathy is now a recognized entity wherein patients with IBS-like symptoms and without evidence of celiac disease get better on a gluten-free diet. Likewise, there is increasing evidence for the benefit of a low-FODMAP diet. Read details in Chapter 20.

EXERCISE

Active lifestyle helps improve symptoms of IBS. Dr. Johannesson and colleagues from the University of Gothenburg in Sweden conducted a randomized controlled trial of 102 IBS patients. They demonstrated that 20-50 minutes of physical activity per day, three to five days per week, was associated with clinical improvement. Only eight percent of the physical activity group got worse during the ensuing 12 weeks, as compared to 23 percent who worsened among controls.

INITIAL MANAGEMENT STRATEGY

The initial management step involves a therapeutic trial based on symptom severity. Fiber is uniformly offered to almost all IBS patients, although its effectiveness in diarrhea-predominant IBS is not clearly established. Patients are encouraged to use a diary to monitor their symptoms for two to three weeks. They should document aggravating or relieving factors and stressors encountered during the period. The role of specific diets and stressors in the patients can then be ascertained.

Patients with mild to moderate symptoms usually can be treated symptomatically with medications targeted at the principal GI symptom.

Dietary fiber (25.0 g/day) with plenty of water is recommended for patients with mild to moderate constipation. However, not all fibers are created equal.

Osmotic laxatives like Phillip's Milk of Magnesia and sorbitol may be used.

MEDICATIONS

Many medications have been developed over the years and then withdrawn from the market due to adverse events. These include Tegeserod and Lotronex.

Antispasmodics

Medications to reduce intestinal spasm are popular but only provide short-term benefit. These include Bentyl and Buscopan and only provide short-term relief. Peppermint oil, used by patients over centuries, is finally a part of evidence-based recommendations of the *American College of Gastroenterology*.

Antidepressants

Most of the 5HT or serotonin, a neurotransmitter in the body, is actually in the gut and not in the brain. This forms an attractive target for intervention in IBS. Antidepressants do not just improve mood but also alleviate pain. Dr. Ford and colleagues performed a meta-analysis of studies to examine the role of antidepressants in IBS. The investigators found that antidepressants are an effective modality, and one in four patients treated with this type of drug will get benefit.

Antidiarrheal agents

Loperamide (Imodium) is a popular remedy. While it improves diarrhea, it does not affect the global symptoms and well-being in patients with IBS. It should preferably be used on an as-needed basis. Likewise, in severe cases of diarrhea, Questran may be tried, especially in patients who have had their gallbladder removed.

Drugs for constipation-predominant IBS

Currently, two drugs are in vogue. Amitiza and Linzess are both effective. However, some practitioners have questioned the value of these drugs. For example, a large trial demonstrated that 18 percent of patients on Amitiza showed improvement, as compared to only 10 percent in the placebo group. While statistically significant, one might wonder if this is clinically significant and worth the cost, as compared to other modalities.

Antibiotics

Gastroenterologists are increasingly appreciating the role of intestinal bacteria in health and disease, and IBS is no exception. Rifaximin (Xifaxan), an antibiotic that selectively works only in the gut is now part of evidence-based recommendations for treatment of IBS.

Anti-anxiety drugs

There is risk for physical dependence when using benzodiazepines (Valium), considering the chronic nature of IBS; as such, they should be only used for brief periods. They may be of short-term benefit in patients with significant anxiety. Antidepressants may, however, be better option in such cases.

SUBSEQUENT MANAGEMENT STRATEGY

FURTHER INVESTIGATIONS

If the above mentioned therapeutic trials fail or the patient's symptoms are severe, further investigation should be considered. Colonic transit X-rays may be required for patients with constipation. If there is difficulty during the bowel movement (obstructive defecation), a check of pressures in the rectum/anal canal (manometry) may be done, along with other imaging studies.

Patients with persistent symptoms of pain-predominant IBS should undergo a plain X-ray of the abdomen during an acute episode to rule out intermittent bowel obstruction or stomach dilatation from swallowing too much air (aerophagia).

Further imaging studies, including a small bowel series, CT scan, and pelvic ultrasound, may be considered for patients with persistent symptoms, especially those with vomiting, weight loss, and abnormal chemistries. In general, expensive and invasive studies should not be solely based on patient reports of symptom severity, but also on clinical suspicion, as determined by alarm signs.

PSYCHOLOGICAL TREATMENTS

Psychological treatments, including psychodynamic therapy, inter-personal therapy, cognitive behavioral therapy, relaxation techniques, and stress management have been shown to improve symptoms. Cognitive behavioral therapy is superior to education or antidepressants for treatment of severe cases. Hypnosis and relaxation decrease pain perception. Group therapy using a team of physicians, nurses, and dietitians is effective.

ALTERNATIVE MEDICINE THERAPIES

An ideal treatment of IBS has been elusive among mainstream medicine options. Among alternative and complementary therapies, Chinese herbal medicine appears a valid alternative for some patients because of the beneficial effect demonstrated in double-blind placebo-controlled trials.

Peppermint oil is now even recognized by the *American College of Gastroenterology* as an evidence-based medicine recommendation for treatment of IBS. Certain probiotics have been shown to be of benefit in early studies, and their role is becoming more and more mainstream.

PLANT-BASED THERAPIES INCLUDING AYURVEDA

Artichoke leaf extract reduces symptoms of IBS and improves quality of life in otherwise healthy volunteers suffering from concomitant dyspepsia. Dr. Walker and colleagues showed that 96 percent of patients rated artichoke leaf extract as better than or at least equal to previous therapies administered for their symptoms.

Bacopa monnieri stabilizes the inflammatory mast cells and has been used in a variety of herbal combinations for IBS.

Belladonna reduces spasms and as such has long been used for IBS. No good studies have examined its efficacy.

Boswellia is an Ayurvedic plant. It reduces diarrhea by normalizing intestinal movements in disease states without slowing the rate of transit in control animals.

Chamomile has long been known for reducing spasms, as well as its soothing and calming properties. However, there is a lack of literature examining this herb in treating IBS.

Fennel seed oil has been shown to reduce intestinal spasms. It is common in India for people to chew a few fennel seeds after dinner as a digestive aid. A randomized placebo-controlled trial found that treatment with fennel oil emulsion eliminated colic in 65 percent of infants, compared to only 24 percent with placebo. Most experts think of infantile colic as analogous to adult IBS.

Marrubiin is a medicinal plant employed in Brazil and other countries. Its bioactive extracts relieve pain. Marrubiin is very effective as an analgesic and for reducing intestinal spasms.

Nutmeg may be useful in treating IBS on account of its antidiarrheal, antihistamine, and sedative properties.

Peppermint oil is effective in treating IBS. Patients on peppermint-oil formulation (Colpermin) experience a significantly greater alleviation of abdominal pain, abdominal distension, stool frequency, abdominal gas, and flatulence, as compared to controls.

Rhubarb has been used to treat intestinal disorders, including IBS. It has been used for constipation since ancient times. Rhubarb can positively modulate the inflammation and promote healthy GI motility.

Turmeric has multiple beneficial properties. However, good clinical studies for its use in treating IBS are lacking.

Padma Lax, a Tibetan medicine, is superior to placebo in relieving symptoms in patients with constipation-predominant IBS. This proprietary multi-herbal blend contains eight different components.

Smooth Move tea contains senna combined with fennel, coriander, and ginger. It is effective in treating constipation and may be of benefit in patients with constipation-predominant IBS.

Compound Ayurvedic Formulation: Dr. Yadav and colleagues compared "standard therapy" (comprised of clidinium bromide, chlordiazepoxide and isaphaghulla), a compound Ayurvedic preparation (*Aegle marmelos Correa* plus *Bacopa monnieri Linn*), and a matching placebo in patients with IBS. The Ayurvedic preparation was effective in 65 percent, standard therapy was beneficial in 78 percent, and the placebo was beneficial in only 33 percent.

STW 5

STW 5 or Iberogast is a complex herbal preparation. It affects transmission of electro-chemical messages across the nervous system and affects the rhythm of intestinal movements. Dr. Madisch and colleagues conducted a double-blind, randomized, placebo-controlled, multi-center trial and found that STW 5 is effective in alleviating IBS symptoms.

The Bottom Line on Herbal Therapies for IBS

A Cochrane database review of herbal therapies in IBS concluded that, as compared with placebo, a Standard Chinese herbal formula, individualized Chinese herbal medicine, STW 5 and STW 5-II, Padma Lax, traditional Chinese formula Tongxie Yaofang Granule, and Ayurvedic preparation (*Aegle marmelos correa* plus *Bacopa monniere Linn*) demonstrate significant improvement of global symptoms in IBS.

MIND-BODY THERAPIES

Psychological stress causes GI distress through changes in intestinal function via the nervous system, immune system, and hormonal system. Numerous studies have examined the role of antidepressants and psychological treatments in treating irritable bowel syndrome. However, the pathophysiological basis of such treatments remains unclear.

Cognitive behavioral therapy (CBT)

CBT appears to have a direct effect on global IBS symptoms without any correlation with psychological distress. Improvement in IBS symptoms is associated with improvements in the quality of life, and the improvement in psychological distress may be a reason for, effect of, or part of IBS improvement.

Dr. Drossman and colleagues from the University of North Carolina conducted a randomized, multi-center trial to examine the effect of CBT versus education and tricyclic antidepressants (desipramine) versus placebo in female patients with moderate to severe functional bowel disorders, including IBS. A significantly higher number of patients in the CBT group responded, as compared to education (70 percent vs. 37 percent), while antidepressants had effects similar to placebo.

Hypnotherapy

Gut-directed hypnosis is most beneficial in patients with predominant abdominal pain and distension. The GI nurses can administer hypnotherapy, which may play a role in the management of IBS.

The use of a specially-devised audiotape for gut-directed hypnotherapy may be equally effective. The beneficial effects of hypnotherapy appear to last at least five years. Dr. Whitehead and colleagues from the University of North Carolina concluded that hypnosis is effective, even in patients refractory to standard therapies.

The use of hypnotherapy in IBS qualifies for the highest level of acceptance as being both efficacious and specific. As such, despite being relatively expensive, it may be a good long-term investment.

Relaxation Therapy and Meditation

Most studies indicate that relaxation therapy and meditation appear to be beneficial over the short and long term in patients with IBS. Dr. Voirol and colleagues investigated the effect of relaxation therapy for six months in patients with IBS. The control group received conventional treatment. While the number of doctor visits in the control group was 53 before and 41 after conventional treatment, the consultations in the relaxation group fell from 74 before to only six after relaxation therapy.

Multicomponent Therapies

Mostly positive results have been obtained from multicomponent therapy use. Dr. Guthrie and colleagues studied patients with medically refractory IBS in a controlled trial of psychological treatment involving psychotherapy, relaxation, and standard medical treatment compared with standard medical treatment alone over a three-month period. The investigators documented a significantly greater improvement on patients' ratings of diarrhea and abdominal pain.

Stress Management

Dr. Shaw and colleagues assigned IBS patients to either a stress management program or usual treatment, including antispasmodics. The stress management program was effective in relieving symptoms in two-thirds of the patients.

The Bottom Line on Psychological Therapies

Dr. Ford and colleagues conducted an expert meta-analysis and concluded that both antidepressants and psychological therapies are equally effective, with the number of patients needed to treat in order to get benefit in one person being four for both strategies.

PROBIOTICS

Data from numerous animal studies suggests that consumption of probiotics can restore gut function back to baseline.

All probiotics are not the same

Many investigators tend to lump all potential probiotics in one group and analyze the effects as if they were one and the same. A clear definition and understanding of probiotic strain selection, dose, and method of delivery are important, just as it is in cases when we use antibiotics. This presents a plausible explanation for the variability in evidence documented by different published trials.

A five-month trial of multispecies probiotic supplementation (*Lactobacillus rhamnosus GG, L. rhamnosus Lc705, Propionibacterium freudenreichii ssp. shermanii JS,* and *Bifidobacterium animalis ssp. lactis Bb12*) results in a significant improvement of the composite IBS score.

Treatment with *Bifidobacterium infantis 35624* is significantly superior to placebo for relief of abdominal pain, bloating, bowel dysfunction, incomplete evacuation, straining, and the passage of gas.

Some authors have reported negative results, including one who documented that *Lactobacillus reuteri ATCC 55730* was similar in efficacy to placebo in patients with IBS. *Lactobacillus plantarum MF1298* may worsen symptoms in patients with IBS.

The Bottom Line on Probiotics

An expert systematic review concluded that probiotics are significantly better than placebo in patients with IBS.

PREBIOTICS

Partially-Hydrolyzed Guar Gum (PHGG)

PHGG is a water-soluble, non-gelling fiber. It increases *Lactobacilli* and *Bifidobacteria* in the gut. Ingestion of PHGG decreases symptoms in both constipation-predominant and diarrhea-predominant forms of IBS associated with improvement of quality of life.

Inulin

Inulin significantly increases healthy *Bifidobacteria* in the gut. There is also reduction of the disease-causing pathogenic bacteria.

Konjac

Konjac glucomannan is used for constipation. Konjac supplementation significantly increases bowel movement frequency and stool weight.

ACUPUNCTURE AND RELATED THERAPIES

Electroacupuncture raises the pain threshold against any provocation by affecting communications between the gut and the brain. Clinical evidence on the use of acupuncture in treating IBS has yielded mixed results.

Transcutaneous electrical acustimulation at the acupoints ST36 and P6 increases the threshold of rectal sensation of gas, desire to defecate, and pain, compared to the period during which no acupuncture therapy was given in IBS patients. However, a prospective, blinded sham-controlled trial (one in which the design is decided upon and then the study is conducted, and where the patient does not know if they are receiving real acupuncture or a sham) of acupuncture in IBS patients found that both groups improved equally at the end of treatment. Acupuncture combined with massage therapy shows a better therapeutic effect than acupuncture alone in IBS patients.

Studies comparing acupuncture to medications for intestinal spasms show that acupuncture is superior. More studies are needed before definitive recommendations can be made.

ROLE OF EXCLUSION DIETS

Increased antibody response to various foods has been found in IBS patients, although a cause-effect relationship remains to be established. Adults with eczema report a high incidence of IBS, suggesting a possible link between atopy and IBS. Food allergy is a common belief among IBS patients. The majority of IBS patients identify two to five foods that upset them, with the overall range being one to 14 foods. More than 50 percent of IBS patients show evidence of sensitization to some food or inhalant without any typical clinical signs.

FOODS IMPLICATED

Patients are usually unable to identify potentially offending foods. Skin prick tests and food-specific antibodies may help in identifying the offending foods. However, there is a lack of correlation between skin prick test results and reported food allergies.

There is higher reactivity to food antigens in diarrhea-predominant IBS patients, compared to those with constipation-predominant IBS and controls, implicating the role of leaky gut. Dr. Zar and colleagues found that IBS patients had significantly higher levels of antibodies to wheat, beef pork, and lamb, as compared to controls. There was no correlation between the pattern of antibody levels and patients' symptoms.

Studies suggest the following order of frequency of food allergens in IBS: milk protein, soybean, tomato, peanut, and egg white.

FOOD IS OFTEN AN OVERLOOKED FACTOR IN IBS

Patients with diarrhea-predominant IBS suffer from more adverse food reactions than healthy controls. Interventions like low- or no-fiber polymeric diet and antibiotic therapy, which reduce colonic bacterial fermentation, improve IBS symptoms.

Although carbohydrate malabsorption can aggravate symptoms in some IBS patients, there is no reliable association. IBS patients frequently suffer from fructose and sorbitol malabsorption, as well. However, symptomatic patients do not differ from asymptomatic patients regarding the presence or absence of fructose and/or sorbitol malabsorption. In general, a low-FODMAP diet helps many patients.

Several studies have documented the benefit of elimination diets in treating IBS. An antibody-guided experimental exclusion diet showed a 10 percent greater reduction in symptom score than the sham diet at 12 weeks, with this value increasing to 26 percent in fully-compliant patients. Appropriate dietary exclusions based on food-specific IgG antibodies in patients lead to a decrease in levels of serum food-specific IgG antibodies, a decrease in frequency and severity of symptoms, and improvement in the quality of life.

A trial of the Six-Food Elimination Diet is easy to implement and may be undertaken as a first step. Some patients may need to go totally gluten-free. A low-FODMAP diet has been shown to ameliorate symptoms in many patients and may be added on for additional benefit.

Further foods may be eliminated based on chemical sensitivity. These include tomatoes, peppers, onions, and soy sauce. See Chapter 21 for more details.

SUPPLEMENTS

Beidellitic montmorillonite

Beidellitic montmorillonite is purified clay containing a double aluminum and magnesium silicate. Dr. Ducrotte and co-investigators assessed its efficacy and safety in IBS patients in a multi-center, double-blind, placebo-controlled study with parallel groups. Significant improvement was seen for patients with constipation-predominant IBS.

L-glutamine

Its role in strengthening the intestinal barrier provides an attractive therapeutic target for intervention in IBS patients.

Zinc

Zinc carnosine steadies small bowel integrity and accelerates gut repair activities. The role of zinc supplementation in treating IBS remains to be established.

MISCELLANEOUS THERAPIES

Yogic intervention or yoga

Dr. Taneja and colleagues conducted a randomized control study to evaluate the effect of yogic and conventional treatment in diarrhea-predominant IBS. Both groups improved to a similar degree over a period of two months. Another comparative randomized trial reported that the yoga group suffers fewer gastrointestinal symptoms, has lower levels of functional disability, and has lower anxiety.

Chiropractic techniques

There is a lack of studies on use of chiropractic techniques in classic IBS. Chiropractic distractive decompression is effective in treating pelvic pain and pelvic organic dysfunction, including bowel problems. Many experts think of infantile colic as an infantile version of IBS. Conflicting results have been reported on the use of spinal manipulation for infantile colic.

Reflexology

Reflexology has not been shown to be of benefit in treating IBS.

Osteopathic treatment

Dr. Riot and colleagues studied patients with levator ani syndrome prospectively over one year. Forty-seven of them also had IBS. Massages were administered with the patient lying on the left side. Appropriate treatment of the pelvic joint disorders was performed at the end of each session. The symptoms were ameliorated in 72 percent of the patients. Most of IBS patients also benefitted from this treatment.

REFERENCES

1. Sarzi-Puttini P, Atzeni F, Di Franco M et al. Dysfunctional syndromes and fibromyalgia: a 2012 critical digest. *Clin Exp Rheumatol*. 2012 Nov-Dec; 30(6 Suppl 74):143-51.
2. Eswaran S, Tack J, Chey WD. Food: the forgotten factor in the irritable bowel syndrome. *Gastroenterol Clin North Am*. 2011 Mar; 40(1):141-62.
3. Dai C, Zheng CQ, Jiang M, Ma XY, Jiang LJ. Probiotics and irritable bowel syndrome. *World J Gastroenterol*. 2013 Sep 28; 19(36):5973-80.
4. Palsson OS, Whitehead WE. Psychological treatments in functional gastrointestinal disorders: a primer for the gastroenterologist. *Clin Gastroenterol Hepatol*. 2013 Mar; 11(3):208-16.

5. Dekel R, Drossman DA, Sperber AD. The use of psychotropic drugs in irritable bowel syndrome. *Expert Opin Investig Drugs.* 2013 Mar; 22(3):329-39.

6. Bensoussan A, Talley NJ, Hing M, Menzies R, Guo A, Ngu M. Treatment of irritable bowel syndrome with Chinese herbal medicine: a randomized controlled trial. *JAMA.* 1998; 280(18):1585-9.

7. Boettcher E, Crowe SE. Dietary proteins and functional gastrointestinal disorders. *Am J Gastroenterol.* 2013 May; 108(5):728-36.

8. Anastasi JK, Capili B, Chang M. Managing irritable bowel syndrome. *Am J Nurs.*2013 Jul; 113(7):42-52.

9. Eswaran S, Tack J, Chey WD. Food: the forgotten factor in the irritable bowel syndrome. *Gastroenterol Clin North Am.* 2011 Mar; 40(1):141-62.

CHAPTER 38

Constipation

KEY POINTS

- Most of the patients diagnosed with severe refractory constipation actually have irritable bowel syndrome or some other more generalized disorder.
- Interventions like dietary changes, fluid intake changes, a bowel retraining regimen, massage, toilet posture, physical exercise, and relaxation exercises provide safe and low-cost options for most patients, at least in early phases of management.
- All fibers are not the same.
- All probiotics are not created equal.
- Biofeedback is effective in defecation problems related to pelvic floor dyssynergia.
- Massage therapy shows promise for management of functional constipation.
- A large number of herbals are being used for relief of constipation across the world, and positive preclinical data lends plausibility to their effectiveness.

Constipation is a symptomatic disorder and not a single disease. A diverse variety of causes play a role in causing and sustaining this disordered bowel function. While laxatives are used frequently, the multifactorial nature of constipation calls for an integrated or holistic approach to the overall management strategies.

SOME CONSTIPATION FACTS TO PONDER

Constipation costs the healthcare system about $235 million per year with the majority of the costs (55 percent) incurred from inpatient care.

The emergency department component of the costs related to constipation is 23 percent, whereas 16 percent and six percent of the expenses involve outpatient physicians and outpatient hospital settings, respectively.

The healthcare cost of children with constipation is $3.9 billion more than those without constipation.

The definition of constipation is open to debate. Experts do not always agree upon what constipation really means; no wonder they keep revising the "consensus" definition and criteria – the standard Rome criteria is now at Rome III.

Stool frequency may be "normal."

PREVALENCE

Constipation is a very common digestive problem, occurring in about 10 to 20 percent of the population. The prevalence of constipation rises with age, with a higher prevalence among elderly people. The term "obstipation" is sometimes used to describe severe constipation.

Constipation as an entity appears esoteric unless you are the one suffering from it. I have seen patients that have gone without a bowel movement for as long as four weeks, all this time feeling miserable because of it!

Constipation is more common in females, non-whites, and individuals of low socioeconomic status. Constipation in the elderly usually correlates with decreased food intake and not with the reduction in fluid or fiber intake.

WHAT IS CONSTIPATION?

Constipation is classically defined as having less than three bowel movements per week. However, different patients, physicians, and scientists think of constipation in different terms. As such, additional criteria have been used.

Features like straining or feeling of incomplete bowel movement, sensation of blockage of rectum, use of manual physical maneuvers to facilitate defecation, or hard or lumpy stools on at least 25 percent of the bowel movements point to functional constipation.

The diagnosis of functional constipation should be entertained after exclusion of organic disorders.

CAUSES OF CONSTIPATION

Common causes for chronic constipation include nervous system diseases (like multiple sclerosis, spinal cord injury, and Parkinsonism), diabetes mellitus, irritable bowel syndrome (IBS), and non-neurogenic diseases (such as underactive thyroid, high or low calcium levels in blood, pregnancy, and scleroderma).

Constipation may also occur as a side effect of numerous drugs, including psychiatric drugs, antispasmodics, antidepressants, iron, aluminum, and calcium containing antacids, sucralfate (Carafate), opiates (like morphine and codeine), and many high blood pressure medicines.

In patients complaining of infrequent bowel movements but normal transit time of food through the digestive system, misperception and a high degree of psychosocial distress are often the cause.

Often, constipation is associated with psychosocial issues and may even be associated with a history of physical or sexual trauma.

WHAT DID ANCIENT MEDICINE THINK ABOUT CONSTIPATION?

Ancient medicine believes that constipation occurs as a result of alteration of the balance of good and bad bacteria in the gut, kinking of the colon, and accumulation of harmful products due to stool stasis, including toxins entering into the body.

In addition to toxins entering across the intestinal barrier into the body, there can be alterations in fermentation patterns, as well as alterations in processing related to altered pattern of the fermenting flora.

BIOPSYCHOSOCIAL MODEL OF CONSTIPATION

No single cause can be pinpointed in the majority of patients. Just like for most functional disorders, the causative mechanisms are explained by a broad biopsychosocial model.

The patient's diseased state is a function of multiple intricate and interrelated factors, including genetic, environmental, and psychosocial factors, like life stress, psychological state, coping, and social support. The interactions between functional, metabolic, and psychological factors are mediated via the gut-brain axis or, even more broadly, by the gut-immune-hormonal-brain axis.

DIAGNOSIS

HISTORY AND PHYSICAL EXAM

The frequency of bowel movements should preferably be documented in a two-week stool diary. Other important points in the history include drug use, systemic and nervous system disorders, recent change in bowel habit, abdominal pain, and bleeding. Physical exam, although usually not useful, is helpful if anal fissures, hemorrhoids, or a gaping anus opening are seen.

Straining during the finger exam of the rectum helps assess contraction of anal sphincter.

ROUTINE STUDIES

Complete blood count, comprehensive metabolic profile, and thyroid tests should be checked and may provide important clues. A plain X-ray of the abdomen may provide evidence of a large amount of stool in the colon.

ENDOSCOPY VERSUS BARIUM ENEMA

Flexible sigmoidoscopy or colonoscopy is undertaken based on clinical presentation and age of the patient. I prefer colonoscopy in most cases, because it provides a greater degree of reassurance to the patient that there is no cancer. In addition, a clean colon after a colonoscopy provides a better opportunity for bowel retraining. Some experts prefer a barium enema in young patients to assess the rectum and colon diameters to exclude megacolon, an abnormally large diameter of the colon.

COLONIC STOOL TRANSIT X-RAYS

Colonic transit studies using radio-opaque markers help distinguish between normal and slow transit constipation. A repeatedly normal study in a patient complaining of infrequent bowel movements suggests misinterpretation or misperception on the part of the patient.

In patients with normal colonic stool transit, a therapeutic trial should be undertaken, and, if there is no improvement, further testing should be undertaken.

ADVANCED STUDIES

Anorectal manometry and balloon expulsion test, barium X-ray defecography, EMG, or MRI may be undertaken in select cases. Abnormality on one single test should be interpreted with caution, since there is a large overlap with the healthy population.

TREATMENT ISSUES

The first step in managing constipation is to exclude a secondary cause for constipation. Both the patient and the physician need to be realistic in their expectations, since a condition that may have evolved over several years and decades may only be partially amenable to any therapeutic strategy in the short term.

Patients whose disorder is complicated by diverse neurologic, biologic, psychological, and social factors present a bigger challenge. Fibromyalgia, chronic fatigue syndrome, interstitial cystitis, autism, or autistic spectrum disorders are included in this category.

MODERN DRUGS VERSUS INTEGRATIVE THERAPIES

Since the modern drug concept of a single targeted molecule is unlikely to have an impact on more than one factor, an integrated approach and/or use of combination therapies (as is common in herbal medicine) is more likely to attain success.

Many of the traditional medications and therapies have not undergone clinical trials; however, this is probably because there is no patent involved that would make such a trial interesting to the pharmaceutical companies. At the same time, it is important to ensure the safety of any therapeutic strategy based on existing empiric evidence, clinical experience, and preferably scientific evidence.

TREATMENT STRATEGY FOR CHRONIC CONSTIPATION

In addition to modern laxatives and prescription drugs, numerous natural products in alternative and complimentary medicine are used to move bowels in patients with constipation.

According to Dr. Wald at the University of Wisconsin School of Medicine, there appears to be an overemphasis on evidence-based analysis rather than on effectiveness of laxative agents. This, coupled with aggressive marketing of pharmaceutical products (many of which have been withdrawn due to adverse events), has created lop-sided recommendations by thought leaders and practice by general practitioners towards more expensive but not necessarily more effective modalities.

There is little shared understanding between patients and medical care providers about what constitutes "normal" bowel function. In addition, there is little consensus on the best treatment strategy for patients suffering from chronic constipation. Let us also not forget that many of the natural and ancient bowel cleansing remedies have been authenticated by clinical trials published in peer-reviewed literature.

Step 1

Initial management includes patient education regarding increase in fluid and fiber intake, as well as attempting to defecate in the morning after breakfast.

- A daily intake of 20.0 to 35.0 g of fiber is recommended.
- Always ensure adequate amount of water intake along with fiber.
- Fiber supplements such as psyllium (Metamucil), methylcellulose (Citrucel), or calcium polycarbophil, along with increased fluid intake, speed up colonic transit.
- The dose of bulk laxatives should be increased slowly, since they can cause gas and bloating.
- Encourage regular exercise.
- Other beneficial fiber supplements include Fiber7, vegetable gum fibers (Benefiber), polycarbophil, cocoa husk, and Glucomannan (Konjac).

All fiber is not the same

Current recommendations suggest consumption of 20-35 g of dietary fiber per day, although the average American's daily intake of dietary fiber is about half of that.

Always consume a variety of fiber-rich foods. The dose of fiber in kids may be based on the formula (age plus 5) g/day.

Fiber is of two types: soluble and insoluble. Neither type is absorbed across the gut. However, they have distinct properties when mixed with water. A 3:1 ratio of insoluble to soluble fiber in the diet is typically recommended.

- Wheat bran is one of the more effective fiber laxatives.
- Among fruits, I recommend mangoes and papaya.

Rich sources of insoluble fiber

- Bran
- Vegetables: bitter gourd, celery, cauliflower, zucchini cucumbers, tomatoes, green leafy vegetables
- Fruits: apple with skin, banana, kiwi, mango, peach, pear, strawberry
- Nuts, broad beans, field beans, cluster beans

Rich sources of soluble fiber

- Psyllium husk
- Vegetables: potatoes, carrots, broccoli, onions, Jerusalem artichoke
- Fruits: kiwi, apples with skin, bananas, blueberries, pears, strawberries, oranges, fruit juices like prune juice
- Nuts, flax seed, dried peas, soybeans and other beans, lentils, seeds

Patients need to take fiber for two to three months before they experience significant relief of constipation.

Step 2

Patients not responding to fiber laxatives may be tried on other laxatives that are not usually harmful, especially if taken two to three times per week under supervision.

Stool softeners like Colace are of limited benefit. Magnesium containing laxatives carry the risk of high toxic levels of magnesium in elderly patients or those with kidney failure.

Caution should be exercised with stimulant laxatives like bisacodyl (Dulcolax) and senna, as they may lead to side effects if used chronically.

Castor oil is not routinely recommended for treating chronic constipation. Lactulose and its cheaper alternative, sorbitol, are both effective and commonly used.

PEG solutions (GoLytely and Miralax) provide relief in most cases. PEG solution (two to four L every one to two weeks) is an effective treatment, especially in patients with severe constipation who are institutionalized or bedridden. Miralax is a powder preparation (17.0 g to 34.0 g per day) that does not contain electrolytes.

Current pharmacological treatments include lubiprostone (Amitiza) and Linaclotide (Linzess).

Step 3

Patients with severe constipation may benefit from bowel retraining, which is initiated by first cleansing the colon completely with an enema twice a day or drinking a gallon of PEG solution until the cleansing is complete.

Subsequently, lactulose, sorbitol, or a solution containing polyethylene glycol (Miralax) titrated can be used to achieve at least one stool every other day.

Defecation should be attempted after breakfast in the morning. The patient should then take an enema or a glycerin suppository if there is no bowel movement after two days.

In demented or bedridden patients with frequent fecal impaction, a regular regimen of enemas once or twice every week or PEG solutions every couple of weeks may be undertaken after the initial cleansing out of the colon.

Step 4

Biofeedback is an effective treatment, especially for patients with pelvic floor dysfunction.

Step 5

Injection of botulinum toxin has been successfully used in patients with difficult defecation due to pelvic floor dysfunction. Surgery involving removal of colon or subtotal colectomy and connecting the small bowel to the rectum may be needed in select patients with chronic severe constipation that is refractory to medical therapy.

ALTERNATIVE MEDICINE STRATEGIES

EXERCISE

While evidence linking lack of physical activity to constipation is conflicting, observational data from across cultures suggests that physical activity and exercise may promote bowel activity.

- Decreased bodily movements add to the development of constipation, at least in a subset of cases.
- Exercise results in an increase in the number of propagated colon contractions, which may accelerate colonic movements of stool.
- Persons with an inactive lifestyle are three times more likely to report constipation.

In Eastern cultures, it is common for people to go out for a walk in the morning to promote defecation.

REGULARIZE BOWEL HABIT

Establishing consistent habits may help in establishing a regular pattern of bowel movement.

- Try to have a bowel movement at least twice a day, usually 30 minutes after meals.
- The best time is in the morning after breakfast and within two hours of waking up.
- Strain for no more than five minutes.

> Toileting posture is a modifiable factor that should be used as part of an overall management strategy. The use of traditional toilet seats has the potential to make the recto-anal angle (the angle between the rectum and the anal canal) more acute, contributing to difficult passage of stools and constipation. Toileting posture is especially of concern in kids who sit with their legs dangling in the air, as constipation can persist throughout life. Physically challenged subjects need to use higher chairs in order to be able to get up after defecations and, as such, have better posture.

Appropriate toilet posture coupled with abdominal exercises and other lifestyle changes helps many patients.

Simple Ways to Mimic Squatting Posture

- Bend forward with elbows resting on thighs.
- Support the feet on a footstool while seated on the toilet, such that the angle at the thighs is acute.

EFFECT OF FLUID INTAKE

While it is true that this issue may be overblown to some extent, it remains biologically plausible that adequate fluid intake is likely a significant factor in normal bowel function.

- The precise amount of adequate fluid intake remains unknown.

- There is a high degree of inter-individual variability, depending on a variety of biological, environmental, and medicinal factors.
- Low fluid intake may be a factor in some cases, leading to a borderline state of dehydration, reduced moisture in stool with altered bacterial flora, and intestinal motility.

Extra fluid intake in normal healthy volunteers does not produce a significant increase in stool output. However, the same may not apply to not-so-healthy subjects or those who may have a borderline case of dehydration.

A daily fiber intake of 20-35 g can increase the number of bowel movements in patients with chronic constipation. The effect of fiber can be significantly boosted by increasing fluid consumption to one-and-a-half to two liters per day.

PREBIOTICS

Prebiotics are substances that provide substrate for the preferential growth of healthy bacteria, thus shifting the balance in favor of good bacteria in the gut. Many of the fibers may be considered prebiotic.

Prebiotics helpful in constipation include inulin, fructo-oligosaccharides (FOS), isomalto-oligosaccharides, barley, and germinated barley foodstuff (GBF).

PROBIOTICS

Dysbiosis or an abnormal pattern of bacteria in the colon occurs in subjects with chronic constipation. However, not all probiotics are the same.

Probiotic strains of benefit in constipation include the following:

- Lactobacillus reuteri (DSM 17938)
- Lactobacillus casei Shirota
- Lactobacillus casei rhamnosus
- Bifidobacterium lactis DN-173-010
- P. freudenreichii

- Bifidobacterium longum
- Escherichia coli Nissle 1917

The commercial formulations that have been subjected to clinical trials and have been found to be helpful include:

- Ecologic Relief
- Activia (*Bifidobacterium animalis DN-173 010* and fructo-oligosaccharide)
- Zir fos

MIND-BODY THERAPIES

Biofeedback

Biofeedback is an effective tool for treatment of defecation problems due to pelvic floor dyssynergia as well as for slow transit constipation.

Stress Management

Chronic stress causes an imbalance of the gut-immune-hormonal-brain axis. Severe constipation may be a defense mechanism, wherein normal physiological and emotional responses to stress are replaced by abnormal bowel movement patterns. Breaking the vicious cycle by appropriate stress management may help many patients.

Art Therapy

This is particularly tailored for kids. One study examined the effects of modeling clay to treat six children between the ages of four to 12 years with a history of constipation refractory to treatment. Clay for art therapy was chosen as a metaphor for feces. Of the six kids studied, four children had no symptoms during two months of therapy.

Miscellaneous Mind-Body Therapies

Other mind-body-based therapies such as hypnotherapy, relaxation techniques, and mental imagery have the potential to be of benefit in functional constipation; however data is lacking.

PLANT BASED THERAPIES

While most of the knowledge has been handed down by word of mouth, much of it can also be found texts written thousands of years ago. The absence of scientific studies does not necessarily mean lack of effectiveness.

Some of the drugs that may be used based on their relaxing and/or antispasmodic effects include chamomile, lavender, and peppermint.

Select plant-based therapies used for constipation across cultures

These include aloe, Ear mushroom, buckwheat, *Cascara sagrada*, *Cassia alata Linn*, *Calotropis procera*, *Croton penduliflorus*, *Carica papaya*, *Cynomorium songaricum*, Colocynth (aka bitter apple; in Sanskrit it is called Gavakshi or Indarvaruni), flaxseed, fennel seeds, *Fumaria indica*, ginger, *Hibiscus rosasinensis*, naringenin flavonoid present in citrus fruits, olive oil, *Peumus boldus* (Boldo), radish seeds, rhubarb, slippery elm bark, *Saussurea lappa*, senna, and yumijangquebo.

Herbal formulations of benefit in constipation

Popular herbal combinations include *Dai-kenchu-to* (DKT or TJ-100), a liquid Ayurvedic preparation called Misrakasneham, SmoothMove, and a Tibetan herbal preparation called Padma Lax.

MANIPULATIVE AND BODY-BASED THERAPIES

Evidence from some but not all studies suggests that massage and aromatherapy alone and in combination help relieve constipation.

Physical therapy incorporating abdominal massage appears to be effective in medically refractory constipation in elderly subjects.

Baduanjin (Eight-Treasured Exercises) is one of the many health-promoting ancient Chinese exercises helpful in indigestion and constipation.

Use of the original Qigong massage technique is effective in children with autism spectrum disorders. Literature on the effect of yoga is mixed.

Chiropractic and osteopathic manipulation

These techniques are popular and usually performed in conjunction with external massage of the abdomen, starting in the right lower quadrant and following the course of the large intestine in a clockwise direction. Such a therapy has been reported to be effective over the long term in patients with chronic constipation.

Reflexology

Reflexology is based on the premise that manual pressure to specific areas or zones of the feet corresponds to different areas of the body and provides healing benefit accordingly. Early data appears promising.

ENERGY-BASED MEDICINE

- Transcutaneous electrical nerve stimulation (TENS) treatment results in amelioration of soiling, along with increase in the frequency of spontaneous bowel movements in kids with medically resistant chronic constipation.
- Electrogalvanic stimulation is a useful adjunct to the therapeutic armamentarium for pelvic floor dyssynergia in normal transit constipation.
- Other energy-based therapies in use for constipation include Reiki and healing touch; however, there is lack of good published studies documenting their effectiveness.

ACUPUNCTURE

Acupuncture may also be considered part of the broader traditional Chinese medicine. Multiple studies have documented its efficacy against constipation in adults as well as kids.

Beneficial acupoints used include Zhigou (TE 6), ST25, CV6, CV4, Tianshu (ST 25), Qihai (CV 6), and Guanyuan (CV 4). Abdominal electroacupuncture (EA) is effective in patients with constipation after stroke.

TRADITIONAL CHINESE MEDICINE (TCM)

TCM considers constipation in terms of a variety of pathologic dysfunctions, including spleen qi deficiency, liver qi stagnation, and yin deficiency. While some of the therapies and studies are outlined below, others are mentioned in other sections because of overlap.

Select TCM formulations for constipation
- Xiao-Chen-Chi-Tang (XCCT)
- Tiao-Wei-Chen-Chi-Tang (TWCCT)
- Ta-Cheng-Chi-Tang (TCCT)
- Maren soft capsule
- Yiqi Kaimi Recipe (YQKMR)
- Shenshen Wan
- Sini Powder (SP)

HOMEOPATHY

This health system is based on law of similar. Treatment of a poison is the poison itself, albeit in such extremely small doses (super-diluted) that it defies biologic plausibility. Nevertheless, it is very popular in Europe and in India. The royal family in the UK is reputed to have a homeopathic physician as well.

Despite a lack of studies examining their efficacy, a variety of homeopathic medications are popular. These include bryonia for dry feces, Nux vomica for incomplete bowel movements, silica for hard stools, and sulfur for hard stool with painful defecation.

REFERENCES

1. Bharucha AE, Pemberton JH, Locke GR 3rd. American Gastroenterological Association technical review on constipation. *Gastroenterology.* 2013 Jan; 144(1):218-38.
2. Lacy BE, Levenick J, Crowell M. Recent advances in the management of difficult constipation. *Curr Gastroenterol Rep.* 2012 Aug; 14(4):306-12.
3. Wald A. Chronic constipation: advances in management. *Neurogastroenterol Motil.* 2007 Jan; 19(1):4-10.
4. Zhang T, Chon TY, Liu B et al. Efficacy of acupuncture for chronic constipation: a systematic review. *Am J Chin Med.* 2013; 41(4):717-42.
5. Stewart ML, Schroeder NM. Dietary treatments for childhood constipation: efficacy of dietary fiber and whole grains. *Nutr Rev.* 2013 Feb; 71(2):98-109.

CHAPTER 39

Ulcerative Colitis

KEY POINTS

- Patients with ulcerative colitis frequently have micronutrient deficiencies.
- Newer biologic drugs have increased the options in our arsenal.
- Surgery is curative for ulcerative colitis but not Crohn's disease.
- Probiotics are helpful in maintaining remission in certain cases of ulcerative colitis.
- Turmeric is effective in maintaining remission in ulcerative colitis.
- The role of omega-3 fatty acids in treating ulcerative colitis appears to be modest at best.

Inflammatory bowel disease (IBD) is a chronic inflammation of uncertain etiology involving the digestive tract. It is primarily divided into ulcerative colitis (UC) and Crohn's disease. About 10 to 15 percent of the cases remain indeterminate.

PREVALENCE OF ULCERATIVE COLITIS

The incidence of UC varies from five to 15 per 100,000 persons; Crohn's disease is found in three to 10 per 100,000 persons. Most cases present between the ages of 15 and 30. There is a second peak incidence manifesting between 50 and 80 years of age.

CAUSATION

There is a genetic predisposition to IBD, although greater than 70 percent of patients have no family history of IBD.

The role of oral contraceptives in the pathogenesis is controversial. Whereas smoking is protective against UC, it tends to worsen Crohn's disease.

Prior appendectomy confers protection against ulcerative colitis but not Crohn's disease.

Nutritional deficiencies do not cause or contribute to the pathogenesis.

The role of infectious agents is controversial and continues to be debated. Studies suggest that "normal" intestinal flora may contribute to the pathogenesis in susceptible individuals.

Non-steroidal anti-inflammatory drugs (NSAIDs) increase the risk for development of IBD or induce flare-up.

Stress does not cause the disease but contributes to exacerbation of symptoms.

DISTRIBUTION OF UC

The inflammation in ulcerative colitis is superficial. It usually starts in the rectum and extends upwards in a continuous fashion. UC may be classified on the basis of location as ulcerative proctitis (involving rectum only), left-sided colitis (involving rectum and left side of colon), or extensive and pancolitis (involving most or the entire colon).

CLINICAL FEATURES

Patients present with intermittent rectal bleeding with mucus, bloody diarrhea, mild abdominal pain, and cramping. Some patients may actually have constipation with bleeding.

Physical examination in UC may be normal or may show mild abdominal tenderness, especially in the left lower abdomen. Patients with severe diverticulitis may be dehydrated with a fast heart rate, fever, and low blood pressure.

The routine blood count may be normal or may show evidence of iron deficiency anemia or mixed anemia related to other nutritional deficiencies. Anemia may occasionally be severe enough to require blood transfusion.

Stool studies are done to exclude infections as the cause of inflammation. Abnormal antibodies can be detected in about two-thirds of the patients. Colonoscopy is the cornerstone of diagnosis.

COMPLICATIONS

- Massive hemorrhage in up to three percent of patients
- Life-threatening colitis in 10 to 20 patients
- Colonic stricture or narrowing in five to 10 percent of the patients. A stricture in patients with UC is considered cancerous unless proven otherwise.

EXTRA-INTESTINAL MANIFESTATIONS

Patients with UC have numerous complications involving other organ systems of the body. These include involvement of the eyes, joints, liver, and skin, and abnormal blood clots in veins.

COURSE OF ULCERATIVE COLITIS

Most patients with UC have intermittent remissions and relapses, although 10 to 20 percent of patients may have prolonged remission after initial presentation.

CURRENT TREATMENT OF ULCERATIVE COLITIS

The goal of treatment is two-pronged: to achieve and maintain remission.

MEDICAL THERAPY

The use of different medications depends upon disease severity.

Treatment with 5ASA aminosalicylate suppositories (Canasa), steroid suppositories, or foam may be all that is needed in those with only rectal involvement or in those with mild symptoms. Patients intolerant to suppositories may benefit from oral 5ASA agents (Asacol, Delzicol, Pentasa, Dipentum, Colazal, Apriso, and Lialda).

Adverse effects of 5ASA formulations include headache, fatigue, cramps, gas, and watery diarrhea. These drugs are considered safe for use during pregnancy and lactation.

Patients with moderate to severe symptoms benefit from 5ASA formulations and sometimes are given steroids (like prednisone), depending upon severity.

Patients not responding to any of the above treatments are usually treated with immunosuppressive drugs like azathioprine (Imuran) and 6MP.

More potent drugs called biologic agents may be used in difficult cases. These include Remicade, Humira, and Cimzia. Even with these expensive and toxic drugs, satisfactory response may occur in only about half the patients. Patients with severe colitis or those not responding to home-therapy require hospitalization.

ADJUNCTIVE MEASURES IN ULCERATIVE COLITIS

- Avoid milk, cheese, raw fruit and vegetables, carbonated beverages, alcohol, fruit juices, spicy foods, ketchup, mustard, high-fiber vegetables (broccoli, cabbage, and cauliflower), red meat, beans, artificial coloring, additives, and artificial sweeteners or sorbitol-containing products during active disease.

- Multivitamins should be taken, along with folic acid. Folic acid supplementation lowers risk of cancer.
- Many patients have micronutrient deficiency, such as vitamin D. Blood levels should be checked and supplements used as needed.
- A bone density scan is done periodically to check on bone health. Patients may need calcium and vitamin D supplements or even formal drug therapy for osteoporosis if present.
- Patients with increased stress may benefit from mild sedatives.

SURGICAL TREATMENT

Surgery can be curative when the rectum and colon are removed. A new rectum (pouch) can be created from the small intestine so that the patient does not need an ostomy with a bag. Inflammation of the pouch or pouchitis occurs in about 10 to 40 percent of patients and is usually a treatable condition.

RISK FOR CANCER

Patients with UC have an increased risk for colon cancer. Periodic colonoscopies are done, depending on the extent and duration of the disease.

ALTERNATIVE MEDICINE THERAPIES

Conventional medical therapy cannot cure UC. In fact, even with the most potent, toxic, expensive drugs like biologics, four patients need to be treated with infliximab (Remicade) to attain satisfactory response in one patient.

An expert review by Dr. Gisbert and colleagues from the La Princesa University Hospital, Autonomous University in Madrid, Spain, concluded that Remicade accomplishes clinical remission only in about 40 percent of patients with moderate to severe ulcerative colitis.

Surgical advancements have brought about a dramatic change in outlook but are accompanied by complications as in any major surgery. As such, many patients flock to complementary and alternative medicine (CAM) therapies.

Thirty to 50 percent of North American patients with UC reportedly use CAM. One study described the relative prevalence of different alternative therapies as follows: homeopathy (55 percent), probiotics (43 percent), classical naturopathy (38 percent), *Boswellia serrata* extracts (36 percent) and acupuncture/Traditional Chinese Medicine (33 percent). Numerous other herbal remedies are being used to treat IBD, including slippery elm, fenugreek, devil's claw, Mexican yam, tormentil, and wei tong ning.

In this chapter, we will focus primarily on UC, even though there is likely to be an overlap with Crohn's disease (CD).

PROBIOTICS

Rationale

Human subjects and their intestinal luminal contents (especially gut bacteria) have evolved together to reach a state of mutual adjustment, adaptation, and tolerance. Colitis does not develop in animal models raised in a germ-free environment.

An unhealthy imbalance of intestinal bacteria flora or dysbiosis, such as reduction in the concentration of *bifidobacteria* and increase of Bacteroides species, is associated with the severity of ulcerative colitis. Consistent abnormalities in intestinal bacterial composition specific to UC have not yet been established, however. Overall, the data is consistent with the concept of abnormal bowel flora or even a specific, albeit unidentified, bacterial pathogen causing UC.

Restoration of balance in the intestinal flora is a plausible strategy for treatment of UC. Components of intestinal bacteria such as *Lactobacillus acidophilus* and *Bifidobacterium bifidus* have long been used as therapeutic agents for bowel disorders.

Epidemiologic data

Consistent with the "hygiene hypothesis" or "old friend hypothesis," IBD is less common in developing countries, which may be due to exposure to parasitic infections, which in turn ameliorate the immune reaction and inflammation.

Consider the fact that administration of *Trichuris suis* parasite eggs to patients with ulcerative colitis over 12 weeks results in improvement in 43 percent of patients, as compared to only 17 percent with placebo. Many Americans actually travel to Southeast Asia for this treatment.

Data from results of fecal transplantation

The most comprehensive mix of probiotic bacteria of human origin is the entire fecal flora. This type of bacteriotherapy has been used effectively for animal health. Infusions of human fecal flora in patients with IBD and IBS have shown promising results. This therapy has been life-saving for many patients with recurrent *Clostridium difficile* colitis.

Probiotics in adults

Dr. Naidoo and colleagues from the Guys and St Thomas' NHS Foundation Trust in London performed a meta-analysis of available literature and reported that probiotics are superior to placebo in maintaining remission. Furthermore, they found that there was no statistically significant difference between probiotics and mesalazine for maintenance of remission in UC. Relapse among those taking probiotics is 40 percent, compared to 34 percent of patients taking the 5ASA formulations. Another review concluded that patients receiving the probiotic (*Bifidobacterium bifidum*) treatment had one-fourth the recurrence rate of those in the non-probiotic group.

Studies on use of probiotics in acute pouchitis have yielded mixed and largely disappointing results. In contrast to treatment of acute pouchitis, the beneficial effects of probiotics for prophylaxis have been documented by multiple studies.

> An expert panel led by Floch and colleagues gave an "A" recommendation for the use of probiotics to prevent and maintain remission in pouchitis. The authors gave "B" recommendations in several other areas of treating IBD.

Probiotics in children

Miele and colleagues from the University of Naples in Italy performed a prospective, double-blind randomized placebo-controlled one-year study, to examine the effect of probiotic blend VSL#3 on induction and maintenance of remission in children with newly-diagnosed active UC. Kids received other treatments, as usual. Ninety-three percent of patients receiving probiotic achieved remission, compared to 37 percent in the placebo group. In addition, only 21 percent of patients in the probiotic group had a relapse of the disease, compared to 73 percent of those receiving the placebo.

PREBIOTICS

Germinated barley foodstuff

Fiber fraction of germinated barley foodstuff (GBF) enhances intestinal production of butyrate, a short-chain fatty acid and a preferred source of nutrition by colon cells. GBF should be avoided by those on a gluten-free diet. Its efficacy in the treatment of UC was examined in a randomized multi-center open controlled trial. In the GBF-treated group, patients received 20-30 g of GBF daily, in addition to the baseline treatment. At four and 24 weeks, the GBF-treated group showed a significant decrease in colitis activity index scores compared with the control group.

Another study using 20 g of GBF daily in addition to conventional treatment reported that the clinical activity index as well as the recurrence rate is better in the GBF group as compared to controls.

Soy and Bowman-Birk inhibitor concentrate (BBIC)

Bowman-Birk inhibitor concentrate (BBIC), a soy extract, is effective in the treatment of colitis in animals.

A randomized, double-blind, placebo-controlled trial investigated the safety and possible benefits of Bowman-Birk inhibitor concentrate for 12 weeks in patients with active UC. The severity of the disease in patients receiving BBIC decreased more than in patients receiving placebo, and there was a trend towards superior rates of remission.

Psyllium

A four-month placebo-controlled trial on the use of ispaghula (commercially-available fiber derived from Plantago seeds) for relief in patients with UC in remission demonstrated that there was a significantly higher rate of improvement (69 percent) in the study group as compared to the placebo group (24 percent).

Plantago ovata seeds

Colonic fermentation of *Plantago ovata* seeds (dietary fiber) yields butyrate, which has been shown to be helpful in treating colitis.

A multi-center, randomized clinical trial compared mesalamine (500 mg three times a day) to *Plantago ovata* seeds plus 5ASA formulations for 12 months. Results showed that the treatment failure rate was 40 percent in the *Plantago ovata* alone group, 35 percent in the mesalamine alone group, and 30 percent in the combined *Plantago ovata* and mesalamine group. Thus, *Plantago ovata* seeds are just as effective as 5ASA for maintenance of remission in ulcerative colitis.

Wheat grass

Wheat grass (*Triticum aestivum*) juice has been used for numerous gastrointestinal and non-GI conditions.

A randomized, double-blind, placebo-controlled study examined the effects of wheat grass juice in active distal UC. Treatment with wheat grass juice was associated with significant reductions in the overall disease activity and in the severity of rectal bleeding. (Note: Wheat grass does not contain gluten.)

Conclusions about use of prebiotics in ulcerative colitis

Use of prebiotics is beneficial in maintaining remission in ulcerative colitis

MIND-BODY THERAPIES

Adjustment to chronic disease is part of a multifaceted need for successful adaptation to disease-specific demands, psychological well-being, functional status, and quality of life. One adaptation is to know where the closest restrooms are when you go to the mall. Another would be to use the restroom before going out for a drive.

Role of stress

Stress and symptom severity (or at least perception of severity) create a vicious cycle and worsen quality of life. While stress can reactivate controlled chronic inflammation, it does not initiate inflammation. As such, stress may be an environmental factor provoking relapses.

Non-medical therapeutic strategies, including cognitive, emotional, and behavioral factors beyond the traditional medical and psychological (depression and anxiety) components, are valuable adjuncts.

> Drs. Maunder and Levenstein from the Department of Psychiatry at Mount Sinai Hospital in Toronto reviewed the epidemiological literature to examine the effect of psychological issues in UC. The authors concluded that there is consistent evidence for a contribution of psychological factors to stress in UC.

- Nurse-delivered counseling is effective in improving mental health.
- Relaxation training is successful in ameliorating pain in patients with UC.
- A protocolized psychological treatment program, including illness information, coping models, problem solving techniques, relaxation therapy, and social skill training, in group sessions results in greater improvement in the quality of life, as compared to usual care.

Cognitive behavioral therapy

Dr. Mussell and colleagues conducted a prospective study aimed at determining whether cognitive-behavioral group treatment accompanying medical standard care is effective. Twelve weekly psychological treatment sessions were undertaken in a group setting. Cognitive behavioral therapy resulted in decreased disease-related worries and concerns.

Hypnosis

Dr. Miller's group from the University of Manchester in the U.K. reported a case series of 15 patients with severe IBD unresponsive to medical drug treatment. Patients received 12 sessions of "gut-focused hypnotherapy" and follow-up for a mean duration of 5.4 years. Hypnosis resulted in improved outcomes, including improved quality of life and significant decrease in need for steroid medications.

PLANT-BASED THERAPIES

Aloe vera gel

A double-blind, randomized, placebo-controlled trial examined the efficacy and safety of aloe vera gel for the treatment of mildly to moderately active ulcerative colitis. Authors concluded that oral aloe vera taken for four weeks is safe and reduces the severity of colitis more often than placebo.

Ambrotose complex and Advanced Ambrotose

Ambrotose complex and Advanced Ambrotose are plant-derived polysaccharide dietary supplements that include aloe vera gel, arabinogalactan, fucoidan, and rice starch, all of which inhibit inflammation in animal models of colitis.

Betel nut

Lee and colleagues conducted a pilot study in Asian patients with UC. Patients and healthy controls filled in questionnaires. Thirteen percent of male patients were found to regularly use betel nut, compared with 20 percent of controls, suggesting a protective role for betel nut.

Boswellia aka frankincense

Results from animal studies have been mixed. Human studies suggest that frankincense is at least equal to or better than therapy with sulfasalazine formulations. According to Dr. Ammon from the Institute of Pharmaceutical Sciences, University of Tuebingen in Germany, preliminary evidence suggests efficacy of Boswellia extracts in Crohn's disease and UC.

Chlorella

Dietary supplements derived from Chlorella pyrenoidosa, a fresh-water green algae, are rich in proteins, vitamins, and minerals. Administration of 10 g of pure chlorella in tablet form and 100 mL of a liquid each day for two or three months speeds up healing in patients with UC.

Curcumin (turmeric)

Curcumin is a biologically-active phytochemical substance present in turmeric, the "yellow curry powder" popular in Indian and other forms of Asian cooking.

A randomized, double-blind, placebo-controlled, multi-center trial assessed the efficacy of curcumin as maintenance therapy in patients with inactive ulcerative colitis. Patients received curcumin or placebo, one g twice a day, plus the usual medical treatment with sulfasalazine or 5ASA for six months. The relapse rate in the curcumin group was 5 percent, compared to 21 percent in the placebo group.

Dr. Kumar and colleagues from the University of Minnesota conducted a meta-analysis of clinical trials on the role of curcumin. They concluded that "curcumin may be a safe and effective therapy for maintenance of remission in quiescent UC when given as adjunctive therapy along with mesalamine or sulfasalazine."

Dandelion

Dandelion (*Taraxacum officinale*) is used in food and in herbal medicines. It is a rich source of micronutrients like vitamins A, B complex, C, D, iron, potassium, and zinc. Both roots and leaves are used. It is available as a tincture, liquid extract, teas, tablets, and capsules. One such supplement containing *Taraxacum officinale* has been studied for treatment of colitis in humans. Authors found the combination formulation treatment to be effective.

Evening primrose oil

A randomized controlled trial found that evening primrose oil significantly improves stool consistency as compared to fish oil (MaxEPA) and placebo for six months; this difference was maintained three months after treatment was discontinued. The study did not find any effect on stool frequency, rectal bleeding, and relapse rate, suggesting only a modest positive effect.

Ginkgo

Ginkgo biloba extract protects against damage due to inflammation in several models of experimental colitis in animals.

Ginseng

American ginseng extract suppresses colitis in dextran sodium sulfate-induced colitis in mice.

Grape seeds

Proanthocyanidins from grape seeds protect against colitis in animal models.

Lemon balm

Citrus fruits are rich in hesperidin, a flavanone-type flavonoid. Hesperidin significantly decreases colitis in animals. Dr. Magee and colleagues from the Ninewells Hospital and Medical School in Scotland studied 81 UC patients recruited at all stages of the disease process, in order to determine what types of foods might be related to UC activity. Foods with beneficial effects in UC included citrus fruits.

One report indicated that treatment using an herbal combination including *Citrus aurantium* and *C. carvi* was effective in chronic colitis.

Scutellariae Radix

Extracts from *Scutellariae Radix* form a part of many traditional Chinese prescriptions. It is effective in treating acute colitis in animals.

Tormentil

Tormentil extracts have antioxidant properties. An open label study examined the role of *Tormentil* extracts (1,200 to 3,000 mg per day for three weeks) in patients with active UC. Treatment reduced the severity of colitis along with laboratory markers of inflammation.

Ayurvedic herbal combinations

An ancient multi-drug Ayurvedic formulation contains four different drugs, Bilwa (*Aegle marmeloes*), Dhanyak (*Coriandrum sativum*), Musta (*Cyperus rotundus*) and Vala (*Vetiveria zinzanioids*). Its effect was found to be equal to that of steroids in animal colitis.

ACUPUNCTURE

An expert meta-analysis and systematic review by Dr. Ji and colleagues from the Shanghai University of Traditional Chinese Medicine reported that acupuncture and moxibustion (acupuncture where heat is applied to the acupoints) therapy are superior to oral sulfasalazine for the treatment of IBD. Literature suggests that the therapeutic effect of acupuncture and moxibustion on UC offers better safety and fewer adverse reactions than conventional treatments.

ENEMA THERAPY

Bovine colostrum enemas

Bovine colostrum is loaded with nutrients, antibodies, and growth factors. Bovine colostrum prevents experimental colitis in guinea pigs.

A randomized, double-blind, controlled trial studied 14 patients with mild to moderately severe distal colitis who received a colostrum enema or placebo for four weeks. Both groups also received the 5ASA medication. The treatment group showed a significant reduction in symptoms and colon damage as compared to the placebo group. This suggests that a bovine colostrum enema may have potential as adjunctive therapy for left-sided colitis with additional benefits over conventional therapy.

Butyrate enema

A randomized placebo-controlled study of butyrate enemas found that enema therapy results in only minor effects on markers of inflammation and oxidative stress. Evidence suggests that such enemas may offer additional benefit in medically refractory cases.

Chinese enema therapy

Zhikang compound liquid (ZKCL) and *Quick-acting kuijie powder (QAKJP)* have been used as enema therapy for UC and found to be of benefit.

Vitamin E enema

An open labeled study in 15 patients with UC found that rectal administration of d-alpha tocopherol (800 units per day) reported a positive response to treatment in 12 of the 15 patients.

SUPPLEMENTS

Dehydroepiandrosterone (DHEA)

Low blood DHEA can be demonstrated in a majority of patients with UC and Crohn's disease. DHEA and 7alpha-hydroxy-dehydroepiandrosterone protect against experimental colitis in rats.

A case of the beneficial effect of 200 mg of DHEA per day for eight weeks in a 35-year-old female patient with chronic active pouchitis has been reported. A pilot study demonstrated that DHEA (200 mg per day) is effective and safe in patients with refractory UC.

Fish oil and omega-3 fatty acids

Patients with IBD frequently suffer from polyunsaturated fatty acid (PUFA) deficiency. The initial excitement about the benefit of their supplementation has been tempered by the results of randomized controlled trials.

Results of studies using fish oil or omega-3 fatty acids have been mixed. According to Dr. Marion-Letellier and colleagues from Rouen University in Rouen, France, "While in vitro and in vivo studies have demonstrated the anti-inflammatory properties of n-3 polyunsaturated fatty acids in experimental models of IBD, results of clinical trials have been disappointing."

Another problem with the use of fish oil is the large amount of fish oil that has to be taken. Compliance becomes a problem because of the fishy odor in the breath.

Glucosamine

Glucosamine, a naturally occurring amino-monosaccharide, is widely used to treat osteoarthritis in humans. It improves disease severity while reducing damage to the colon in animal models of colitis.

Dr. Salvatore and colleagues from the University Department of Pediatric Gastroenterology, Royal Free in London conducted a pilot study of N-acetyl glucosamine (three to six g orally) as adjunct therapy for treatment of severe treatment-resistant IBD in kids. Some kids received enemas of this product. Eight of the 12 children given glucosamine treatment showed significant improvement.

Melatonin

Melatonin is one of the most versatile and ubiquitous hormonal molecules in the body. It is present throughout the gut. It regulates inflammation and movements in the gastrointestinal tract. It has antioxidant and anti-inflammatory properties. Studies in animals suggest beneficial effects against colitis.

Limited data in humans suggest that supplemental melatonin administration may ameliorate effect on colitis. Studies by Dr. Chojnacki and colleagues suggest that adjuvant melatonin therapy may help in sustaining remission in patients with UC.

Paradoxically, melatonin administration may trigger Crohn's symptoms.

Muscovite

Muscovite is a common rock-forming mineral also known as common mica or potash mica. It is made up of aluminum and potassium. Rectal administration of muscovite decreases weight loss and improves gross and microscopic colitis severity in mice.

Propionyl-L-carnitine (PLC)

L-carnitine plays a critical role in fatty-acid metabolism and short-chain fatty acids such as butyrate and propionate, which are important for colon health. Dr. Mikhailova and colleagues from the State Scientific Centre of Coloproctology, Rosmedtechnology in Moscow conducted a double-blind trial to study the effect of PLC on patients receiving stable treatment of UC. Seventy-two percent of the PLC group attained clinical response, as compared to 50 percent in the placebo group. The remission rate with one gram of PLC per day was 55 percent, as compared to 35 percent in the placebo group.

VITAMINS AND MINERALS

Special attention should be paid to the nutritional status of patients with IBD. Abnormalities of the trace elements can be demonstrated in pediatric patients, probably as a result of inadequate intake, reduced absorption, and increased intestinal losses.

Zinc

Zinc strengthens the intestinal barrier, making it less leaky. Zinc supplementation ameliorates damage to the colon in animal models of colitis.

A four-week placebo-controlled double-blind cross-over trial explored the effect of oral zinc supplementation in patients with inactive to moderately active IBD. Plasma zinc levels increased during the supplementation. However, there was no effect on the disease activity of the patients.

> Patients with IBD frequently develop iron deficiency and are prescribed oral iron therapy. It should be pointed out that oral iron can, in some cases, potentiate the severity of colitis. In cases of intolerance or severe iron deficiency and in acute exacerbations, intravenous iron may be the preferred option.

REFERENCES

1. Lissner D, Siegmund B. Ulcerative colitis: current and future treatment strategies. *Dig Dis.* 2013; 31(1):91-4.
2. Danese S, Colombel JF, Peyrin-Biroulet L et al. Review article: the role of anti-TNF in the management of ulcerative colitis -- past, present and future. *Aliment Pharmacol Ther.* 2013 May; 37(9):855-66.
3. De Greef E, Vandenplas Y, Hauser B et al. Probiotics and IBD. *Acta Gastroenterol Belg.* 2013 Mar; 76(1):15-9.
4. Floch MH, Walker WA, Madsen K et al. Recommendations for probiotic use-2011 update. *J Clin Gastroenterol.* 2011 Nov; 45 Suppl:S168-71.
5. Hanai H, Iida T, Takeuchi K et al. Curcumin maintenance therapy for ulcerative colitis: randomized, multi-center, double-blind, placebo-controlled trial. *Clin Gastroenterol Hepatol.* 2006 Dec; 4(12):1502-6.

CHAPTER 40

Crohn's Disease

KEY POINTS

- Surgery is curative for UC but not Crohn's disease.
- Corticosteroids are effective for inducing remission but should not be used for maintaining remission.
- Patients with Crohn's disease should be screened for micronutrient deficiencies.
- Data supporting the use of CAM in Crohn's disease is scanty.
- Clinical studies using probiotics have been disappointing.

Crohn's disease, like UC, is one of the components of chronic idiopathic IBD. In contrast to UC, which is limited to the colon and rectum, Crohn's may involve any part of the GI tract from mouth to anus. The small intestine is involved in as many as 80 percent of Crohn's patients, while 50 percent have both colon and small intestine disease.

Upper GI disease can be seen in less than 15 percent of those with Crohn's disease. Due to the variability of symptoms, diagnosis is frequently delayed.

> There is no medical or surgical cure for Crohn's disease. Treatment is aimed at suppressing the disease and making the patient better. Most patients with Crohn's disease require at least one surgery during the lifetime.

OCCURRENCE

The prevalence of Crohn's disease is 201 per 100,000 persons in the U.S. IBD is less common in Asia and South America. It is more prevalent in the northern hemisphere than the southern.

Most cases present between the ages of 15 and 30. There is a second peak incidence manifesting at 50 to 80 years of age. Crohn's is more common in females. It is more common in persons of Jewish ancestry. In contrast, IBD tends to be less frequent among Hispanics and African-Americans.

CAUSATIVE FACTORS

INCREASED RISK IN FAMILIES

There is an increased genetic predisposition to IBD, although greater than 70 percent of patients have no family history of IBD. Multiple gene mutations are seen in patients with Crohn's disease. These mutations may also be present in healthy subjects, suggesting that additional gene mutations and environmental factors are important in determining who ultimately develops the disease.

DIET

Dietary factors are widely believed to be involved in causing disease. While the precise factors have not been specifically determined, a Western diet is associated with an increased risk.

History of cow's milk allergy is common in patients with Crohn's. Refined sugar, high fat, low fiber, low vegetable diet, and milk proteins are associated with higher risk of Crohn's. While nutritional deficiencies do not appear to have a role, higher omega-3 fatty acid intake reduces the risk.

ORAL CONTRACEPTIVES

A meta-analysis by Dr. Cornish and colleagues provides evidence that oral contraceptives increase the risk of Crohn's disease.

However, the risk is small and does not tend to affect disease activity in patients who already have documented Crohn's disease.

POSTMENOPAUSAL HORMONAL THERAPY

The effect of hormone therapy in women after menopause remains to be established. The risk, if any, is small.

USE OF ANTIBIOTICS

Antibiotics can disrupt the normal healthy bacterial pattern in the gut. Use of antibiotics two to five years prior to diagnosis has frequently been noted. NSAIDs may increase the risk for development of IBD or induce flare-up.

DYSBIOSIS

Literature suggests an imbalance of intestinal bacteria or dysbiosis contributes to causing and sustaining the disease. The role of infectious agents is controversial and continues to be debated. The intestinal bacterial pattern does not have to be abnormal. Studies suggest that "normal" intestinal flora may initiate and/or promote Crohn's disease in genetically predisposed subjects.

EARLY LIFE EVENTS

While the data on the relationship between breastfeeding and Crohn's disease has been inconsistent, studies indicate that health and sickness events in early infancy play a role.

MISCELLANEOUS FACTORS

- Whereas smoking is protective against UC, it tends to worsen Crohn's disease.
- Prior appendectomy confers protection against UC, but not for Crohn's disease.
- Stress does not cause IBD but contributes to exacerbation of symptoms.

CLINICAL FEATURES

Clinical presentation depends upon the intestinal location of the disease and the type of disease. Clinical features include abdominal pain, fever, diarrhea (which may be bloody), weight loss, and low-grade temperature. Patients with predominant upper GI involvement have indigestion, pain in mid-upper abdomen, and feeling of fullness/bloating on eating.

Difficult or painful swallowing and chest pain may occur if the esophagus is involved. A fistula may occur around the anus. Some patients may present for the first time with bowel obstruction.

Most children with Crohn's disease present with weight loss, which may precede intestinal symptoms.

Physical findings in Crohn's disease are variable and include elevated temperature, weight loss, muscle wasting, and abdominal tenderness, especially in the right lower abdomen, mimicking acute appendicitis. Small ulcers may be seen in the mouth.

DIAGNOSTIC TESTING

A complete blood count may be normal or show evidence of anemia. White blood cells (WBC) may be increased because of the inflammation or infection. A complete metabolic panel may show low levels of albumin, abnormal electrolytes, and abnormal liver tests.

Stool studies should always be performed to exclude infections as the cause of inflammation and any recurrence.

Anti-Saccharomyces cereviciae antibody (ASCA) is positive in about two-thirds of the patients with Crohn's disease and in about 10 percent of the patients with UC.

Colonoscopy is the cornerstone of diagnosis. The terminal small bowel can be examined during the same test. Findings include redness, swelling, and ulcers. Involvement of the gut can be patchy. Involvement of the upper GI tract can be confirmed or excluded by upper GI endoscopy.

The correlation between findings on upper and lower GI scope and the clinical effects on the patient is suboptimal.

A plain X-ray series of the abdomen is helpful in acute cases to exclude any acute emergency. Small bowel X-rays can help document the small intestinal involvement as well as to look for narrowing and fistulae. Abdominal ultrasound and CT scans are helpful in excluding abscesses and documenting any blockage or fistula.

Microscopic exam of the biopsies done during endoscopy are helpful in confirming diagnosis and excluding other diagnoses.

CROHN'S DISEASE MAY MIMIC OTHER CONDITIONS

Crohn's disease should be distinguished from other causes of inflammation in the gut, including infections, microscopic colitis, diverticulitis, drug-induced colitis (NSAIDs, gold), ischemic colitis, radiation colitis, appendicitis, and even cancer.

NSAIDs can cause inflammation and ulceration throughout the GI tract. Effects of radiation on the bowel may manifest even years after the radiation therapy.

CROHN'S DISEASE ILLNESS BEYOND GUT

Patients with Crohn's may suffer one or many complications beyond the gut. These include involvement of eyes, skin, joints, liver, gallbladder stones, and kidney stones, osteoporosis, and clot formation in blood vessels. Just like cancer, metastatic Crohn's disease may occur.

MEDICAL TREATMENT OF CROHN'S DISEASE

Medical management of Crohn's disease depends on the disease location and severity. Two approaches to treatment of Crohn's are used, step-up or top-down. The former implies using less potent and less toxic medications initially and to move up to more potent/toxic drugs if the initial treatment is not effective. The top-down approach involves using the most potent/toxic drugs first and then phase out as appropriate.

Drug treatment in step-up approach involves starting with 5-aminosalicylates class of drugs (Pentasa, Asacol) although the data on their efficacy in Crohn's is controversial. Failures may then be treated with steroids (like prednisone). Steroids like budesonide (Entocort) are less toxic. Patients with fistula may be treated with antibiotics (Flagyl, Cipro).

Ulcers in the mouth are treated with local application of hydrocortisone or sucralfate (Carafate). Patients with stomach disease may benefit from acid blockers (Prilosec, Protonix, Nexium, Prevacid) and sucralfate (Carafate). If there is no response to these drugs, other medical therapy for Crohn's may be added.

The treatment of Crohn's may further be escalated to immunosuppressive drugs like azathioprine (Imuran) or 6MP and biologic drugs like Remicade, Humira, or Cimzia. Biologic drugs have a high risk of life-threatening infections.

Dr. Ford and a panel of several other international Crohn's experts conducted an expert literature review with meta-analysis and published their findings in the *American Journal of Gastroenterology* (2011). These investigators concluded that as many as eight patients with Crohn's would need to be tried on this treatment (number needed to treat) in order to accomplish successful remission in one patient. Of the patients in whom drug treatment is effective in achieving remission, only one in four who continued on the medication would maintain remission.

SURGICAL TREATMENT OF CROHN'S DISEASE

Surgery is very common in patients with Crohn's disease. Over a period of 15 years after diagnosis, almost 75 percent of the patients will have had at least one operation, with over 50 percent having had multiple operations. The choice of operation depends upon the underlying problem.

Common reasons for surgery include Crohn's disease not responding to medical treatment, development of complications like abscess, blockage, perforation, severe bleeding, or even cancer.

As a rule, minimalist surgery is the preferred option.

FERTILITY

Fertility in men and women with IBD is not decreased.

- Factors affecting fertility may include drugs, presence of active disease, and prior surgery.
- Sulfasalazine (Azulfidine) causes low sperm count in men, which is reversible within two months of discontinuation. Newer 5ASA formulations do not affect sperm count.

- Azathioprine (Imuran) does not reduce the quality of semen. Anatomic defects like blockage of fallopian tubes may occur in females.
- Painful sex may be a barrier in efforts to conceive.

RISK FOR CANCER

Both UC and Crohn's disease have an increased risk for cancer. The risk increases with the extent of involvement of the gut and duration of the disease.

ALTERNATIVE MEDICINE THERAPIES

Thirty to 60 percent of patients with Crohn's use complementary and alternative medicine options. A Canadian study found that the most often used alternative medicine therapies are massage therapy (30 percent), chiropractic therapy (14 percent), physiotherapy (4 percent), acupuncture (3.5 percent), and naturopathy/homeopathy (3.5 percent).

Another study reported the relative prevalence of different therapies was as follows:

- Homeopathy (55 percent)
- Probiotics (43 percent)
- Classical naturopathy (38 percent)
- Boswellia serrata extracts (36 percent)
- Acupuncture and Traditional Chinese Medicine (TCM) (33 percent)

Other herbal remedies being used across the world include slippery elm, fenugreek, devil's claw, Mexican yam, tormentil, and wei tong ning, a traditional Chinese medicine.

In this chapter, we will focus primarily on Crohn's disease (CD) even though there is likely to be an overlap with UC. The latter is discussed in Chapter 39.

PROBIOTICS

A dysfunctional intestinal barrier can allow intestinal bacteria or bacterial proteins to initiate chronic inflammation in Crohn's disease. Probiotics studied include *Lactobacillus johnsonii*, *Lactobacillus GG*, and *Saccharomyces boulardii*.

In a recent review, Drs. Whelan and Quigley from the King's College London School of Medicine concluded that current evidence of the role of probiotics in Crohn's has been disappointing.

PSYCHOTHERAPY

Psychotherapy does not have an impact on the course of the Crohn's disease, although patients with psychological issues may find that it enhances adjustment and coping mechanisms.

ACUPUNCTURE

Limited evidence supports the use of acupuncture in Crohn's disease. Dr. Schneider and colleagues from the University Medical Hospital in Heidelberg, Germany concluded in a systematic review that real acupuncture is effective in improving Crohn's disease activity, as compared to sham acupuncture.

SUPPLEMENTS

Dehydroepiandrosterone

Dehydroepiandrosterone sulfate concentrations are decreased in patients with IBD. A pilot study from the University of Regensburg in Regensburg, Germany reported that dehydroepiandrosterone is effective and safe in patients with refractory Crohn's disease or UC.

Melatonin

Preliminary data regarding the utility of melatonin in the treatment of Crohn's disease is ambiguous or negative. A case of melatonin triggering Crohn's disease symptoms has been reported.

Omega-3 fatty acids

A systematic review and meta-analysis done at the Hebrew University of Jerusalem concluded that that there was statistically significant advantage for omega-3 fatty acids in Crohn's disease. However, the studies were heterogeneous and, as such, there is insufficient data to make a firm recommendation about its use.

Glucosamine

N-acetyl glucosamine may lead to enhanced tissue repair mechanisms. A pilot study reported that N-acetyl glucosamine treatment results in clinical improvement in kids with IBD.

Glutamine

Glutamine-enriched diets decrease intestinal damage and disease severity while improving nutritional status in animal models of IBD.

A randomized controlled trial from the All India Institute of Medical Sciences in New Delhi found that glutamine supplementation improves structural damage and reduces leakiness of the bowel in patients with Crohn's disease.

Butyrate

Short chain fatty acids are a source of nutrition for colon cells and are essential for a healthy colon. Laboratory experiments done on tissue samples from patients with Crohn's disease suggest that butyrate, a short chain fatty acid, reduces intestinal inflammation caused by bacterial toxins. The beneficial effect is mediated via its antioxidant actions.

An open-labeled study conducted at the University of Pavia in Italy found that taking butyrate tablets (4g per day for eight weeks) results in improvement in 69 percent of the patients, including 53 percent who achieved remission.

Colostrum

Administration of multiple nutritional elements (consisting of fish peptides, bovine colostrum, boswellia serrata, curcumin and a multivitamin), probiotics, and recombinant human GH (rhGH), along with exclusion of dairy products, certain grains, and carrageenan-containing foods results in prolonged remission and restoration of weight in subjects with Crohn's disease. There is a lack of data for the use of colostrum alone in Crohn's disease.

Insulin-like growth factor-1

Low serum levels of insulin-like growth factor- 1 have been implicated in stunting of growth in pediatric Crohn's. There is a lack of evidence documenting its beneficial role in patients.

Vitamins and minerals

Although most patients with IBD are well-nourished, there is a decrease in muscle cell mass and handgrip strength in patients compared to controls. Micronutrient deficiency is common. Vitamin D deficiency is common in the population at large and more so in patients with Crohn's disease. It should be checked and corrected as needed.

> Studies conducted by Dr. Ananthakrishnan and colleagues from the Massachusetts General Hospital in Boston suggest that vitamin D deficiency is associated with increased risk of hospitalization, surgery, and cancer.

- Normalization of vitamin D levels results in decreased risk of Crohn's-related surgery.
- Over two-thirds of Crohn's disease patients have low levels of vitamin C, vitamin B3, and zinc. This may occur due to decreased food intake, diminished intestinal absorption, and loss from inflamed gut.
- Reduced levels of vitamin C, zinc, and selenium may contribute to weaker antioxidant defense apparatus of the gut, leading to perpetuation of the disease activity.

> Zinc supplementation strengthens a "leaky gut" in Crohn's disease and potentially can reduce relapse.

HERBAL THERAPIES

There is a huge overlap the between UC and Crohn's disease, especially in experimental evidence related to herbal therapies.

Artemisia absinthium (wormwood)

A double-blind randomized controlled trial conducted by the Yale University School of Medicine examined the effect of an herbal blend containing wormwood (500 mg three times a day or a placebo for 10 weeks) in patients with Crohn's disease. Ninety percent of patients in the treatment group improved; 65 percent achieved full remission within eight weeks. In contrast, none of the patients in the placebo group achieved remission.

Tripterygium wilfordii

A single-blinded trial compared the use of polyglycosides of *Tripterygium wilfordii* (GTW) to conventional treatment with mesalazine (5ASA) for the recurrence of Crohn's disease in patients after surgery. Patients treated with GTW suffered significantly fewer recurrences than the group treated with the standard 5ASA formulation.

Turmeric (curcumin)

There is a paucity of human studies for the use of curcumin (turmeric) in treating Crohn's disease. One open labeled pilot trial from Columbia University used 360 mg of curcumin three times a day for one month, followed by same dose four times a day for an additional two months. Four of the five patients completed the study. Treatment resulted in decreased severity of Crohn's, along with improvement in symptoms and blood markers of inflammation.

Boswellia

Results of studies of the use of Boswellia in animals and humans with Crohn's disease have been mixed. A recent randomized, controlled trial from Hospital Porz am Rhein in Cologne, Germany demonstrated that the use of *Boswellia serrata* extract (Boswelan, PS0201Bo) was no better than placebo for maintaining remission in patients with Crohn's disease.

Miscellaneous herbal treatments

- *Uncaria tomentosa*, also known as cat's claw, has been used to treat chronic disorders, including IBD and arthritis since ancient times. There is a lack of data for its use in treating Crohn's disease.
- Berberine is an active constituent of several botanicals. It protects against experimental colonic tissue damage in animal models of colitis. There is a lack of human studies documenting its benefit in treating Crohn's disease.

DIETARY MANAGEMENT

Results using elimination diets in Crohn's disease have been mixed.

Low-fat diet

Avoid high-fat diets, especially high-fat, non-vegetarian diets. Multiple studies have documented the increased risk of Crohn's in patients on such diets.

Role of food sensitivities

Food sensitivities have been implicated in the pathogenesis of Crohn's disease. Patients may identify potential symptom-provoking foods using a food-symptom diary and then try elimination diets for two to four weeks at a time, to see if any part of elimination diet is helpful. Of note, a case-controlled study of nutritional factors found a negative correlation of citrus fruits and Crohn's disease.

Paleolithic diet

Efficacy of a paleo diet in alleviating symptoms of Crohn's disease has not been studied.

FODMAP diet

High-FODMAP diets have been implicated in the rise of Crohn's disease and celiac disease in recent times.

Adopting a low-FODMAP diet (see chapter 20) might be an easier strategy with greater success for compliance and may be undertaken as the first step in patients whose symptoms are disproportionately greater than intestinal damage would indicate. Such patients frequently have IBS, as well.

One retrospective study of 72 patients with IBD found that all 70 percent of patients who continued on a low-FODMAP diet had improvement in symptoms. Note that a low-FODMAP diet is somewhat the opposite of Specific Carbohydrate Diet (SCD) diet described below.

Exclusive enteral nutrition (EEN)

Beneficial effect of exclusive enteral nutrition (tube feeding) in children with Crohn's disease has been well established. Normal foods by mouth are completely excluded. A liquid nutritional formula is used instead.

Protocols on how to give it vary. It may be given by mouth or tube feeding into the stomach or small intestine. Water is permitted, as is some chewing gum. Some experts administer partial enteral nutrition (PEN), whereby most of energy needs are met by liquid nutritional formula and a small component may be consumed as food. Considerable success has been achieved with PEN, depending on the protocol used.

Ideal duration of exclusive enteral nutrition remains to be established. The food is slowly restarted with a meal every three to four days and gradually scaled upwards.

EEN results in healing of gut damage, as well as better nutritional status and bone health. The disease can be controlled in as many as 90 percent of the kids with Crohn's.

A recent study by Dr. Soo and colleagues reported in the *Journal Digestive Diseases and Sciences (2013)* concluded that EEN is equal to, and should be preferred over, steroid treatment of kids with newly-diagnosed Crohn's disease.

EEN is more widely used in Europe than North America. Literature suggests that over 90 percent of Swedish pediatric gastroenterologists use it regularly for their patients, as compared to only 12 percent of doctors in the United States.

Drs. Day and Burgess argued in a recent expert review, "This therapy is no longer on the side-lines, but is ready for prime time."

Semi-vegetarian diet (SVD)

Patients with active disease are usually prescribed a low-fiber diet, so as not to exacerbate symptoms. However, this precludes the beneficial effect of undigested fiber on gut bacteria.

Dr. Chiba and colleagues from Japan compared the efficacy of a semi-vegetarian diet to an omnivorous diet for prevention of relapse in Crohn's disease over two years. The semi-vegetarian diet was designed on the premise that compliance with an exclusively vegetarian diet would be difficult. Ironically, this diet included numerous components excluded by FODMAPs and/or Specific Carbohydrate Diets. These allowed foods in the semi-vegetarian diet included brown rice, soybeans, yam, potatoes, and onions.

Remarkably, 92 percent of the patients in the Chiba study sustained on a semi-vegetarian diet maintained remission, compared to only 33 percent of patients on an omnivorous diet.

Specific Carbohydrate Diet (SCD)

Specific Carbohydrate Diet (SCD) was popularized by its documentation in a book, "Breaking the Vicious Cycle." This diet restricts all but simple carbohydrates. No grains are allowed. Lentils and split peas are allowed, while chickpeas and soy beans are not. All fresh fruits and vegetables except potatoes and yams are permitted. Canned fruits and vegetables are excluded. Similarly, canned, processed, and smoked meats are not allowed. Milk is not allowed, but patients may consume lactose-free cheeses.

Dr. Suskind and colleagues from the University of Washington studied the role of SCD in seven kids with Crohn's disease. The investigators found that all symptoms had resolved within three months of initiating the diet. Of note, patients on an SCD diet are at risk for vitamin D deficiency, and it needs to be checked and supplemented as appropriate.

The fiber paradox

Interestingly, both SCD and Paleolithic diets are high in fiber, while excluding fiber derived from cereal grains. On the other hand, cereal grain-based fiber, like oat bran and germinated barley foodstuff, has been shown to be helpful in treating UC. This paradox raises many more questions than we have answers for at this time.

Bottom-line on efficacy of dietary management of Crohn's disease

Literature points to the role of intestinal contents as playing a critical role in Crohn's disease. Evidence supports the use of exclusive enteral nutrition support, exclusion diets, and semi-vegetarian diets for patients with Crohn's disease. There is a paucity of evidence from randomized controlled trials in favor of or against the use of SCD, FODMAP, and Paleolithic diets, although many patients swear by them. Irrespective of any specific diet, much more research needs to be done on all these dietary interventions.

REFERENCES

1. Whelan K, Quigley EM. Probiotics in the management of irritable bowel syndrome and inflammatory bowel disease. *Curr Opin Gastroenterol.* 2013 Mar; 29(2):184-9.
2. Day AS, Burgess L. Exclusive enteral nutrition and induction of remission of active Crohn's disease in children. *Expert Rev Clin Immunol.* 2013 Apr; 9(4):375-83; quiz 384.
3. Baumgart DC, Sandborn WJ. Crohn's disease. *Lancet.* 2012 Nov 3;380(9853):1590-605.
4. Rogler G. Top-down or step-up treatment in Crohn's disease? *Dig Dis.* 2013; 31(1):83-90.
5. Schneider A, Streitberger K, Joos S. Acupuncture treatment in gastrointestinal diseases: a systematic review. *World J Gastroenterol.* 2007 Jul 7; 13(25):3417-24.
6. Ng SC, Lam YT, Tsoi KK et al. Systematic review: the efficacy of herbal therapy in inflammatory bowel disease. *Aliment Pharmacol Ther.* 2013 Oct; 38(8):854-63.

CHAPTER 41

Diverticulosis and Diverticulitis

KEY POINTS

- Diverticulosis is primarily a disease of the West.
- Most patients with diverticulosis do not have any problems due to it. Only a small fraction develops acute diverticulitis.
- Diverticular bleeding is uncommon during an episode of diverticulitis.

The diverticulum is a sac or pouch-like structure that forms in the wall of the colon, usually at points where the wall is the weak. These points usually correspond to points of entry of blood vessels into the colon. Although diverticuli may occur anywhere in GI tract, diverticulosis in the colon is the most common.

Diverticular disease comprises mainly of diverticulosis and diverticulitis. Diverticulosis implies presence of diverticuli, while diverticulitis indicates inflammation or infection of the diverticulum due to a microscopic or overt hole or puncture in the colon.

OCCURRENCE

Diverticulosis is a disease of the modern civilization. The first operation for diverticular disease was performed by Dr. Mayo in 1907.

It is primarily a disease of the West, with prevalence rates as high as 45 percent, whereas in Africa and Asia, the prevalence is less than 2 percent. It is uncommon before the age of 40. By 80 years of age, as many as 80 percent of Americans may have diverticulosis. It affects both sexes equally.

Risk factors include low dietary fiber intake, obesity, and lack of physical exercise. Obese patients are more likely to suffer from diverticulitis and diverticular bleed. An association with smoking, alcohol, or caffeine has not been clearly established. There may be a correlation with colon cancer; however, a cause and effect relationship has not been established.

HOW DOES DIVERTICULOSIS AFFECT BODY?

Most people with diverticulosis do not have any problems because of it.

PAINFUL DIVERTICULAR DISEASE

The existence of painful diverticular disease is controversial. Patients complain of intermittent pain in the abdomen, irregular bowel movements, and passage of pellet-like stools, with occasional diarrhea. Such patients may have co-existing IBS. Antibiotics are not helpful. Medications to reduce bowel spasm (like Bentyl), along with a high-fiber diet, plenty of fluids, and exercise are recommended. Some of these patients eventually have an episode of acute diverticulitis.

DIVERTICULITIS

Diverticulitis is caused by a microscopic or a gross hole of the diverticulum pouch, along with spillage of fecal material into the abdomen. Most cases are mild, because the hole is quickly walled off by the body's defense mechanisms.

Clinical Features

Patients complain of pain in the left lower abdomen. Pain may be smoldering for several days. Associated complaints may include nausea, vomiting, constipation, diarrhea, and painful and frequent urination. Bleeding is uncommon in the presence of diverticulitis.

The abdomen may be distended and painful to the touch or pressing on the left side. Patients frequently have a low-grade fever. Presence of severe symptoms is a worrisome sign.

Diagnosis

A complete blood count (CBC) shows increased white blood cells in most cases. Most of the other routine labs are usually normal. The diagnosis is usually made on clinical grounds.

Abdominal X-rays may help exclude an intestinal blockage or gross puncture of the bowel. Further testing is only needed if the symptoms are severe, if the diagnosis is in doubt, or if patients do not respond to antibiotics. The CT scan of the abdomen is accurate in 95 to 100 percent of the cases.

Diseases mimicking diverticulitis

Many diseases may mimic acute diverticulitis and confound the diagnosis. These include:

- Acute appendicitis (pain is usually on the right side)
- Crohn's disease
- Endometriosis
- Pelvic inflammatory disease
- Ischemic colitis, which occurs due to a transient drop in blood supply to part of the colon, causing damage, much like a heart attack does to the heart
- Stomach ulcers

Treatment

Young, healthy patients with mild symptoms may be treated as outpatients with antibiotics (like Cipro bid plus Flagyl). Patients with severe cases, especially the elderly, are usually admitted to the hospital and treated with intravenous antibiotics. Most patients start improving within two to three days.

Failure of treatment

Risk factors for failure of medical treatment include immune-suppressed patients, like those with a history of diabetes, chronic kidney disease, collagen vascular diseases like lupus, and those undergoing chemotherapy or taking steroids.

Clinical deterioration or lack of improvement suggests that an abscess has been formed in the abdomen outside the colon. These can be drained under guidance with CT scan or by performing surgery.

Post-healing management

About one-third of patients will suffer recurrent episodes after resolution of the first episode. About five percent will continue to suffer chronic smoldering abdominal pain.

The role of dietary therapy after resolution is controversial. Most physicians recommend a high-fiber diet. Avoiding foods like seeds, corn, and nuts is controversial.

A colonoscopy should be undertaken about four to eight weeks after resolution to rule out the possibility of colon cancer.

Recurrence occurs in about 30 to 40 percent of the cases. Surgery is recommended after the first attack of complicated diverticulitis. Elective surgery should be considered after the second episode, in most cases. The role and timing of surgery in young patients remains controversial. Many experts recommend surgery in young patients after the first attack of uncomplicated diverticulitis.

DIVERTICULAR BLEEDING

Bleeding from the diverticulum pouch may occur in about five percent of patients. It is usually seen in elderly subjects with significant other diseases.

Clinical features

Bleeding is painless, massive, and usually requires blood transfusions. A minor or microscopic bleed is unusual. There may be nausea, weakness, dizziness, and rapid heartbeat. Abdominal pain is absent, except for abdominal cramps related to the laxative effect of the blood trying to expel the contents of the bowel.

General management

In addition to initial resuscitation with IV fluids and blood as needed, patients usually undergo a colonoscopy. Colonoscopy is performed to establish the cause of bleeding. Therapeutic measures to control the bleeding can sometimes be undertaken during colonoscopy.

Colonoscopy may be difficult in patients with active and severe bleeding. Arterial scan is recommended in such cases. If a bleeding site is identified, the bleeding can be stopped during the same procedure.

An RBC bleeding scan may be performed in patients in whom the bleeding site cannot be localized by colonoscopy and the bleeding is suspected to be slow or intermittent.

Elective surgery is recommended after two or more transfusion-requiring episodes of bleeding or if the source of the bleed has not been identified.

Prognosis

A recurrence of bleeding occurs in 20 to 30 percent of the patients after the first episode, which rises to 50 percent after the second episode of bleeding.

SEGMENTAL COLITIS

Patients with left-sided diverticulosis may develop segmental colitis mimicking IBD. The causative factors have not been clearly established. Patients complain of abdominal pain, diarrhea, bleeding, and even weight loss. Optimal treatment has not been clearly determined and may include antibiotics, anti-inflammatory agents (like 5ASA drugs), and even steroids.

ALTERNATIVE MEDICINE THERAPIES

PREBIOTICS

Fiber, which frequently acts as a prebiotic, also plays an important role in management of diverticular symptoms. Several large studies have reported that fiber in the diet reduces risk of diverticular disease.

PROBIOTICS

Several studies have examined the role of probiotics in diverticular disease. Drs. Frick and Zavoral from the Central Military Hospital and Postgraduate Institute of Medicine in Prague conducted an open labeled trial to examine the effect of the probiotic *E. coli strain Nissle*. The probiotic treatment increased the duration of remission with a significant improvement of abdominal symptoms of painful diverticular disease.

Another study by Dr. Tursi and colleagues from Italy studied the effect of a 5ASA drug mesalazine alone, the probiotic *Lactobacillus casei DG* alone, or both combined. Both mesalazine as well as the probiotic prevented recurrence of symptoms of painful diverticular disease in 77 percent of patients. The combined treatment was even better.

REFERENCES

1. Mann NS, Hoda KK. Segmental colitis associated with diverticulosis: systematic evaluation of 486 cases with meta-analysis. *Hepatogastroenterology*. 2012 Oct; 59(119):2119-21.
2. Boynton W, Floch M. New strategies for the management of diverticular disease: insights for the clinician. *Therap Adv Gastroenterol*. 2013 May; 6(3):205-13.
3. Tursi A, Brandimarte G, Elisei W et al. Randomised clinical trial: mesalazine and/or probiotics in maintaining remission of

symptomatic uncomplicated diverticular disease—a double-blind, randomised, placebo-controlled study. *Aliment Pharmacol Ther*. 2013 Oct; 38(7):741-51.

SECTION X
Dr. M's Seven-X Plan for Digestive Health

CHAPTER 42

Overview of Dr. M's Seven-X Plan

KEY POINTS

- You are healthy until you are unhealthy.
- Using the Seven-X Plan for healing is good – adopting it for prevention is even better.

Now is the time when rubber hits the road. You have presumably gone through the background material I have provided in the previous chapters. And I am sure most of you already have a pretty good idea of the health problems you face, the things that might be doing wrong, all the challenges you face, and the opportunities for improvement.

In a nutshell, there are some core elements of the program that everyone needs to adopt. And then there are some specific modifiable elements. The latter pertain to the specific type of nutrition based on your genetically-engineered and environmentally-transformed intestinal metabolic constitution.

My goal thus far in the book has been to empower you with knowledge so you may judge for yourself what is good for you. Since the science is not advanced enough to test for it, we just have two main elements to guide us:

- Overall health of the person and presence or absence of diverse illnesses.
- Reaction of the person's body to any single food or the type of foods – for example, most people with lactose intolerance can

easily handle one glass of milk per day especially if consumed in split doses. However, a person with irritable bowel syndrome may not be able to tolerate even that.

So who are the candidates for Dr. M's Seven-X Plan? Is it for everyone to some extent or just for those with perceived unhealthy digestion?

Let's just divide the readers into four broad categories.

- Patients with an unhealthy gut, digestion problems like irritable bowel syndrome, chronic heartburn, etc.
- Patients with multiple illnesses, where unhealthy gut might be one component related to the primary illness, such as GI problems in patients with diabetes.
- Patients with neurobehavioral problems and chronic pain syndromes where GI symptoms may be present and the unhealthy gut may be playing a critical role in sustaining the pain and brain and gut dysfunction.
- Ostensibly healthy persons who look and feel great and of whom many of us feel jealous.

PERSONS WITH AN UNHEALTHY GUT

Not much write-up is needed here to justify the need for such patients to follow the gut-healthy Seven-X Plan. While following the general principles outlined in the succeeding chapters, the patient must take into account the information in previous chapters where I may have provided disease-specific information. This will allow the person to modify the Seven-X Plan specifically to the illness.

One example would be patients with IBS. Such patients would benefit from the use of specific probiotic strains targeted at IBS and mentioned in Chapter 37.

Another example is gastroparesis or slow stomach. There is not just a decreased ability to tolerate food, but patients may have many other associated problems, including but not limited to malabsorption of nutrients and overgrowth of bad bacteria in the gut. In cases of gastroparesis, unlike many other GI disorders, we frequently recommend a low-fiber diet! This is just one example of how one needs to modify the Seven-X Plan based on the individual GI disorders described earlier.

PERSONS WITH NON-GI PRIMARY ILLNESS OR MULTIPLE ILLNESSES

Subjects with multiple bodily illnesses (such as diabetes and lupus) frequently have GI problems.

And if it is not due to some illness, the GI symptoms may also arise as a result of medications being used to treat the illness. You just have to look at the package insert of any of your medicines and you will find that GI side effects are almost always listed as a possibility.

Patients with such conditions develop unhealthy gut due to their primary disease or the medicine they are taking. For example, when diabetes is associated with leaky gut and inflammation as causative factors, the diabetes may result in slowing down the gut or cause diarrhea. Medications like NSAIDs can cause indigestion and even ulcers anywhere in the gut.

> Side effects of many acid-blocking medicines include weakened absorption of nutritional elements, small intestinal bacterial overgrowth, and increased risk of infections, including GI and non-GI infections.

PERSONS WITH NEUROBEHAVIORAL AND CHRONIC PAIN SYNDROMES

Notwithstanding the fact that the majority of such patients have concurrent GI issues, an unhealthy gut is one of the critical elements at the root of the perceived main problem.

GI problems are a significant part of life for the vast majority of such patients, whether the diagnosis is autism, ADHD, OCD or one of the chronic pain syndromes, like fibromyalgia, chronic fatigue syndrome, or restless leg syndrome.

The preceding chapters on intestinal bacteria, leaky gut, inflammation, and oxidative stress have gone into the rationale behind this assertion. Needless to say, a full-throated adoption of Dr. M's Seven-X Plan will likely help soothe the illness.

ARE THERE ANY "PERFECTLY" HEALTHY PERSONS

A person is only healthy until he or she becomes unhealthy. Dr. M's Seven-X Plan serves as an insurance policy that will help any hidden problems that might be lurking inside the bowels of our body (no pun intended).

Let me explain this with an example. Former President George W. Bush has always been fit as a fiddle and passed his physicals done by the best physicians with flying colors. He continued his strenuous exercise routine after leaving the White House. Then one day, he was admitted to the hospital, where in he was found to have a life-threatening blockage of his arteries of his heart. Obviously, this blockage did not arise overnight. All through the years, there had been no alarm bells of anything ominous going on. Had he not received prompt medical attention, he could have died.

Another example you might know: Former President Bill Clinton always looked great and had regular check-ups. Although he had an aggressive exercise routine, he was notorious for his love for fast food. Years after he left the White House, he had to be admitted to the hospital, where a critical blockage of his arteries in heart was found. He underwent emergency bypass surgery. Subsequently, he adopted a vegan lifestyle, lost his excess body weight, and continues to work on his Clinton Global Initiative. By the way, Mr. Clinton did not change his religion when he switched to a vegan lifestyle; he just did it for his health and feels proud of it. Obviously, Mr. Clinton was thinking on the lines of experts like Dr. Jane Ferguson from the Perelman School of Medicine at the University of Pennsylvania, who has written a report titled, "Meat-loving microbes: Do Steak-Eating Bacteria Promote Atherosclerosis?" She then goes on to provide evidence for an affirmative answer to this question.

A note of caution

One should not expect an overnight cure. Let perfection not be a barrier to good. A condition, perhaps with roots implanted in the womb and simmering for years, is unlikely to be reversed in short order. We need to be pragmatic. Patience is required! At the very least, based on what I know, I believe that Dr. M's Seven-X Plan will stem the downward slide of health and facilitate the body's natural processes to get on the path to mending.

CHAPTER 43

Dr. M's Approach to Healing Leaky Gut

KEY POINTS

- Pharmaceutical companies are working feverishly to develop medications aimed at strengthening the gut barrier.
- Simple lifestyle and dietary measures can help reduce leakiness and restore the barrier.

While there are no specific medications to augment the intestinal barrier, some of the commonly used drugs used to treat inflammation also strengthen the intestinal barrier. These include steroids, aminosalicylates, and biologics like Remicade. However, there are steps we can take, both for ourselves as well as our children, before the problem requires medication.

LIFESTYLE CHANGES

The basic framework of our intestinal barrier is established in early formative years and then continues to undergo transformational changes based on how we live our lives.

Note that any changes in medications or significant changes in lifestyle and diet need to be undertaken under appropriate physician supervision. Following are some of the steps we can take to help ourselves.

- First and foremost, we should avoid factors that worsen a leaky gut as much as possible (See Section Four).

- Breastfeed in early infancy, if possible, or use milk banks, as appropriate.
- Expose kids to farm animals. If you live in a city, check out some nearby petting zoos, where they allow kids to pat the animals. Driving around in a Jeep with hay on a farm is a plus.
- Avoid animal-derived milk, especially milk fat.
- Consume a low-sodium diet and low-glycemic foods.
- Eat a high-fiber diet. Include fresh fruits and vegetables in every meal, as much as possible. Note that an increase in fresh fruits and vegetables may sometimes worsen symptoms in some subjects. Read about FODMAPs in Chapter 20.
- Good oral and dental hygiene, including regular dental visits, for prevention and treatment. This minimizes the chance of low-grade infection and inflammation affecting our entire body, including the intestinal barrier.
- Avoid and treat constipation.
- If you have irregular bowel habits, try an elimination/exclusion diet as detailed in Chapter 21.
- Quit smoking. Drink alcohol in moderation, as long as it does not bother your system.
- Avoid and treat infection. For example, zinc supplements have been shown in multiple studies to decrease the duration and severity of respiratory infections.
- Micronutrient deficiency plays a role in leaky gut. Check vitamin A and D levels. Talk to your doctor about supplements that may benefit your health. Read about my personal choices of supplements in Chapter 49.
- Optimize stress coping mechanisms. If stress seems to be a big part of life, learn about relaxation training, breathing exercises, and meditation.
- Take gut-selective antibiotics and herbal antimicrobials (under medical supervision), as appropriate, if small intestinal bacterial overgrowth ensues.

PROBIOTICS

The beneficial effects of probiotics during health and sickness occur in part due to their effects on strengthening the intestinal barrier, making it less leaky. This also allows probiotics to temper the inflammatory reaction in response to intestinal contents, including bacteria, proteins, and toxins.

Multiple studies have documented that probiotics reduce the risk of recurrence in pouchitis. The effect on the intestinal barrier is thought to be one of the mechanisms involved. Studies conducted by Dr. Persborn and colleagues from Linköping University in Sweden indicate that probiotics restore intestinal barrier in patients with pouchitis.

VSL#3, a multi-strain probiotic combination, modifies the intestinal bacteria and tight junctions of the intestinal barrier, making the gut less leaky, thus reducing passage of bacteria and toxins from the gut into the body. It reduces colitis in animals and protects against atherosclerosis in animals. It reduces inflammation and the inflammation-induced resistance to insulin, which precedes onset of diabetes. It also reduces gut leakiness induced by alcohol intake.

Studies from Dr. Takadanohara's laboratory in Japan have shown that a symbiotic preparation with *S. boulardii* reduces stress-induced gut leakiness in rats.

PREBIOTICS

The effect of prebiotic inulin-type fructans on the intestinal bacterial balance and intestinal permeability has a favorable impact on body's immune system. Such changes have been associated with several health benefits, including the prevention of infections and inflammatory diseases in animal colitis, as well as in humans.

- The intestine of animals fed a fiber-free diet is more leaky than those fed fiber.

- A mixture of prebiotics is frequently used in infant formulas. Studies suggest that these enhanced formulas alter the bacterial flora by increasing healthy Bifidobacteria and reducing harmful Clostridia. This is associated with decreased gut leakiness, along with a decrease in gastrointestinal and respiratory infections, as well as skin eczema.

> Green banana and pectin fibers reduce intestinal permeability and improve diarrhea in kids in developing countries.

TRADITIONAL CHINESE MEDICINE

Randomized controlled trials have shown that *Dachengqi decoction* decreases intestinal permeability and blood levels of bacterial toxin, along with reduced bacterial infections and multi-organ dysfunction in patients with acute pancreatitis, as compared to controls.

SUPPLEMENTS

BOVINE COLOSTRUM

Multiple studies have documented that bovine colostrum strengthens the intestinal barrier and reduces passage of intestinal bacteria across the gut wall into the body.

GLUTAMINE

It is a useful nutrient for gut wall cells, as well as gut-associated immune cells. It promotes growth of intestinal cells with potential to strengthen gut barrier function. It maintains and/or restores the intestinal barrier and healthy balance of permeability in critically ill patients and improves their prognosis by reducing frequency of infections. It reduces chemotherapy-induced disruption of the gut barrier.

TAURINE

Human milk is rich in the free amino-acid taurine. Relative taurine deficiency in early infancy has been implicated in adverse long-term neuro-developmental outcomes in preterm infants. As such, it is present as a supplement in formula milk and parenteral nutrition solutions for infants.

SPRAY-DRIED PROTEINS OR PLASMA PROTEIN FRACTIONS

Plasma protein supplements improve the structure as well as function of the intestinal barrier system. They are associated with modification of the gut immune reaction and inflammation, protecting it from possible excessive activation by the toxins. Animal data suggest that these diets improve growth performance of farm animals.

ALANYL-GLUTAMINE SUPPLEMENTED FORMULA

Kids taking alanyl-glutamine supplemented enteral formula (24g per day for 120 days) have a greater weight-for-age and height-for-age than controls. This is accompanied by a significant improvement in the lactulose/mannitol urinary excretion ratio, as compared to controls, suggesting that improved intestinal permeability is involved.

ENZYME-MODIFIED CHEESE

In vitro data suggests that enzyme-modified cheese inhibits passage of allergenic proteins across the gut wall into the body. Studies in rats with drug-induced intestinal damage confirm these effects on gut leakage.

IMMUNE-NUTRITION

Feeding formula supplemented with immunoglobulin A suppresses bacterial entry from the gut into the body while preserving the structure and function of the intestinal barrier.

A large meta-analysis examining the role of immune-nutrient feeds found that they decrease the risk of infectious complications, suggesting that beneficial function involves improvement in intestinal permeability.

BUTYRATE

Colon cells derive their nutrition in part from short chain fatty acids (mainly propionate, butyrate, and acetate) produced by bacterial fermentation in the colon.

- Butyrate strengthens the colonic defense barrier, reduces oxidative stress, and protects colonic mucosa against inflammation, programmed cell death, and cancer in animals.
- Bacterial fermentation of ingested germinated barley foodstuff results in increased butyrate production, strengthened intestinal barrier, and healing in rats.
- Butyrate (60 ml enema per day for 32 weeks) calms oxidative stress processes in the healthy human colon.

N-ACETYL CYSTEINE

Administration of N-acetyl cysteine protects animals against drug-induced intestinal damage and leakiness.

AGED GARLIC EXTRACT

It prevents programmed cell death. It decreases disruption of the intestinal barrier and protects the intestine from damage due to cancer chemotherapy.

VITAMIN A

It plays a role in maintaining healthy cell linings, including the intestinal barrier. It also promotes immune function. Supplementation to kids in developing countries helps reduce frequency of infections and promotes growth. Vitamin A levels should be checked before taking supplements.

ZINC

Zinc deficiency causes disruption of tight junctions of the intestinal barrier. It aggravates the gut leakiness caused by alcohol.

- High-dose zinc reduces the disruption of tight junctions of the intestinal barrier in animal colitis.
- Zinc supplements improve markers of intestinal permeability in patients with diarrhea.
- Zinc supplementation in controlled Crohn's reduces gut leakiness in subjects, as evident on a lactulose/mannitol ratio test. This improvement in barrier function is associated with a decrease in relapses.

CALCIUM

Multiple controlled animal and human studies suggest that dietary calcium improves intestinal resistance and strengthens the intestinal barrier. Such an improvement of barrier function is associated with improvement of colitis in animals.

HERBS AND HERBAL EXTRACTS

A variety of plant-based supplements can strengthen intestinal barrier. Examples include crude rhubarb and berberine.

NUTRITIONAL APPROACH TO STRENGTHEN BARRIER

Animal milk avoidance may help, since it alters the intestinal bacteria. Animal milk fat promotes inflammation in animal colitis. In contrast, fermented milk has beneficial effects against inflammation.

A nutritional approach to restore impaired intestinal barrier function and growth can be accomplished by using an adapted diet containing specific long-chain polyunsaturated fatty acids, prebiotics, and probiotics. Studies of stressed baby rats suggest that this diet reverses the negative effects of stress on the intestinal structure and body growth. Such data perhaps can be extrapolated to humans, and evidence indicates biological plausibility.

According to Drs. Rapin and Wiernperger from the University of Bergundy in France "intestinal permeability should be largely improved by dietary addition of compounds, such as glutamine or curcumin, which have the mechanistic potential to inhibit the inflammation and oxidative stress linked to tight junction opening."

REFERENCES

1. Ohland CL, Macnaughton WK. Probiotic bacteria and intestinal epithelial barrier function. *Am J Physiol Gastrointest Liver Physiol.* 2010 Jun; 298(6):G807-19.

2. Sturniolo GC, Di Leo V, Ferronato A et al. Zinc supplementation tightens "leaky gut" in Crohn's disease. *Inflamm Bowel Dis.* 2001 May; 7(2):94-8.

3. García-Ródenas CL, Bergonzelli GE, Nutten S et al. Nutritional approach to restore impaired intestinal barrier function and growth after neonatal stress in rats. *J Pediatr Gastroenterol Nutr.* 2006 Jul; 43(1):16-24.

4. Rapin JR, Wiernsperger N. Possible links between intestinal permeablity and food processing: A potential therapeutic niche for glutamine. *Clinics (Sao Paulo).* 2010 Jun; 65(6):635-43.

CHAPTER 44

Dr. M's Probiotic Tips to Defeat Bad Gut-Bacteria

KEY POINTS

- All probiotics are not created equal.
- Effects of probiotics are strain-specific.

TIPS ON USE OF PROBIOTICS

Medical science related to probiotics is still in its infancy. It is not surprising that many of the pharmaceutical companies have come up with their own formulations, mostly arbitrary, containing different probiotics strains. Based on the limited clinical literature available, I offer the following recommendations:

- I suggest avoid taking the probiotic with food, so as not to subject the probiotic bacteria to peak digestive acids and juices.
- Since the administered probiotic bacteria are transient inhabitants in the gut, I recommend taking the probiotic twice a day, in order to maintain steady probiotic levels in the gut and to avoid sharp fluctuations.
- Data suggests that even killed probiotic bacteria may provide some health benefits.
- Multi-strain formulations may be superior to single-strain products.

Studies have shown that the information provided by manufacturers may not be entirely accurate, so do your own due diligence.

My opinion on the benefits of selected probiotic species (list is NOT complete):

- *B. infantis*: Treats IBS and constipation
- *L. casei*: Boosts immunity, relives digestive distress and constipation
- *L. reuteri*: Boosts immunity to fight infections, prevents infant colic, tames constipation
- *L. rhamnosus*: Reduces skin eczema
- *Saccharomyces boulardii*: Treats antibiotic-induced diarrhea
- VSL#3: Treats UC
- *B. infantis 35624*: Heals abnormal/uncontrolled inflammation
- *Bifidobacterium lactis DN-173-010*: Treats constipation
- *Escherichia coli Nissle 1917*: Heals inflammation and treats constipation

The contents of the various formulations are based on information provided by the manufacturer with the product or on the Internet and is NOT guaranteed by the author. Since these are poorly regulated by the Food and Drugs Administration, the type of bacterial strain (as well as the strength) is liable to change without notice. Do your own due diligence.

Please also refer to individual chapters for greater number of selections. For instance, Chapter 38 on constipation lists a whole range of probiotic strains shown to be of benefit specifically in treating constipation.

A wide variety of probiotics is currently available on market. Development of tailor-made probiotics, designed for specific aberrations that are associated with microbial dysbiosis, continues worldwide. The young science of proteonomics is being increasingly used in research for the future.

Buyer beware: Studies have shown that the formulation may not contain the particular strains or the strength that has been advertised. As such, it is prudent to purchase from a reputable manufacturer. The probiotic formulations mentioned in this book have not been evaluated by or endorsed by the author.

> Dr. Minocha's personal opinion: Unless a particular formulation has been shown in clinical trials to be effective, I prefer a formulation to be multi-strain, containing at least five billion live bacteria (CFUs).

LISTING OF SELECT PROBIOTICS ON MARKET

Accuflora Advanced CD Probiotic Acidophilus

- Probiotic Blend of Lactobacillus Acidophilus, Lactobacillus Rhamnosus, Bifidobacterium Bifidum, Lactobacillus Salivarius, and Streptococcus Thermophilus.
- Two caplets have one billion live bacteria at the time of manufacture.
- Other ingredients include turmeric (Curcuma Longa).
- Recommended dose: two caplets twice a day

Activia yogurt (4 oz. single serving cups, also available as 24-oz. tubs)

- Manufactured by Dannon, Inc.
- Multiple related products, like Activia Light, Activia Fiber, Activia drinks, and Activia Dessert
- Contains *Bifidobacterium animalis DN-173010*, also known as *Bifidus regularis*, in addition to *Streptococcus thermophilus* and *Lactobacillus bulgaricus*.
- Contains 2.5 g of saturated fat per 4 oz.
- Each serving contains 10 billion CFUs of live bacteria.

Adult Formula CP-1

- Manufactured by Custom Probiotics, Inc.

- Five probiotic strains: *L. Acidophilus, L. Rhamnosus, L. Plantarum, B. Lactis,* and *B. Bifidum.*
- Each capsule has 50 billion CFUs.

Advanced Probiotic 10

- Manufactured by Nature's Bounty, Inc.
- 10 strains of bacteria: *Lactobacillus Plantarum, L. Rhamnosus, L. bulgaricus, L. salivarius, L. acidophilus, L. casei, L. paracasei,* and *Bifidobacterium bifidum.*
- 10 billion live cultures per capsule.
- Recommended dose: two capsules per day.
- Other probiotic products by the manufacturer have different ingredients.

Align capsules

- Manufactured by Proctor & Gamble Inc.
- Contains *Bifidobacterium infantis 35624* in a vegetarian capsule shell.
- Each capsule contains one billion bacteria per capsule.
- Manufacturer recommends one capsule per day.

Attune nutrition bars

- Manufactured by Attune Foods, Inc.
- Contains Kosher *Lactobacillus acidophilus NCFM, L. casei Lc-11,* and *Bifidobacterium lactis HN019*
- Comes in several flavors.
- Contains 3g of fiber.
- Each serving contains 6.1 billion CFUs.
- Note: This is different from granola munch also made by this company, which contains one billion CFUs of *L. acidophilus.*

BifoViden ID

- Manufactured by Metagenics.

- A proprietary blend of *Bifidobacterium lactis Bi-07, Bifidobacterium lactis Bi-04,* (formerly known as *BI-01*), and *Streptococcus thermophilus St-21.*
- 15 billion live organisms per capsule.

Bio-K+ cultured milk based probiotic

- Manufactured by Bio-K+ International, Inc. (Also makes flavored as well as rice and soy fermented products).
- Contains *L. acidophilus CL1285* and *L. casei LBC804.*
- Contains total of 50 billion CFUs.

Bio-K+ probiotic capsules (regular and Rx extra strength)

- Manufactured by Bio-K+ International, Inc.
- Contains *L. acidophilus CL1285* and *L. casei LBC804.*
- Contains 30 billion CFUs per capsule (Rx extra strength has 50 billion CFUs).

Colon Health capsules

- Manufactured by Proctor & Gamble, Inc.
- Probiotic bacteria include a proprietary blend of *Lactobacillus gasseri KS-13, Bifidobacterium bifidum G9-1,* and *Bifidobacterium longum MM-2.*
- Each capsule contains 1.5 billion cells.
- Capsules are also available as a symbiotic formulation called Colon Health Probiotic + fiber that contains 3g of inulin in addition to the probiotic blend.

Culturelle capsules

- Manufactured by Amerifit Nutrition, Inc.
- Contains *L. rhamnosus GG.*
- Each capsule contains 10 billion CFUs.

DanActive cultured milk (100 ml bottles)

- Manufactured by Dannon, Inc.

- Marketed in Europe as Actimel
- Contains *S. thermophilus* and *L. bulgaricus*, in addition to *L. casei DN-114 001*. The latter is also marketed as *L. casei Defensis* or *Immunitas*.
- Different flavors are available.
- Each serving contains 10 billion CFUs.

Digestive Advantage probiotic

- Manufactured by Schiff Nutrition International, Inc.
- Contains BC30 (*Bacillus coagulans GBI-30, 6086*)
- Contains two billion CFUs.
- Once-a-day dosing.
- Different products made by the company have additional non-probiotic ingredients based on indication.

Florastor capsules (250 mg)

- Manufactured by Biocodax, Inc.
- Contains *Saccharomyces boulardii.*
- Each 250 mg capsule contains five billion CFUs.
- Dose 500 mg twice a day.

Gerber Good Start Protect Plus powdered infant milk formula

- Manufactured by Nestle, Inc.
- Contains *B. lactis Bb-12*.
- Each 4 oz. serving contains 10 million CFUs.

Good Belly fruit drink

- Manufactured by NextFoods, Inc.
- Contains *L. plantarum 299v*.
- Each serving contains 20 billion CFUs.

Kefir drinks

- One brand is Lifeway Foods, Inc.
- Contains 10-12 different probiotics.

- Has 7-10 billion CFUs per cup.

LactoFlamX

- Manufactured by Metagenics, Inc.
- Contains *L. plantarum 299v*.
- Contains 18 billion live organisms per capsule.

LactoViden ID

- Manufactured by Metagenics, Inc.
- A multi-strain proprietary blend of *Lactobacillus acidophilus NCFM Strain, Lactobacillus salivarius Ls-33, Lactobacillus paracasei Lpc-37 Lactobacillus plantarum Lp-115*, and *Streptococcus thermophilus St-21*.
- Contains 15 billion live organisms per capsule.

OWP probiotics

- Manufactured by One Wellness Place, Inc.
- Multi-strain blend of *B. longum, B. breves, B. infantis, L. plantarum, L. rhamnosus*, and *L. acidophilus*.
- Each capsule has 15 billion CFUs.

Phillips Colon Health

- Manufactured by Bayer, Inc.
- Probiotic blend has 1.5 billion bacteria, comprised of three probiotic strains.
- *Lactobacillus gasseri (KS-13), Bifidobacterium bifidum (G9-1)*, and *Bifidobacterium longum (MM-2)*.
- Once a day dosing regimen.

Proboulardi

- Manufactured by Metagenics, Inc.
- Contains *S. boulardii* plus *B. lactis HN019* and *L. rhamnosus HN001*.

- A 3:1 blend of *Bifidobacterium lactis HN019* and *Lactobacillus rhamnosus HN001*, with four billion live organisms and *Saccharomyces boulardii.*
- Each capsule provides 5.5 billion live organisms.
- Capsule size: 275 mg.

StonyField Farm Yogurt (also makes other probiotic products like Oikos and Soy yogurt)

- Manufactured by Stonyfield Farms, a subsidiary of Dannon, Inc.
- Available in 4 oz., 6 oz., and 32 oz. containers. Flavored and plain varieties are available.
- Contains multiple strains of bacteria like *L. rhamnosus HN001, B. lactis, L. acidophilus* and *L. casei,* in addition to *S. thermophilus* and *L. bulgaricus.*

TruBiotics

- Manufactured by Bayer, Inc.
- Blend of two probiotics — *Lactobacillus acidophilus LA-5* and *Bifidobacterium animalis BB-12.*
- Contains 1.5 billion live cultures per capsule.
- Recommended dose: once a day.

Ultimate Flora Extra Care Daily Probiotic

- Manufactured by Renew Life, Inc.
- 10 strains of bacteria (three Bifido strains and seven Lacto strains).
- Contains 30 billion live probiotic cultures per capsule, including 18 billion *Bifidobacteria* and 12 billion *Lactobacillus* cultures.
- Other products by the same company have fewer live cultures, varying from 10-25 billion.

Ultimate Probiotic Formula

- Manufactured by Swanson Health Products, Inc.

- Probiotic strains: *B. lactis, B. longum, L. plantarum, L. acidophilus, L. casei, Kyo-Dophilus blend, L. salivarius, L. rhamnosus, L. bulgaricus, L. sporogenes.*
- Contains 60 billion CFUs per capsule, plus 100 mg of prebiotic NutraFlora short chain FOS.

VSL#3 sachets

- Manufactured by Sigma-Tau Pharmaceuticals, Inc.
- Contains eight different strains of bacteria (*B. breve, B. infantis, B. longum, L. acidophilus, L. bulgaricus, L. casei, L. plantarum,* and *Streptococcus thermophilus*).
- Each sachet contains 450 billion CFUs.
- Dose: Manufacturer recommends different doses for different disorders. For IBS patients, 0.5-1 packet per day are recommended, ulcerative colitis 1-2 packets per day, and pouchitis 2-4 packets per day. In patients whose remission from UC is difficult to maintain, 4-8 packets per day are recommended.
- Doses are reduced in kids based on age.
- Capsule formulations are also available.

Yakult cultured milk

- A Japanese probiotic milk product manufactured by Yakult Honsha Co.
- Probiotic *L. casei Shirota.*
- Each serving contains eight billion CFUs.
- Manufacturer recommends one to two bottles per day. It also cautions that you may experience bloating initially.
- Each 2.7 oz. bottle contains 11 g of sugar.

Yo-Plus yogurt

- Manufactured by Yoplait, Inc.
- Contains *B. animalis subsp lactis Bb-12* in addition to *S. thermophilus* and *L. bulgaricus*, plus prebiotic and inulin 3 g per serving.

- Each serving contains greater than five billion CFUs

REFERENCES

1. Aureli P, Capurso L, Castellazzi AM et al. Probiotics and health: an evidence-based review. *Pharmacol Res.* 2011 May; 63(5):366-76.
2. Gerritsen J, Smidt H, Rijkers GT, de Vos WM. Intestinal microbiota in human health and disease: the impact of probiotics. *Genes Nutr.* 2011 Aug; 6(3):209-40.
3. Aires J, Butel MJ. Proteomics, human gut microbiota and probiotics. *Expert Rev Proteomics.* 2011 Apr; 8(2):279-88.

CHAPTER 45

Dr. M's Recommendations for Controlling Inflammation and Potentiating Antioxidant Defenses Naturally

KEY POINTS

- Inflammation can have adverse effects far beyond the local site of injury.
- Aspirin is an anti-inflammatory drug. It not only control pain and inflammation of arthritis but also protects against heart disease and cancer.
- Some fruits and vegetables are richer in antioxidants than others.
- Multiple factors are involved in perceived lack of benefit of specific antioxidant supplements in many diseases associated with oxidative stress.

We learnt earlier that chronic inflammation has been identified as a significant risk factor for many chronic diseases like heart disease, diabetes, obesity etc. as well as cancers like liver cancer due to chronic viral hepatitis B or C, lung cancer due to chronic inflammation due to chronic irritant effect of smoking.

Inflammation has also been implicated in neurobehavioral and neurodegenerative disorders like autism, schizophrenia and Alzheimer's.

CURBING INFLAMMATION

Importance of harmful effects of inflammation can be gauged by the fact that a simple aspirin is not just effective against chronic inflammatory diseases like arthritis; it can also reduce not only heart disease as well as many cancers. However medications like aspirin have increased risk for complications like ulcers and bleeding etc. and may not be appropriate for everyone. At the same time, I would like to point out that advantages of aspirin outweigh risks in most people and these issues should always be discussed with the physician.

MEDICATIONS TO TREAT INFLAMMATION

- NSAIDs, like aspirin
- Corticosteroids, like prednisone
- Biologic anti-TNF (an inflammation-promoting biochemical) drugs, like Remicade

NATURAL WAYS TO CURB LOW-GRADE CHRONIC INFLAMMATION

These strategies apply to the constant low-level inflammation our body is subjected to, due to the constant barrage of dietary and environmental stimuli surrounding us. These must not to be understood as a substitute for otherwise treatable causes, like antimicrobials for infections like tuberculosis or orthopedic treatments for fractures. Be sure to talk to your doctor.

WEIGHT CONTROL

Obesity is both a cause and result of chronic low-grade inflammation. Breaking this cycle by proper weight control makes for a healthy body and lower risk of chronic diseases.

DIETARY MODIFICATIONS

- Eat a healthy diet. The Mediterranean diet has been shown to provide the most benefit among the widely prevalent dietary patterns.
- Increase intake of antioxidant-rich foods.
- The modern Western diet has an over-abundance of pro-inflammatory omega-6 fatty acids, whereas ancient diets had equal proportions of omega-3 to omega-6 fatty acids in diet. Increase omega-3 fatty acids and decrease omega-6 fatty acids.
- Cow milk avoidance may help. Animal studies suggest that administration of cow's milk to rats results in development of arthritis.

LOW-CHOLESTEROL DIET

- Consume low glycemic index foods. A high-glycemic diet promotes inflammation.
- A high-fiber diet is low-glycemic plus has prebiotic effects.
- Eat a diet rich in argenine, vitamins B, C, D, E, and magnesium.
- Eat foods rich in carotenoids, lycopene, and astaxanthin. Foods rich in lycopene include tomatoes, red grapefruit, and guava. Astaxanthin is mainly derived from seafood like salmon and shrimp.
- Focus on flavonoids-rich diet like green tea, polygonum cuspidatum (also known as Japanese knotweed) containing 20 percent resveratrol, ginger, and garlic.
- Use turmeric for cooking. It is also known as the yellow curry powder.
- Reduce saturated fats and trans-fats in your diet.

LOW-STARCH DIET

Drs. Ebringer and Wilson from King's College in London devised a low-starch diet comprised of lower amounts of bread, potatoes, and pasta and studied it in healthy subjects and patients with ankylosing spondylitis. They reported their findings in the journal *Clinical Rheumatology*. The investigators found that a low-starch diet reduces antibody levels against Klebsiella proteins. Furthermore, the low-starch diet resulted in decreased inflammation, improved symptoms, and reduced need for anti-inflammatory drugs at nine month follow up in patients with ankylosing spondylitis.

NATURAL DIETARY SUPPLEMENTS

- Multi-vitamin, multi-mineral, and antioxidant supplements
- Curcumin

Read more about my personal choices of supplements in Chapter 49. Overall, it is much better to eat a diet rich in the above nutrients than to just take the supplements!

LIFESTYLE CHANGES

- Moderate drinking
- Smoking cessation
- Regular physical exercise, although too much strenuous exercise is actually pro-inflammatory. Incorporate multi-dimensional yoga in your exercise program to diversify the benefit. Read more about yoga in Chapter 47.
- Good orodental hygiene is a must. Bad teeth are associated with an increased risk of chronic ailments, like heart disease.
- Avoid constipation. Use strategies to prevent and overcome constipation, including proper toileting posture.

ENHANCE ANTIOXIDANT DEFENSES

The literature is clear that use of an antioxidant-rich diet consisting of appropriate fruit and vegetables protects against numerous diseases, including heart disease and cancer. Results of the studies using antioxidant supplements have, however, not been encouraging for most part.

Below are some of the strategies to enhance the body's antioxidant defenses. Since many of the natural products contain multiple compounds rather than a single one (as in most drugs), it is understandable that they might have multiple health-supporting properties and may appear on more than one list of things to do.

FOODS RICH IN ANTIOXIDANTS

Fruits: acai, apple (especially red apple), red grape, prune, orange, berries (especially wild blueberry and cranberry), plum, peaches, watermelon, kiwi

Vegetables: garlic, broccoli, tomatoes, artichokes, spinach

Beans and legumes: kidney beans, pinto beans, black beans

Nuts and raisins: pistachios, pecans

Herbs, spices, and condiments: cinnamon, sage, turmeric, cloves, chili pepper, mustard, basil, parsley

NATURAL COMPOUNDS WITH PROVEN ANTIOXIDANT ACTIONS

Vitamins and minerals: vitamins C and E, selenium, zinc

Miscellaneous: resveratrol, mangiferin, L-carnosine, methionine, polyphenols, D-ribose, fruit seed extracts like D-ribose, glutathione, rottlerin (used as food additive across cultures), ginsenoside Rb1

EFFECT OF ANTIOXIDANTS IN DISEASE STATES

Data from animal experiments clearly shows the benefit from antioxidant supplements. However, most randomized controlled trials trying to prove the benefit of antioxidants have come up short.

For example, vitamin E is effective in healing non-alcoholic fatty liver disease. However, this vitamin appears to be associated with negative outcomes in many other conditions, including heart disease.

Many population-based studies have shown a reduced risk of heart disease among people with high consumption of fish and fish oil. However, data from use of supplements has been contradictory. Many physicians recommend taking a daily fish oil supplement to protect against heart disease.

In general, however, evidence suggests that most pure, isolated antioxidants used as supplements do not improve health outcomes. In fact, some studies suggest an increased risk of disease.

Reconciling contradictory evidence

The conflicting evidence of the benefit from antioxidant rich fruits and vegetables, but not from some antioxidant supplement trials, may be explained by multiple factors:

- Too late.
- Too little.
- Too non-specific. Specific reactive oxygen species play a role in specific functions. Lack of effect of non-specific use of antioxidants should not be construed as lack of effect of antioxidants overall.

There is redundancy in the biologic system, such that reactive species may not always be the sine qua non of the harmful effects.

> Overall, the sheer number of reactive oxygen species, their chemical structure, and the ability of any single gene to affect multiple functions makes it difficult to localize, quantify, and manipulate these reactive oxygen species for therapeutic intervention.

CONCLUSIONS ABOUT ANTIOXIDANTS

- The healthiest option is to meet all your needs by consuming a healthy, antioxidant-rich diet. This option is not a practical alternative for many people in this fast-paced life.
- An alternative may be a happy medium of a healthy, antioxidant-rich diet as much as possible, plus antioxidants with some proven benefit for health in some conditions. This includes dietary adjustment, even at a fast-food restaurant.

For example, when you order a sandwich, instead of ordering French fries, order a side of antioxidant-rich green apples. Yes, such sides are available even at McDonald's!

The potential supplements that can be easy and practical include turmeric (yellow curry powder) and perhaps a glass of red wine a day, if allowed by the physician.

Specific antioxidants that have been shown to be of benefit under certain circumstances include zinc, L-carnosine, N-acetyl cysteine, D-ribose, and vitamin C. The use of vitamin E as a supplement is best restricted to patients with non-alcoholic fatty liver disease and used under strict physician supervision, because of studies showing harmful effect in other conditions.

REFERENCES

1. Nagareddy P, Smyth SS. Inflammation and thrombosis in cardiovascular disease. *Curr Opin Hematol*. 2013 Sep; 20(5):457-63.
2. Barbaresko J, Koch M, Schulze MB, Nöthlings U. Dietary pattern analysis and biomarkers of low-grade inflammation: a systematic literature review. *Nutr Rev*. 2013 Aug; 71(8):511-27.
3. Soory M. Nutritional antioxidants and their applications in cardiometabolic diseases. *Infect Disord Drug Targets*. 2012 Oct; 12(5):388-401.
4. Bulló M, Lamuela-Raventós R, Salas-Salvadó J. Mediterranean diet and oxidation: nuts and olive oil as important sources of fat and antioxidants. *Curr Top Med Chem*. 2011; 11(14):1797-810.
5. Kahleova H, Matoulek M, Malinska H et al. Vegetarian diet improves insulin resistance and oxidative stress markers more than conventional diet in subjects with Type 2 diabetes. *Diabet Med*. 2011 May; 28(5):549-59.

CHAPTER 46

Dr. M's Strategies for Healing Nutrition

KEY POINTS

- Avoid the foods that our ancestors avoided – they also stayed clear of chronic diseases like heart disease, diabetes, and cancer.
- Persons prone to allergies or with neurobehavioral concerns should adopt a gluten-free, casein-free, plus SFED diet strategy.
- A vegetarian diet is the least irritating to the gut; a semi-vegetarian diet may be a pragmatic substitute in kids at risk for chronic illness.

This is perhaps one of the most important, and yet the most difficult chapter to enunciate my views. Why? Because your nutrition needs to be highly individualized, based on your unique metabolic constitution.

NUTRITION UNIQUE TO GENETIC CONSTITUTION AND METABOLISM

This concept is not new. The oldest system of medicine, Ayurveda, broadly divides people into three classes, on the basis of *doshas* or inner constitution. They are further classified into sub-doshas. The diet that a person should consume is based on his inner constitution. Eating foods inconsistent with the body's constitution and metabolism makes the person sick.

We are all different. Our genes are different. Our metabolism is different. Even with the same disease, the underlying factors that led to and may be sustaining the disease may be different. Bottom line, we got to the current state of health via different metabolic pathways, even though the symptoms may be similar. One size does not fit all.

One of the problems I see in many books is that they offer a "one size fits all" approach. It may be easy to do so for a weight loss book, where the main focus is to consume fewer calories without any focus of effects on health.

Nutrition for chronic sickness is another matter. To offer a "one size fits all" approach would be like living in a fool's paradise. A stereotyped approach to nutrition in such cases decreases the chances of successful healing to the core.

So what is a layperson to do?

APPLY PRINCIPLES
OUR ANCESTORS LIVED BY

The clues about dietary manipulation also come from our studies of tribes continuing to practice a paleo diet. The key is to look at not what was included in ancient diets, but what was absent in those diets. Grains were conspicuously absent. Milk was not as frequently used either.

Follow paleo diet principles. I don't mean strictly paleo diet, because that would not just be impractical but may not be totally healthy with the lifestyles we follow and foods that are available in market.

Depending on the clinical situation, I would suggest reduction of glutenous grains as much as possible. Vulnerable or already-unhealthy patients should go gluten-free. Remember, it's not just the toxin itself, but also the amount of toxin that determines state of health.

Most people with lactose intolerance can tolerate one glass of milk per day, whereas persons with IBS cannot. Concentrate more on healthy, gluten-free alternative foods like quinoa and buckwheat that are described elsewhere in the book.

Within the context of this diet, it would be prudent to go the extra mile, especially with children, even if all is well. For example, eat organic plant foods or organic lean meat.

If the person is healthy overall and the Seven-X Plan is being followed to stay healthy, you may, if you wish, continue to drink cow's milk, with an emphasis on its fermented products. On the other hand, persons with an unhealthy gut and/or body should avoid cow's milk altogether and go to other milk alternatives.

PERSONS PRONE TO ALLERGIES OR INTOLERANCES

Subjects with a history of allergies need more exclusions in the diet. In addition to the gluten-free and casein-free diet (GFCF), I would recommend the Six-Food-Elimination-Diet (SFED) that involves elimination of the six most common allergens: milk, soy, egg, wheat, peanut/tree nuts, and seafood, including all fish. The SFED program is described in more detail in Chapter 21.

> There is, of course, some overlap between the GFCF diet and SFED. SFED is simple to follow and excludes the most common allergenic provocations to the gut and have been proven to help patients with eosinophilic esophagitis, a chronic inflammation of esophagus with links to food allergies.

PERSONS WITH IRRITABLE BOWEL OR IBS-LIKE SYMPTOMS

Patients can have adverse reaction to multiple foods. Sometimes, the SFED is just not enough. Adopt a low-FODMAP diet. This diet has been shown in multiple trials to help patients with IBS.

Are you sensitive to a lot of foods?

Exclusion of foods based on chemical sensitivities is frequently learned by trial and error and less so by the doctor's testing. Again, I have provided lists of the foods most likely to cause chemical sensitivity and less-sensitive options in earlier chapters.

Always remember, a carefully-designed organic gluten-free vegetarian diet is least likely to aggravate or irritate the gut. And, of course, it is healthier than the non-vegetarian option. There are several kinds of vegetarians, depending on the foods excluded. These are described in greater detail in Chapter 23.

The most common question I get asked is, "Then where do I get my protein?"

It is no secret that many of us would like to have muscles like a bull. All of us would like to be "healthy as a horse." Have you ever asked where the bulls, horses, or elephants get their protein muscles?

> Bottom-line, you can get a healthy, nutritious diet from vegetable sources. The key is to carefully choose your foods. Not every meal of the day needs to have every nutrient, but the key is that they should complement each other.

Talk is cheap. It may be easier for a motivated adult to go vegetarian, but to expect a child to switch altogether is another matter. Semi-vegetarian diet to the rescue!

SEMI-VEGETARIAN DIET

Recognition of the potential for the vegetarian diet to heal intestinal inflammation, coupled with the harsh reality that it may be impractical for kids, has prompted experts to suggest a semi-vegetarian diet. This allows 10-20 percent of the nutrition to be derived from meat sources. The small, non-vegetarian component increases the appeal of this diet. Kids can be convinced to adopt a vegetarian diet with a weekly reward of a meat dish.

> Carefully-done clinical trials have shown that the semi-vegetarian diet is successful in healing inflammation and damage of the gut wall in patients with Crohn's disease.

PERSONS WITH CHRONIC PAIN OR NEUROBEHAVIORAL CONCERNS

I firmly believe that our gut plays a critical role in our overall health, based on the now well-recognized concept of the gut-immune-hormonal-brain axis. An extension of this is the gut-immune-hormonal-brain-skin axis as evident by involvement of psychological factors, altered intestinal bacteria, and leaky gut in skin diseases like psoriasis and acne. Science on this issue is evolving quickly. It is critical that we modify our nutrition and eliminate the components that can adversely affect us in order to improve chronic pain, like fibromyalgia, CFS, migraines, or restless leg syndrome. The same principle holds true for those suffering from neurobehavioral syndromes like autism, ADHD, or OCD. Patients with psoriasis and difficult-to-manage acne may benefit from this strategy, as well.

> Persons with such complex issues have multiple metabolic challenges in different pathways of the brain-gut axis, including but not limited to intestinal bacteria, leaky gut, abnormal immune reactions, abnormal antibodies, and inflammation. With so many challenges and so many redundancies in the intricately-balanced metabolic systems, one has to go out all the way in the nutritional strategy.

All three below must be followed:

- Gluten-free Casein-free diet (See Chapter 17)
- SFED (see Chapter 21)
- Vegetarian diet, or at least semi-vegetarian diet (Read Chapter 23).

The recommendation of a vegetarian diet is not made in the context of religion. I am not and do not profess to be your spiritual advisor.

> My recommendation for a vegetarian diet is rooted in hard science. It is for your health! A recent study by Dr. Orlich and colleagues from the Loma Linda University, published in the prestigious *JAMA Intern Med* journal, reported that a vegetarian diet results in a significant reduction in all-cause mortality. They stated, "These favorable associations should be considered carefully by those offering dietary guidance."

Results of studies from patients with Crohn's disease make the beneficial effect of such a diet abundantly clear, particularly when it comes to controlling inflammation.

RISKS OF ELIMINATING DIFFERENT FOODS FROM DIET

Whenever there are exclusions from the diet, there is potential for nutritional deficits. The more the exclusions, the greater the risk. These issues have been discussed in earlier chapters. This problem can be easily overcome with a consultation with a dietician who can then design a diet and menu specifically tailored to your needs. This has been also discussed in earlier chapters, along with how to deal with these issues.

REFERENCES

1. Chiba M, Abe T, Tsuda H, Sugawara T et al. Lifestyle-related disease in Crohn's disease: relapse prevention by a semi-vegetarian diet. *World J Gastroenterol*. 2010 May 28; 16(20):2484-95.
2. Gonsalves N, Yang GY, Doerfler B et al. Elimination diet effectively treats eosinophilic esophagitis in adults; food reintroduction identifies causative factors. *Gastroenterology*. 2012 Jun; 142(7):1451-9.

3. Orlich MJ, Singh PN, Sabaté J et al. Vegetarian dietary patterns and mortality in Adventist Health Study 2. *JAMA Intern Med.* 2013 Jul 8; 173(13):1230-8.

CHAPTER 47

Dr. M's Suggestions for Daily GI Upkeep

KEY POINTS

- A seemingly simple problem like infection/inflammation in the gums can have adverse consequences in distant organs, including the heart and brain.
- The only cure for sleep deficit is sleep.
- Exercise and meditation, especially yoga, have beneficial effects on our heart, brain, and metabolism.

In order to keep the computer running smoothly, it is recommended that we keep the computer clean, not have clutter surrounding it to allow proper aeration and venting, and dust it regularly. We should also do a "disk clean" every day or every couple of days, depending upon the amount and type of usage.

Our gut and body is far more complex than even the fastest of computers available. It also needs a daily upkeep, more aggressive weekly "colon cleanse and detox," and monthly "shock and awe" to keep it going well. See Chapter 48.

The daily upkeep component is multi-dimensional and equivalent to "disk clean" at physical, mental, and spiritual levels.

DO NOT ALLOW CONSTIPATION TO GET AHEAD OF YOU

It is never normal not to have a bowel movement for several days at a time. Yet, it is not as uncommon as you might think.

> One should have a good bowel movement at least once every couple of days. Do not let constipation get the better of you. While it may seem to be a tall order to some, a simple change such as eating papaya and mango salad in lieu of the usual vegetable salad, good hydration, and good toileting posture alone can work wonders for many.

I would refer the reader to Chapter 38 for more details.

BRUSHING TEETH AND FLOSSING ARE A MUST

The mouth is involved in our first encounter with foreign bodies and disease-producing organisms going into our body. No wonder the oral-dental region represents the tip of the spear for most things, good and bad (food, drugs, toxins, pathogens), that enter our body.

The status of our mouth and our teeth may reflect our overall health, including nutritional and immunological status. The concept of involvement of the mouth as a result of GI diseases is well-established. Examples include inflammatory bowel disease and celiac disease. The reverse is also true. Mouth sickness can cause illness far and wide as well.

BACTERIA IN MOUTH

The oral cavity is "dirty." A variety of bacteria is present, including the inflammation- and disease-producing ones. Some of them are capable of local and body-wide health repercussions.

Orodental activities, as simple as chewing, flossing, brushing, and minor procedures like scaling, result in the release of bacteria into the blood stream, although they are in the blood only transiently before being taken care of by the body's immune system, at least in most cases. However, the release of bacteria or their toxic product into the circulation has potential to seed more infection or inflammation, setting off a deleterious chain reaction.

In the presence of a weakened immune system, even the non-disease producing bacteria can act brave and produce harm. This can be seen as chronic inflammation in teeth or gums, which in turn can affect health throughout the entire body.

IS A SMALL FOCUS OF INFECTION ANYWHERE SIGNIFICANT?

Poor oral-dental health implies a localized focus of infection. The word "localized" may be a misnomer, since a localized focus of infection need not have effects at the local site only.

Not unlike cancer, metastasis of bacterial infection may occur in the form of bacteremia, which is the release and spread of bacteria into the blood circulation.

Metastatic inflammation describes the phenomenon wherein a bacterial toxin released into circulation interacts with an antibody, resulting in immune complexes. This process can results in its own disease process.

LOCALIZED INFECTION CAN CAUSE BODY-WIDE DISEASE: A HISTORICAL PERSPECTIVE

The concept of focus of infection in one part of the body and its effect on the remainder of the body is not new; in fact, it has been part of the history of medicine since ancient times.

Hippocrates successfully treated a case of arthritis by performing tooth extraction. Dr. C.H. Mayo in 1914 declared in the *Journal of American Medical Association* that "root abscesses and pus pockets connecting them are often the source of acute and chronic rheumatism."

LOCALIZED ORODENTAL INFECTION FOCUS

Much of the research has focused on gum disease and its effects beyond the mouth. Dental caries is also increasingly attracting attention. The World Health Organization considers caries a global health problem.

EFFECT OF POOR TEETH AND GUMS ON HEALTH

Laboratory experiments suggest that when we inject components of normal mouth bacteria into mice suffering from brain infection, the injection worsens their brain inflammation.

In this context, an additional concept gaining traction is the involvement of RAGE.

THE EMERGING RAGE CONCEPT (ANGER AT CELLULAR LEVEL)

RAGE (Receptor for Advanced Glycation End Products) has been implicated in multiple disorders. RAGE are plentiful in the gums and are released into circulation when gums are inflamed.

Biochemical messaging through RAGE is thought to be involved in many diverse disorders. According to Dr. Katz and colleagues, the AGE-RAGE axis may be involved as the mechanism in the association between orodental diseases and diseases beyond the oral cavity, including heart disease and Alzheimer's disease. An excess of AGEs has been documented in numerous organ systems, including the brain of patients with autism.

Bottom line: Brush your teeth at least in the morning and at bedtime, and preferably after each meal. In addition, floss regularly and religiously.

SLEEP IS ESSENTIAL TO REVITALIZE THE BODY

Sleep is an active and dynamic process different from wakefulness.

SLEEP AND DIGESTIVE SYSTEM

The biological rhythms in the digestive system are usually synchronized with the master clock in the brain that determines our sleep. A disrupted sleep pattern can thus dissociate the GI rhythms.

- Poor sleep increases risk of acid reflux or gastro-esophageal reflux disease (GERD).
- Incidence of peptic ulcers is higher among shift workers than daytime workers.
- Patients with IBS report higher incidence of sleep problems, like trouble with sleep initiation and frequently waking up at night.
- Sleep deprivation causes worsening of inflammation in animal models of colitis.
- Sleep deprivation affects the brain, including thinking, reflexes, and neuromuscular performance.
- Being awake for 24 hours is akin to being legally drunk.
- Adults need an average of eight hours of sleep to satisfy the body's functional needs.
- There is little variation in sleep need between individuals.
- The body is physically and mentally impaired if sleep is less than five or six hours a day.
- Sleep debt from sleeping five hours per night accumulates over time. The person becomes less aware that he or she is sleep deprived. They can't even recognize that they are pathologically sleepy.
- Interaction between alcohol and sleep is deadly.

WHY DO WE FEEL SLEEPY?

Two processes determine inclination to and duration of sleep:

- Amount of wake time. One gets more sleepy and tired with each passing hour.
- Biological rhythm driven by our biological master clock residing in our brain.

PREVENTATIVE NAPS

Napping helps provide an alertness boost, but it should be short. Naps longer than one to two hours produce deeper sleep. Rather than waking up fresh, people wake up groggy with sleep lethargy.

- A one-hour nap prior to working the graveyard shift increases attentiveness and vigilance and reduces stress. The job is felt to be less burdensome.
- Even a 10-20 minute nap prior to a night shift or during a night shift provides benefit.
- The key is length of nap and time of day. Do not get into the habit of napping closer to your regular sleep-time. It reduces the sleep instincts that you will need later to get to the regular sleep. Doing this on a routine basis creates an abnormal sequence of nighttime wakefulness and daytime sleepiness, creating a vicious cycle of escalating daytime napping and decreased sleep at night.
- Napping becomes a hindrance when your daytime nap disrupts your regular nighttime sleep pattern.

According to Dr. Horne from the Sleep Research Centre at Loughborough University in Loughborough, U.K., "Sleep range is approximately six to nine hours, although a timely, short (less than 20-minute) nap can equate to one hour 'extra' nighttime sleep."

COUNTERMEASURES TO SLEEPINESS

- Caffeine boosts alertness, but tolerance develops quickly. It disrupts quality of sleep and has unfavorable effects on mood.
- Do not use caffeinated products shortly before the end of a night shift.
- Drugs to counter sleep are not generally recommended.

While there are short-term countermeasures available, the only cure for sleep deprivation is sleep itself.

MEASURES TO FACILITATE SLEEP

- Make the sleeping place favorable to sleep by reducing light, noise, and temperature.
- Alcohol is a poor choice as sleep aid. While it initially makes the person sleepy, it causes sleep fragmentation.
- Short-acting prescription drugs medications may be used as sleep aids under physician supervision.

> A great sleep-aid: Melatonin is not just for sleep, it helps with the digestive system too. It is especially helpful when sleep patterns are disrupted due to travel, especially jet lag.

Bottom-line on sleep: There is no substitute for sleep!

EXERCISE TO KEEP THE BODY COMPUTERS RUNNING SMOOTHLY

Regular exercise is important for keeping all the bodily biological rhythms in sync, including the gastrointestinal rhythm. However, very strenuous exercise disproportionate to the person's normal routine can have unfavorable effects at least transiently. GI changes include reduced blood flow to the gut and sometimes even bleeding. Such is a situation frequently seen among marathon runners.

- Lack of time or money to go to the gym is a poor excuse. The exercise part of daily upkeep does not just involve going to the gym. You can do simple things at work like:
- Park the car farthest from the office and walk to the office.
- Take the stairs rather than elevators as much as possible.
- Perform intermittent movements at ankles and knees when involved in a prolonged sitting job.

Outdoor exercises are a plus, since they allow one to be in natural synchronism with the nature. This has additional calming effect on the mind. Examples include swimming, jogging on the trails, and gardening.

> My personal favorite recommendation is yoga, since it has been documented to have multiple health benefits in a variety of illnesses, including high blood pressure, heart disease, diabetes, irritable bowel syndrome, and chronic pain syndromes. Yoga in a group setting may be better than doing it alone, since the peaceful relaxing impact in a group is very pacifying and tends to melt the stresses away.

DE-STRESS EVERYDAY
TO START AFRESH THE NEXT DAY

MIND-BODY MEDICINE

Our brain and gut are intimately intertwined and they both affect each other, both in positive and negative ways. Stress is a negative influence, no matter what. Stressful situations are not avoidable; however, our responses that cause distress are.

The key is to learn how to cope with stress in order to minimize the negative impact and maximize the positive advantages. For example, even the birth of a child is a stressful event. The positive goal in this case would be to maximize the joy of new arrival and the happy family life.

> A therapist usually tends to focus on a single therapy and a specific outcome. On the other hand, the mind-body therapeutic approaches tend to consider the role of human, environmental, and social factors in the overall healing processes. Mind-body techniques tend to improve the patient's well-being at physical, mental, emotional, and spiritual levels.

SIMPLE WAYS TO DISTRESS

- Exercise, at least part of which should be outdoors (like swimming or jogging) so you may be one with nature.
- Regular rest and relaxation.
- Allow yourself short breaks during the day.
- Take a 10 to 15-minute nap during the afternoon, if possible.
- Practice deep breathing.
- Spend some time on outside interests like gardening.
- Avoid stressful situations, if possible. Examples include arriving for a meeting a few minutes early so you may use the restroom.
- Make a list of things to accomplish during the day and keep crossing them off as you finish the task. This is one of my favorites and de-stresses me when I feel overwhelmed.
- Don't forget to meditate!

Don't go to bed angry. Personally, I try to talk to the person that I may have had conflict with and apologize for my part in the disagreement. Frequently, the other side apologizes, as well. Both end the day in a better shape!

MEDITATION

Meditation has a profound impact on our metabolic functions, including favorably modifying the heart rate, blood pressure, breathing rate, and blood flow.

While some look at meditation as cleansing of the mind, others look to it for a systematic focus on a particular issue or experience without scattering thoughts or indulging in internal struggle.

If you already have a preferred method of meditation that works for you, that is great. If not, read on.

Mindfulness Meditation

Mindfulness practice is the form of technique that *empties the mind* without constraining thoughts or attention to any unique sensation, emotion, or perception. However, it does involve strong focus and attentiveness. This allows the person to become more aware of his or her inner self.

I recommend Mindfulness-Based Stress Reduction (MBSR), which is a clinical equivalent of mindfulness meditation.

Mindfulness-Based Stress Reduction (MBSR)

MBSR is a physical-mental program of attitude adjustment at multiple levels. The person learns to calm his or her mind by examining the situation carefully in a non-judgmental manner. The person does not restrict or avoid any thoughts. It offers the person various options on how to respond and affect the distressful circumstances, rather than acting in an impulsive, emotional manner to the currents of stress.

MBSR was originally developed as a group program for pain management and owes its origins to the University of Massachusetts Medical Center.

- It is a secular clinical practice.
- It does not require any particular religious beliefs.
- The person needs to be motivated and determined.
- Both formal and informal meditation are integrated into the program.
- On the physical front, correct posture and breathing technique are required.
- MBSR practice leads to beneficial changes in brain density in regions involved in learning, memory, and emotion.
- No adverse side effects from MBSR have been documented.
- It is helpful also for healthcare providers and results in improving their interactions with patients.

Improved psychosocial well-being following the MBSR program results in beneficial effects on the immune system. It has been shown to be a viable treatment for insomnia and hot flashes. It helps patients with failed back surgery and has the potential to help treat fibromyalgia. An expert meta-analysis of clinical studies concluded that MBSR has positive effects on depression, anxiety, and psychological distress in patients with chronic somatic diseases.

PRAYER AND SPIRITUALITY

An overwhelming number of people across various cultures believe in the Higher Power. Religion is a matter of and sustained by belief. Prayer is part of religious practices. It may be individual or done as a group and performed at home or in community settings, such as church or temple.

WHAT IS PRAYER?

The National Center for Complementary and Alternative Medicine (NCCAM) defines prayer as an active process of communicating with and appealing to a higher spiritual power.

Prayer is a matter of personal preference and should not be prescribed.

FORMS OF PRAYER

- Conversational prayer where a person seeks advice from and expresses gratitude to God.
- Meditation involves reflection and contemplation of spirituality in context of the life and the divine power.
- Ritual prayer involves singing, chanting, or just reciting established prayers, hymns, or mantras.
- Intercessory prayer involves prayer on behalf of others for their healing and overall well-being.

POTENTIAL MECHANISMS OF PRAYER

- Relaxation response
- Placebo effect
- Expression of positive emotions
- Supernatural intervention, although frequently invoked, is highly speculative and not scientifically verifiable.

Data on the effect of spiritual interventions in health and sickness is mixed. Some of the literature suggests that spirituality has beneficial effects on patients' quality of life and stress response.

Many of the studies of spirituality have been conducted in the context of yoga and MBSR and have shown encouraging results. Some experts recommend extending the biopsychosocial model to the biopsychosocial-spiritual model of sickness and therapeutic interventions.

> There is very limited data examining the effect of distant prayer in healing disease. Caution is advised, since a couple of studies have reported adverse effects.

It is my personal belief and shared by a lot of experts that prayer, irrespective of the religion, plays a beneficial adjunct role in healing sickness, as well as in helping the patient with adjusting and coping mechanisms, which contribute to healthy healing.

REFERENCES

1. Shangase SL, Mohangi GU, Hassam-Essa S, Wood NH. The association between periodontitis and systemic health: an overview. *SADJ*. 2013 Feb; 68(1):8, 10-2.
2. Wells ME, Vaughn BV. Poor sleep challenging the health of a Nation. *Neurodiagn J*. 2012 Sep; 52(3):233-49.
3. Patel NK, Newstead AH, Ferrer RL. The effects of yoga on physical functioning and health related quality of life in older adults: a systematic review and meta-analysis. *J Altern Complement Med*. 2012 Oct; 18(10):902-17.

4. Seybold KS. Physiological mechanisms involved in religiosity/spirituality and health. *J Behav Med*. 2007 Aug; 30(4):303-9.

CHAPTER 48

Dr. M's Plan for Weekly Colon Cleanse and Body Detox

KEY POINTS

- Protein restriction in animals results in a 20 percent increase in lifespan, in contrast to fat or carbohydrate restriction that has no such effect.
- One must talk to their doctor before initiating any changes in diet or embarking on calorie restriction or fasting.

Humans live on one-quarter of what they eat; on the other three-quarters lives their doctor." - Egyptian pyramid inscription, 3800 B.C.

Every few days, we are asked to do a "disk clean" to keep our computer working smoothly. Our super-charged GI superhighway is no exception.

Our gut is subjected to loads of different foods, drugs, pollutants, and toxins every day. When I was growing up, the focus on Sunday was cleaning up the house, and our meals were smaller, simpler, and easier. In addition to a weekly jolt, our digestive system needs a different and simpler food intake along with a cleanliness drive. I call it a weekly colon cleansing and detox, using a fruit or juice fast to clean the gut, get rid of any toxins, and allow it to reset its bacterial patterns.

I am sure you have heard a lot about colonics, colon flushes, and colon cleansers that are advertised and are meant to be done every few months. In my opinion, not only are they using harsh and unnecessary methods and laxatives, they miss the point. While the gut gets cleaned out, evidence suggests that the gut bacteria reverses back to its fingerprint quickly within a couple of days or so. The body then has to live with the unhealthy gut all over again for all the months waiting for the next unpleasant colonic experience.

In my opinion, the process needs to be gentle and more frequent, so as not to allow bad bacteria/toxins to hunker down in the gut and cause damage. For example, studies have shown that a change of vegetarian to meat diet just for two days can have a profound impact on intestinal bacteria by increasing the numbers of bad bacteria that promote inflammation.

FASTING

Fasting involves a voluntary avoidance or restriction of food, with or without fluids. A person may undertake a partial or total abstention from all foods, or a select abstention of specific foods.

- Absolute fasts are usually undertaken for one day or a few days at a time, although fasts lasting several weeks may be undertaken for religious reasons or as part of civil disobedience.
- Intermittent fasts may also be undertaken. Liberal consumption of water is usually allowed during all times in alternate fasting and intermittent diet.
- Partial fasts restrict only specific foods.
- Fasting can be a therapeutic strategy.

Fasting has been promoted as a medical treatment against disease across cultures since ancient times. It was advocated by the forefathers of medicine, including Hippocrates, Galen, and Paracelsus. Modern proponents of fasting include the famous Dr. Andrew Weil of the University of Arizona. Practitioners of integrative medicine prescribe fasts for detoxification and cleansing the body for health maintenance as well as a treatment for disease.

HEALTH EFFECTS OF FASTING

Fasting has been examined for its role in health maintenance, disease prevention, and enhancing longevity. Much of the data is derived from animals. Human data is largely derived from supervised and recorded fasts. In addition to observation of religious diets, data about health effects in humans has been derived from three types of diets:

- Caloric restriction, which involves reduction of calories by 20-40 percent
- Alternate-day fasting with consumption as much you like on eating days
- Dietary restriction, which involves reduction of a dietary component, usually a macronutrient

Animal studies reveal that feeding regimens, caloric restriction, and intermittent fasting every other day result in increased longevity and improved health. The mechanism may include resetting the GI circadian clock to get in sync with the rhythm of other organs, including the biological clock in the brain. This results in a healthy synchronized metabolism across the entire body.

BENEFITS OF CALORIE RESTRICTION

In addition to enhanced longevity, health benefits of calorie restriction include delayed onset of numerous chronic disorders. These include autoimmune diseases, heart disease, cancer, diabetes, chronic kidney disease, and obesity.

DOES INTERMITTENT FASTING PROVIDE HEALTH BENEFITS?

Fasting on alternate days, while consuming twice the amount of food on non-fasting days, improves glucose control and longevity. This is accompanied by an upgrading of biochemical markers of improved health. The effects are actually similar to calorie restriction every day.

> Fasting for even one day per month may improve the markers for risk of cardiovascular disease.

HEALTH IMPLICATIONS OF RESTRICTION OF DIETARY COMPONENTS

Dietary restriction involves consumption of a reduced amount of one or more components of food without significantly reducing total caloric intake.

> Protein restriction in animals results in a 20 percent increase in lifespan, in contrast to fat or carbohydrate restriction, which has no such effect.

FASTING TO LOSE WEIGHT

Fasting on alternate days allows the person to lose weight over the short to medium term, although it is not sustained over the long term. On the other hand, the alternate day diet is superior to daily restriction for retaining lean mass.

Note: Punctuated fasting is superior to continued calorie restriction for weight reduction and increasing lifespan.

SAFETY OF FASTING

Healthy persons can fast for a few days without any adverse long-term effects, as long as adequate hydration is maintained. However, long-term absolute fasting is harmful and can lead to severe organ disease and death. Children, women who are pregnant or breastfeeding, or anyone undernourished should not practice fasts. Excessive fasting like anorexia nervosa may cause severe body-wide metabolic and functional problems. Wide fluctuations in blood levels of glucose and requirements for insulin can occur in those taking insulin. Undernourished persons must not undertake fasting of any kind.

WEEKLY COLON CLEANSE AND DETOX WITH JUICE AND SOUP FAST

Our gut needs a regular cleanliness overhaul, accompanied by different and simpler nutritional intake. There needs to be some rest. There needs to be a change. In short, some R&R is a must for our digestive system. I call it a weekly colon cleanse and detox using Juice & Soup fast. This will clean your gut, detoxify your system, and allow the gut to reset to a healthy bacterial pattern and metabolic sync.

Before you jump to the conclusion that such a fasting regimen is impossible to do, just think about when you or someone you love had a colonoscopy. Clear liquids for a day or two prior to the colonoscopy, depending upon the patient's needs, are not unusual. As long as you are focused on getting it right and becoming healthier, it would be easy to manage.

PRINCIPLES OF JUICE AND SOUP FAST

Be sure to discuss your plans for any fast with your doctor, especially if you are taking prescription medicine.

- The duration of this weekly colon cleanse and detox fast is one to two days, depending on health and medical status. This weekly reboot should not be extended beyond two days.

- The juice should be fresh (pulp free) and extracted from a juicer. Use organic products only.
- While fruit-only or vegetable-only juices are a reasonable option, it is better to have mixed juices, since the phytochemicals in vegetables and fruit are somewhat different and complementary.
- Avoid commercially available juices.
- Avoid commercial ready-to-drink juice cleansers.

While you may chill the juice somewhat in the refrigerator for taste, do not use ice as part of the juice. I am sure you have heard of or have yourself used the expression, "Brain freeze." It's not just that the brain is affected by ingestion of cold stuff. Cold temperature tends to slow the biologic processes at the very time we want the transformational metabolic processes to be active.

ADVANTAGES OF WEEKLY JUICE AND SOUP FAST
- Ready source of energy, but overall calorie restriction
- Easier to digest and absorb
- Rich in micronutrients
- Rich in antioxidants

AN EXAMPLE OF THE WEEKLY COLON CLEANSE & DETOX

If early-morning caffeine is a must, you may have a cup of hot green tea and then begin the fast.

- Start the breakfast with three bowls or one quarter to one half of a small seedless watermelon.
- Drink a glass of juice every two to four hours.
- Eat one half of a ripe small papaya for lunch.
- Enjoy two ripe mangoes (skinned and without the seeds) for supper. In addition, you may have a vegetarian bouillon soup for supper. Use oil and salt sparingly in the soups. The soup should be strained before consuming.

DURING THE FAST

- Pace your activity and rest during the reboot period.
- While you should not perform strenuous exercise during this period, you should not become a couch potato either. Do yoga exercises to maintain the skeletal muscle flexibility and intestinal smooth muscle balance.
- Continue to do normal activities, including running errands. It is always advisable to know where the nearest restroom is when you are out of your home.
- In addition to the juices, drink three to five glasses of water during the day.
- As can be expected, it is not uncommon to feel hungry. Motivation to stay healthy is always a great driving force.

You may take an over-the-counter melatonin at bedtime. It is not just good for sleep; it plays a critical role in digestion and metabolism, including the synchronization of the biological clock in the brain and the GI circadian clock.

EXAMPLES OF HEALTHY JUICE COMPONENTS

JUICE ONE FOR FASTING

- 3 carrots
- 1 one-inch slice of skinned ginger
- ½ medium green apple
- ½ small papaya

JUICE TWO FOR FASTING

- 1 mango (peeled and pitted)
- 1 pear
- 3 kale leaves
- 3 pitted dates
- 3-6 fresh cilantro leaves

- 1 half-inch slice of fresh ginger

JUICE THREE FOR FASTING

- 4 carrots
- 1 large beet
- ½ pear
- ½ small papaya
- 3-6 fresh mint leaves

JUICE FOUR FOR FASTING

- 1 yam
- 2 carrots
- 3 kale leaves
- 1 medium orange
- 2 whole kiwis

JUICE FIVE FOR FASTING

- 2 red grapefruits
- 1 large beet
- 3-6 fresh cilantro leaves
- 1 red apple

JUICE SIX FOR FASTING

- 2 peaches
- 2 plums
- 2 whole kiwis
- 1 orange
- 3-6 fresh mint leaves

JUICE SEVEN FOR FASTING

- ½ small papaya
- 2 tbsp flaxseeds
- 1 apple
- 1 teaspoon honey

- 1 pitted, peeled ripe mango
- 4-6 cilantro leaves

JUICE EIGHT FOR FASTING

- ½ cup of cranberries
- ½ cup blueberries
- 1 cup green apple
- ½ freshly squeezed lemon
- 1 teaspoon honey

JUICE NINE FOR FASTING

- 1 cup lychee
- 2 tbsp flaxseeds
- ½ whole pomegranate
- 1 teaspoon honey
- 1 whole small beet
- 3-6 fresh mint leaves

JUICE TEN FOR FASTING

- 1 whole sweet (not sour) ripe mango
- 3-6 mint leaves
- ½ whole pomegranate
- 1 ripe pear
- 1 small beet

BREAKING THE FAST

There is no particular transition needed for a one-day fast. Resume eating healthy foods the next day.

A two-day fast should be broken with a light, healthy soup. My favorite is a light pumpkin soup made in a standard fashion using three to four cups of mashed cooked pumpkin. Minimize the additives to healthy ingredients, like a tablespoon of extra-virgin olive oil, one to two minced white bulb of leek, a tablespoon of powdered fenugreek leaves, one tablespoon of minced cilantro leaves, and one teaspoon of ground cumin. Although canned pureed pumpkin may be used, a fresh one is always preferable. Do not use milk, meat, or meat broth.

Note: Rebooting a computer improves the functioning of the computer by resetting it. Similarly, while the basic framework of your body stays the same, the weekly colon cleanse and detox intends to make your gut (and indirectly the entire body) healthier via actions on the gut-immune-brain axis.

WEEKLY COLON CLEANSE AND DETOX TO MONTHLY SHOCK AND AWE

Your digestive system may need more than a weekly colon cleanse and detox described above to keep it running in a healthy fashion. Enter the monthly Shock & Awe strategy. It means doing the weekly colon cleanse and detox on a grander scale. People doing a weekly one day juice fast should step up to two-day juice and soup.

Those that are accomplished in the weekly two-day juice and soup stage should do a water-only fast (Saturday) followed by juice and soup (Sunday) for one weekend every month. Transition to normal intake on Monday.

Some persons may need the shock and awe twice a month rather than once a month, depending on their health and digestive condition needs.

Reminder: Always talk to your doctor before changing any dietary regimen, including embarking on any fast.

REFERENCES

1. Cava E, Fontana L. Will calorie restriction work in humans? *Aging (Albany NY)*. 2013 Jul; 5(7):507-14.
2. Fontana L. The scientific basis of caloric restriction leading to longer life. *Curr Opin Gastroenterol*. 2009 Mar; 25(2):144-50.

CHAPTER 49

Dr. M's Personal Choices for Supplements

KEY POINTS

- Vitamin D is involved in numerous critical metabolic functions in the body. At the same time, vitamin D deficiency is widespread. If you don't check your levels, you will not know it.
- Numerous studies have documented the protective effect of zinc supplementation against respiratory infections.
- Turmeric, the yellow curry powder, is a must-have medicinal spice in the kitchen.

The human body, when unhealthy, is riddled with imperfections. Further complicating matters is that our modern lifestyle does not allow for a perfect diet at every meal, if there ever was one.

The above scenario is ripe for exploitation by taking nutritional supplements. However, it is not as simple as it sounds. The scientific literature is full of inconsistencies and contradictions. Furthermore, supplements that show benefit in laboratory studies of animals may not show benefit in human clinical trials. At the same time, the market is burgeoning with increasing number and type of supplements to choose from, without any sane guidance. Everyone has his or her own favorites.

Rather than confuse the readers with data on the clinical trials and the pros and cons of each and every supplement available, I would just share with you the supplements I personally take.

RATIONALE FOR MY CHOICES
OF SUPPLEMENTS

The supplements I take are meant for general gut-health maintenance only. One could easily argue and make a case for some other supplements as a routine. However, at some point, one has to draw the line rather than let the stomach become a pharmacy!

BEYOND MY CHOICES OF SUPPLEMENTS

In addition to the ones I take, there are additional supplements effective in specific disorders that one could take with potential for benefit. Examples include D-ribose and L-carnitine for autism and ADHD. Patients with frequent urinary tract infections may be helped by cranberry juice and mannose.

TURMERIC

Turmeric, derived from the plant *Curcuma longa*, is a golden yellow-colored spice used in Indian and Chinese cultures since ancient times. Because of its numerous diverse clinical uses without any known adverse effects, it has been labeled by many as the "spice of life" It is known as *Haldi* in India.

In several thousand years of Ayurveda use, turmeric has been used for a wide variety of diseases and conditions, including asthma and wound healing, respiratory disorders, gastrointestinal and liver disorders, non-specific aches and pains, dementia, and Parkinson's disease.

The yellow color is due to its active component, curcumin, which constitutes two to five percent of turmeric.

TRADITIONAL USES
- Medicinal
- Culinary
- Religious ceremonies

- Dye

HISTORICAL PERSPECTIVE

While it has been used in India for thousands of years, turmeric is also mentioned in the writings of the famed explorer, Marco Polo, discussing his voyage to China and India in the thirteenth century. The West got its first taste of turmeric in the thirteenth century through Arab traders. The term "curry powder" was coined during the British rule of India.

MECHANISM OF ACTION

General

- Antioxidant properties
- Reduces inflammation
- Protects against infections
- Stomach acid blocker
- Improves blood glucose control
- Inhibits growth and spread of cancer cells
- Potential evidence-based clinical uses

Ulcers

- Protects against development of experimental stomach ulcer in animals
- Reduces drug-induced damage in the rat small intestine
- Reduces *H. pylori* infection in animals

Adjuvant for chemo-radiation therapy in cancer

- Curcumin sensitizes cancer cells to the effect of chemotherapy and radiation therapy, while protecting normal cells.

Colon cancer

- Protects against inflammation-induced colon cancer in mice
- Reduces migration of human colon cancer cells

Ulcerative colitis and Crohn's disease

The role of curcumin as maintenance therapy for ulcerative colitis was examined in a randomized, multi-center, double-blind, placebo-controlled trial. The relapse rate in the curcumin group over six months was five percent, compared to 21 percent in the placebo group.

Liver protection

- Protects animals against liver damage due to acetaminophen (Tylenol)
- Reduces liver damage in rats consuming alcohol
- Prevents fatty liver in animals

Viral hepatitis

- Inhibits hepatitis C virus multiplication
- Inhibits hepatitis B viral production.

Pancreas

- Protects against experimental pancreatitis in animals
- Inhibits growth of pancreatic cancer cells

Immune booster

- Turmeric is frequently consumed in India (about 2.5 to 4 g per day) in order to boost immunity and ward off infections, especially during the winter season.

ZINC

FUNCTIONAL SIGNIFICANCE

- Present throughout the body, mostly inside skeletal muscles and bones
- Involved in numerous critical metabolic pathways
- Plays an important role in maintaining our immune defense system

MANIFESTATIONS OF ZINC DEFICIENCY

- Growth retardation
- Sexual dysfunction
- Hair loss
- Bad taste in the mouth
- Immune dysfunction with impaired healing

ROLE OF ZINC SUPPLEMENTATION

- Enhances growth, especially in kids with zinc deficiency
- Multiple studies have documented the beneficial role in reducing both respiratory and gastrointestinal infection-related morbidity and mortality in kids and the elderly.
- Frequently used as part of treatment for the common cold
- Reduces risks of premature or prolonged labor and premature birth
- Improves sperm counts
- May protect against cancer
- Preventative zinc supplementation improves morbidity and mortality due to diarrhea, pneumonia and malaria in developing countries

Drs. Singh and Das from Chandigarh, India, recently conducted an expert meta-analysis of randomized controlled trials investigating the effect of zinc supplementation on the common cold. They concluded, "Zinc administered within 24 hours of onset of symptoms reduces the duration of common cold symptoms in healthy people."

Data suggests that taking zinc during a common cold reduces the duration of symptoms by an average of over a day and a half.

ZINC REQUIREMENTS AND TOXICITY

- Daily requirements for zinc vary with age, gender, pregnancy, and lactation.

- Zinc toxicity is rare and manifests with GI problems as abdominal pain, nausea, vomiting, and diarrhea.

Personal note: I take over-the-counter zinc at a dose of 50 mg per day.

VITAMIN D

SOURCES OF VITAMIN D

These include vitamin D produced in the skin, as well as that absorbed from the diet.

Food

Very few foods contain sufficient quantities of vitamin D. In addition to vitamin D-fortified milk, the dietary sources rich in vitamin D include fatty fish, cod-liver oil, and eggs. Vitamin D2 is a plant steroid used for milk fortification. Other products that may be fortified include cereals and breads. The diet usually provides vitamin D3.

Skin

Because of the paucity of vitamin D in foods, the human body depends upon skin exposure to sun, which leads to production of vitamin D in body.

FUNCTIONAL SIGNIFICANCE OF VITAMIN D

Vitamin D and its metabolites are intricately related to calcium homeostasis and bone metabolism. It is involved in multiple other metabolic processes directly or indirectly.

VITAMIN D DEFICIENCY

Vitamin D stores decline with age, especially in the winter, because of reduced sun exposure. Vitamin D deficiency can be seen in as high as 57 percent of hospitalized patients in some studies, 22 percent of whom are severely deficient.

While many argue that vitamin D deficiency is a growing epidemic around the world, the Institute of Medicine suggests that the majority of people are doing well. This also means that a significant portion of the population (albeit a minority) is vitamin D-deficient.

CONSEQUENCES OF VITAMIN D DEFICIENCY

Although rickets is rare these days, subclinical vitamin D deficiency is common. Such a deficiency assumes an important role because of involvement in balancing numerous metabolic functions. Disease states linked to vitamin D deficiency include:

- Weakening of bones, which is very common. That is why you see so many TV commercials for drugs to treat osteoporosis.
- Weak immune system
- Increased risk of various cancers, including colon cancer
- Increased risk of heart disease
- Increased risk of falls and fractures

> Low levels of vitamin D are an increased risk of all-cause mortality, whereas supplementation of vitamin D results in reduction of all-cause mortality.

VITAMIN D REQUIREMENTS

- Healthy adults: A minimum of 200 IU per day
- Pregnant and lactating mothers: 400 IU per day.
- Elderly: 800 IU per day, plus at least 1.2 g of elemental calcium per day
- Infants who are exclusively breastfed: 400 IU per day. Since infant formulas are fortified with vitamin D, formula-fed infants require supplementation if they consume less than 1000 mL daily of formula.

A toxic dose is greater than 2000 IU per day over the long term. It should be noted that sometimes physicians do prescribe as high as 50,000 IU as single dose.

TOXICITY OF VITAMIN D

Vitamin D is not innocuous. Excess ingestion can lead to vitamin D intoxication. Subjects prone to toxicity include not only those who consume mega-doses of supplements, but may also occur in patients on vitamin D replacement therapy for a variety of disorders.

Symptoms of vitamin D toxicity may include brain dysfunction, increased urination, vomiting, muscle weakness, and bone pain.

MULTIVITAMIN-MINERAL FORMULATIONS

Multivitamin formulations contain 100-150 percent of the recommended daily allowance. They may not be needed in subjects consuming a healthy diet every day.

SUBJECTS LIKELY TO BENEFIT FROM MULTIVITAMIN SUPPLEMENTS

- Those with unhealthy eating habits
- Vegans
- Alcoholics
- Subjects who had major GI surgery
- Patients with IBD
- Hemodialysis

HEALTH BENEFITS OF MULTIVITAMIN-MINERAL SUPPLEMENTATION

According to Dr. Grima and colleagues from the Monash University in Australia, multivitamin supplementation improves immediate memory recall.

Data on the effect of multivitamin-multimineral combinations is mixed. According to an expert systematic review of literature by Dr. Alexander and colleagues from the Exponent Inc. Health Sciences in Colorado, these formulations may provide modest protective benefit against cancer, death due to heart disease, and all-cause mortality.

While earlier studies included formulations with just three or more ingredients, more recent studies have the formulations containing 10 or more components. Dr. Comerford from the University of California at Davis Medical Center points out that many recent trials focusing on adult mental health concerns have yielded positive results. He suggests that there is moderate to strong evidence that multivitamin-multimineral formulations "should be considered first line of defense...against recently recognized wave of mental health issues such as anxiety, stress, depression, and cognitive or memory complaints."

VITAMIN C

Vitamin C does not reduce the chance that you will get a cold, and, as such, routine daily supplementation for this purpose is not appropriate.

Vitamin C does appear to reduce the duration and severity of cold symptoms.

Drs. Hemila and Chalker from the University of Helsinki in Finland conducted an expert meta-analysis of placebo-controlled trials examining the efficacy of vitamin C for treatment and prevention of cold. They concluded that there is "consistent effect of vitamin C on the duration and severity of colds in the regular supplementation studies."

In view of the low cost and good safety profile, it may be appropriate for patients to try it for themselves, if vitamin C provides benefit to them.

While vitamin C does not appear to have benefit in treating cancer and stroke, results of studies examining its effect in treating coronary heart disease have yielded conflicting results.

> Intake of vitamin C over a 10-year period is associated with a small reduction in total death rate.

Personal Note: I take vitamin C only during episodes of colds in winter. I believe that the vitamin C supplementation during my episode of common cold, in addition to the other supplements I take, does reduce the severity and duration of my cold symptoms. Touch wood!

REFERENCES

1. Binkley N, Ramamurthy R, Krueger D. Low vitamin D status: definition, prevalence, consequences, and correction. *Endocrinol Metab Clin North Am.* 2010 Jun; 39(2):287-301.
2. Alzaim M, Wood RJ. Vitamin D and gestational diabetes mellitus. *Nutr Rev.* 2013 Mar; 71(3):158-67.
3. Tabesh M, Salehi-Abargouei A, Tabesh M, Esmaillzadeh A. Maternal vitamin D status and risk of pre-eclampsia: a systematic review and meta-analysis. *J Clin Endocrinol Metab.* 2013 Aug; 98(8):3165-73.
4. Shen LR, Parnell LD, Ordovas JM, Lai CQ. Curcumin and aging. *Biofactors.* 2013 Jan-Feb; 39(1):133-40.
5. Singh M, Das RR. Zinc for the common cold. Cochrane Database Syst Rev. 2013 Jun 18; 6:CD001364.
6. Grima NA, Pase MP, Macpherson H, Pipingas A. The effects of multivitamins on cognitive performance: a systematic review and meta-analysis. J Alzheimers Dis. 2012; 29(3):561-9.

Section XI

Going beyond the Optimal Digestion of Seven-X Plan: A Digestive Wellness Potpourri

CHAPTER 50

Gallstones: Should You be Worried?

KEY POINTS

- Most patients never have any problems related to their gallstones.
- Routine use of prophylactic cholecystectomy is not recommended.
- Data suggests that acupuncture is widely used for bile duct diseases in many parts of the world. However, there is a lack of high-quality trials.
- Probiotics may alter the bile composition and potentially the lithogenic potential of bile.

OCCURRENCE

Gallstones occur in 10 to 20 percent of the population. These are rare in Asia, while North Europeans have higher prevalence than Southern Europeans. They tend to occur more among females. Native American women are particularly at risk.

TYPES OF GALLSTONES

Gallstones may be of three types: yellow or cholesterol stones (80 to 85 percent), black pigment stones, and brown pigment stones.

Mixed patterns may be seen. Fifteen percent of patients with gallstones also have stones in the bile duct connecting the gallbladder to the small bowel.

Precipitation of concentrated cholesterol or bilirubin leads to stone formation. Sludge in the gallbladder is an intermediate step in the process of stone formation. However, sludge leads to stone formation only in a minority of cases.

Some stones have calcium in them also. Although normally sterile, stones may be associated with infection.

RISK FACTORS

Risk factors for cholesterol stones include multiple pregnancies, use of oral contraceptives, obesity, rapid weight loss, low vegetable protein intake, sedentary lifestyle, high fat levels, diabetes, insulin resistance, and spinal cord injuries.

Black stone formation is determined by the amount of breakdown of red blood cells. Risk factors for black stones include hemolytic anemia (sickle cell disease, beta thalassemia), chronic liver disease, Crohn's disease, and total parenteral nutrition.

Brown stones are usually seen in the bile duct and occur as a result of bacterial infection of foreign substance, such as a suture or retained stone after gallbladder surgery. Parasitic infections are the cause of brown stones in East Asia.

DIAGNOSTIC MODALITIES

Less than 25 percent of gallstones can be seen on plain X-ray. Ultrasound is the test of choice. However, CT scan is superior for visualization of stones in the bile duct. A HIDA scan of the gallbladder is 95 percent accurate for the diagnosis of acute cholecystitis (inflammation of gallbladder).

An endoscopic retrograde cholangiopancreatography (ERCP) scope test is useful for diagnosis of bile duct stones; the stones can also be removed during the exam. An MRCP scan (an MRI of bile ducts and pancreatic ducts) is as accurate as ERCP, but it is only an imaging study, and stones cannot be removed during the scan.

CLINICAL FEATURES

Gallstones remain silent without any symptoms in about 75 to 85 percent of the cases. Complications of gallstones occur in less than 0.2 percent of patients per year. The most common problem associated with gallstones is biliary colic, which occurs at the rate of 2 percent per year. The incidence of cancer is 0.02 percent per year.

BILIARY COLIC

Biliary colic is right upper abdomen pain that occurs when a gallstone gets impacted in the duct. Once a patient has an episode of biliary colic, recurrence occurs in 30 percent of patients per year. The pain is a steady, constant pain radiating to the back or right shoulder and subsides in a few hours. Nausea and vomiting may be present.

A physical exam in cases of biliary colic is normal, as are the laboratory studies. Ultrasound is the test of choice.

ACUTE CHOLECYSTITIS

Patients complain of right and mid-upper abdomen pain, radiating to the shoulder blade. Surgical consultation is warranted. Ultrasound is excellent for the diagnosis of gallstones. A CT scan is frequently done to discern the cause of pain. The patient is usually admitted to the hospital and given intravenous fluids and antibiotics. Usual treatment is removal of gallbladder or cholecystectomy. This can usually be undertaken by making tiny incisions in the abdomen.

CHRONIC CHOLECYSTITIS

It is more of a pathologic than a clinical entity occurring as a consequence of acute cholecystitis or recurrent biliary colic. There may not be prior history of abdominal pain.

MEDICAL TREATMENT OF GALLSTONES

STRATEGY FOR SYMPTOMS SUGGESTIVE OF PROBLEM DUE TO GALLSTONES

- Patients undergo a gallbladder ultrasound. In case of normal gallbladder, a repeat examination or another imaging may be done. Checking pressures in the bile duct is controversial, and select cases may benefit from it.
- Patients with gallstones on ultrasound who are good surgical candidates should undergo gallbladder removal via tiny incisions in the belly.
- Patients who are poor surgical candidates and have a small stone burden without calcification may be considered for medical dissolution treatment with or without breaking the stones using lithotripsy.

Actigall can be an option in select patients who have small cholesterol stones and a functioning gallbladder. It is considered only for symptomatic patients with small stones that have not caused complications. Complementary lithotripsy may be undertaken along with oral dissolution therapy in select patients.

ROLE OF PREVENTATIVE GALLBLADDER REMOVAL

Routine cholecystectomy for an incidental finding of gallstones is not recommended. Candidates for prophylactic surgery include:

- Patients with high risk of gallbladder cancer (such as patients with a large gallbladder polyp or calcified gallbladder, and Native American females)
- Young sickle cell disease patients
- Patients on the waiting list for organ transplant
- Patients travelling to remote areas or space for prolonged periods

ALTERNATIVE MEDICINE THERAPIES

LIFESTYLE CHANGES TO PREVENT GALLSTONES

Changes in lifestyle are especially important in high-risk patients, including after gallbladder surgery. The following factors help reduce the risk of gallstones:

- Low-fat, high-fiber diet
- Vegetarian diet
- Diet containing onions and garlic
- Diet low in refined sugar
- Consumption of caffeinated products (but not decaffeinated coffee) tends to reduce the risk
- The role of lentils and legumes is mired in debate
- Weight reduction if overweight. However, it should be gradual since rapid weight loss can increase the risk of stones, as well.

NUTRITIONAL SUPPLEMENTS

Several supplements, such as vitamin C, lecithin, and Rowachol (comprised of plant terpenes) have been known to reduce the risk.

GALLBLADDER FLUSH

A gallbladder flush is a popular remedy practiced around the world. A variety of versions have been recommended. The protocol typically includes a period of fasting and then consumption of oil (like olive oil) along with juices (like lemon juice, apple juice, or vegetable juice) without eating solids. One study demonstrated reduction of gallstones, as seen on ultrasound imaging. However, there is a lack of randomized controlled trials studying the role of gallbladder flush in treatment or prevention of gallstones.

CHINESE HERBAL MEDICINE

- Muh-Shiang-Bin-Lang-Wan, which modulates the sphincter of Oddi function.

- Yiqi-Yangyin is a prescription which attenuates the lithogenic potential of bile in patients with gallstones.
- Jinquiancao Gao reduces rate of growth of gallstones in animals and has a high clinical effective rate in humans in uncontrolled studies.

ACUPUNCTURE

Acupuncture reduces the rate of gallstone formation and the number of gallstones in animals. It stimulates gallbladder contractions, facilitating stone expulsion.

A controlled trial of 1,291 patients found that the treatment results in the total effective rate of 99.7 percent, with a total stone excretion rate of 20 percent. No stone excretion occurred in the control group.

Another randomized controlled trial of 120 patients examined the effect of electro-acupuncture in patients with gallstones. Controls received a comprehensive stone treatment in the form of Chinese medicine Paishi Decoction, magnesium sulfate, hydrochloric acid and fat diet, and a Tuian Yunjing Instrument. The acupuncture group demonstrated a significantly higher total effective rate of 87 percent, as compared to the 68 percent in the controls receiving Chinese medical therapy.

> Preliminary data indicates potential for use of acupuncture in treating gallstone disease. However, good randomized controlled trials are needed before a firm recommendation can be made.

PROBIOTICS

Probiotics may alter the composition of bile and improve bile flow, thus reducing the risk for gallstones. There is a lack of trials studying the role of probiotics in gallstone disease.

Note: The usual treatment of patients with problems due to gallstones is removal of the gallbladder; other therapies should be undertaken only if that is not an option.

REFERENCES

1. Duncan CB, Riall TS. Evidence-based current surgical practice: calculus gallbladder disease. *J Gastrointest Surg.* 2012 Nov; 16(11):2011-25.
2. Shaffer EA. Gallbladder sludge: what is its clinical significance? *Curr Gastroenterol Rep.* 2001; 3(2):166-73.
3. Gaby AR. Nutritional approaches to prevention and treatment of gallstones. *Altern Med Rev. 2009 Sep; 14(3):258-67.*
4. Xu X. Acupuncture in an outpatient clinic in China: a comparison with the use of acupuncture in North America. *South Med J.* 2001 Aug; 94(8):813-6.
5. Savage AP, O'Brien T, Lamont PM. Adjuvant herbal treatment for gallstones. *Br J Surg.* 1992 Feb; 79(2):168.

CHAPTER 51

Hiccups

KEY POINTS

- Most hiccups are short-lived and resolve spontaneously or in response to simple home remedies.
- Hiccups, while usually benign, can be a harbinger of serious underlying illness.
- An underlying cause of chronic hiccups cannot be identified in a majority of cases.

WHAT ARE HICCUPS?

Hiccups or singultus (from singult in Latin meaning catching breath while sobbing) is an involuntary nuisance-type bodily action of no functional value. They do not occur as part of any bodily function.

- Hiccups may occur even prior to birth and may be programmed as a fetus during the pregnancy. Just like computer programming, hiccups can get programmed into the fetal mind-body system and persist later.
- The mechanisms involved in hiccups remain unclear. Hiccups occur as a result of intermittent and involuntary spasmodic contraction of in-breathing respiratory muscles associated with abrupt airway closure at the glottis, which produces the audible sound.

CAUSATIVE FACTORS

Hiccups are common after a large meal or alcohol ingestion. Other factors include excessive smoking, intake of mints, and drinking carbonated beverages.

Patients with anxiety and emotional stress are especially at risk. They are not uncommon when excessive air gets insufflated into the gut during an upper or lower GI scope.

The frequency varies amongst different individuals, ranging from four to 20 per minute and going as high as 60 per minute in some cases. Similarly, the duration of hiccups is variable from a few minutes to hours, days, and even weeks.

Prolonged hiccups may be caused by foreign bodies in the ear canal, cervical tumors, neurologic disorders, diabetes, uremia, alcoholism, and diseases in the chest like tuberculosis, pleurisy, and cancer. Medications like corticosteroids and benzodiazepines have been implicated, but convincing evidence is lacking.

GI causes include acid reflux and stomach obstruction. GERD is frequently the result—and not the cause—of hiccups.

Hiccups, while usually benign, can be a harbinger of serious underlying illness. Occurrence of hiccups during sleep suggests an underlying cause that must be investigated.

CHRONIC HICCUPS

Chronic hiccups are defined as those persisting for longer than 48 hours. Prolonged hiccups can persist for days and even months or years. They can result in multiple problems, such as chronic fatigue, sleep disturbances, depression, weight loss, and even suicide.

DIAGNOSTIC TESTING

Tests are tailored to the patient based on the overall presentation. Most patients do not require any testing. However, patients with prolonged and intractable hiccups are candidates for thorough investigations.

Tests may include complete blood count, comprehensive metabolic profile, upper GI endoscopy, laryngoscopy, X-rays, and CT of the chest and abdomen. Fluoroscopy should be performed to evaluate movements of respiratory muscles (diaphragm). An MRI scan of the brain may occasionally be undertaken. Even more extensive testing may be needed in certain cases, depending upon presentation. For example, a physician may recommend a spinal tap to check the spinal fluid to exclude meningitis.

No cause is found in majority of the cases.

TREATMENT OF HICCUPS

Treatment should be directed at the cause. However, no cause can be identified in many cases. Hiccups are frequently subjected to numerous home-remedies. Most hiccups are short-lived and resolve spontaneously without any active intervention.

Physical maneuvers are based on tradition and have not been subjected to rigorous clinical trials. Nevertheless, they are recommended as first-line therapy by most medical providers. The potentially helpful actions include:

- Take a deep breath and hold it as long as you comfortably can.
- Close ears with fingers/hands while drinking cold water with a straw.
- Re-breathe into a bag.
- Drink cold water.
- Gargle with cold water.
- Perform the Valsalva maneuver.
- Eat a spoonful of dry sugar.
- Pull knees to the chest while leaning forward.
- Pull your tongue.
- Bite on a lemon.

MEDICAL TREATMENTS

There is paucity of evidence-based medical therapies. Throat stimulation with a nasogastric tube may be of benefit. Patients with suspected acid reflux may benefit from acid blockers like Zantac and Prilosec. Other medications options include baclofen, metoclopramide (Reglan), chlorpromazine (Thorazine), haloperidol (Haldol), amitriptyline (Elavil), carbamazepine (Tegretol), Dilantin, and nifedipine (Procardia).

One AIDS patient used marijuana to get rid of his hiccups. Alternate medicine options include hypnosis and acupuncture.

SURGERY

Devices may be implanted to suppress hiccups. These include breathing pacemakers and vagus nerve stimulators. Surgery may be performed as a last resort.

REFERENCES

1. Bredenoord AJ. Management of belching, hiccups, and aerophagia. *Clin Gastroenterol Hepatol*. 2013 Jan; 11(1):6-12.
2. Moretto EN, Wee B, Wiffen PJ, Murchison AG. Interventions for treating persistent and intractable hiccups in adults. *Cochrane Database Syst Rev*. 2013 Jan 31; 1:CD008768.
3. Dobelle WH. Use of breathing pacemakers to suppress intractable hiccups of upto thirteen years duration. *ASAIO J*. 1999 Nov-Dec; 45(6):524-5.

CHAPTER 52

Making Smart Choices When Buying Yogurt

KEY POINTS

- The live culture seal is voluntary.
- All yogurts are not the same.
- Some brands subject yogurt to heat treatment, resulting in the killing of bacteria in an attempt to boost the shelf life. This step gets rid of many potential benefits of these bacteria.

The knowledge that yogurt, with its probiotic bacteria, provides healthy nutrition has been passed on through generations. It was Dr. Metchnikoff who, in the early 20th century, publically espoused the benefits of yogurt for health. In fact, he attributed his own health and longevity to yogurt.

YOGURT CONSUMPTION IN THE UNITED STATES

An average American eats four to six pounds of yogurt per year. The commercial market for yogurt exceeds $2.2 billion in the US. It is expected to grow to $9.3 billion by 2017.

The texture of different yogurts is obviously different and depends on a variety of factors. Greek yogurt is perhaps the most popular.

YOGURT VERSUS MILK

A big advantage of yogurt over milk and its other products is that yogurt contains lactase derived from the bacteria. Yogurt may be better tolerated by those with lactose intolerance, although the data is mixed. Yogurt is considered especially beneficial for health.

LIVE ACTIVE CULTURES

Some brands subject yogurt to heat treatment in an attempt to boost the shelf life. This results in the killing of bacteria and may get rid of some of the benefits of these probiotic bacteria.

A brand of yogurt containing live cultures has a logo or seal (in the form of "AC," which stands for active cultures) on the container. Yogurt may be made by active cultures but may or may not have the bacteria, depending upon the brand.

The seal is voluntary, and its presence implies that the yogurt contains at least 100 million bacteria per gram at the time of manufacture. Standard yogurt contains *Lactobacillus bulgaricus* and *Streptococcus thermophilus*, but their beneficial probiotic effect, especially in doses present in usual yogurt, is controversial and limited at best.

KEFIR

Conceptually similar to yogurt, Kefir is a fermented milk drink that usually contains multiple diverse species of probiotic. The number of probiotics may vary from 10 to as many as 30 species/strains. For example, *Lifeway Organic Probiotic Kefir* (plain) contains 12 probiotic strains of bacteria.

HEALTH-ORIENTED YOGURTS

Yogurt appears to fulfill basic criteria for probiotic. Many immune-enhancing benefits have been ascribed. Health-oriented yogurt brands tend to contain one or more bacteria in addition to the two standard ones outlined above.

In addition, the number of bacteria per serving is higher, making it likely that enough bacteria can survive all the way to the colon and exert their beneficial effects to the highest potential. Some of these brands are mentioned in Chapter 10.

FACTS TO CONSIDER
WHEN PURCHASING YOGURT

- Some of the products from popular brands may contain gelatin, which is derived from animal skin and bones. Refrain from such products if you are on a strict vegetarian diet based on religious, cultural, or health convictions. This may not always be mentioned on the label, so check out the company Web site.
- Some but not all yogurt products are gluten-free.
- Prefer plain yogurt over sweetened yogurts or those with fruit, which tend to have a much higher sugar content. Add your own fruit to the plain yogurt just before eating. Sugar alternatives like Stevia may be used as sweetener, if needed.
- Prefer plain yogurt over frozen yogurts if your goal is the highest health benefit.
- Yogurt without live cultures has a low likelihood of providing the significant health benefits of probiotics.

REFERENCES

1. Weissmann G. It's complicated: inflammation from Metchnikoff to Meryl Streep. *FASEB J.* 2010 Nov; 24(11):4129-32.
2. Chagas CE, Rogero MM, Martini LA. Evaluating the links between intake of milk/dairy products and cancer. *Nutr Rev.* 2012 May; 70(5):294-300.
3. Adolfsson O, Meydani SN, Russell RM. Yogurt and gut function. *Am J Clin Nutr.* 2004 Aug; 80(2):245-56.

4. de Vrese M, Stegelmann A, Richter B, Fenselau S et al. Probiotics--compensation for lactase insufficiency. *Am J Clin Nutr*. 2001 Feb; 73(2 Suppl):421S-429S.

CHAPTER 53

Antibiotics in Meat Animals: Implications for Your Health

KEY POINTS

- Antibiotics are used for growth in animals raised for meat.
- The presence of antibiotics in meat has been documented and has potential to alter the gut bacteria of the person eating the meat.
- How much do you know about the meat you consume on a day-to-day basis?

ROUTINE ANTIBIOTIC USE IN ANIMALS IS NOT TO TREAT INFECTIONS

Consider that antibiotics are routinely used in animals, not to treat infections but to promote growth, so the ultimate product would yield more profits. As much as 300 mg of antibiotics are used in production of every kilogram of meat and eggs. Wow!

IMPLICATIONS OF USE OF ANTIBIOTICS IN MEAT ANIMALS

The use of sub-therapeutic doses of antibiotics not only has the potential to alter the meat itself, but also what comes along with it, i.e. antibiotic-resistant bacteria. By the way, small amounts of antibiotics can still be detected in the meat that is ready for you to buy and then eat!

No wonder there has been an exponential rise of antibiotic-resistant bacteria that have the potential to cause disease. It could be especially dangerous for those who have suboptimal immune status and risk of frequent infections!

To be fair, the rise of antibiotic-resistant bacteria has been much more due to use of antibiotics by humans rather than the use in farm animals.

Wait, there's more!

A Consumer Reports study found presence of the drug ractopamine, indicating that it is again being used to promote growth in animals to make them bigger for bigger sale. Although banned in many countries, it is permissible in the United States.

POTENTIAL CONSEQUENCES OF DRUG/ANTIBIOTIC USE IN MEAT ANIMALS

- There is potential for increased prevalence of antibiotic-resistant bacteria.
- Meat may be altered. We do not know if antibiotics and altered bacteria produce changes in the meat. We do not know for sure if there is exchange of genetic material between bacteria and animals. Such changes may be very gradual.
- There is potential for an altered intestinal bacterial environment with disrupted bacterial patterns in the person consuming meat.
- The consuming person may become host to potentially disease-producing bacterial patterns in the gut.

> Studies suggest a bidirectional exchange of bacteria between animals and humans. An unwise use of antibiotics in animals or humans is not just a public health problem for us as humans, but it also alters health of animals. Consumption of such meat may have unknown consequences on humans and animals over the long term.

BENEFITS OF ORGANIC MEAT RAISED WITHOUT DRUG/ANTIBIOTIC USE

No studies have examined a direct benefit, hence we have to go by circumstantial evidence, connect the dots, and try to do what may be safer for at least these select populations:

- Infants and children in early life
- Kids and adults with psychological issues, since some of the drugs (like ractopamine) may have an effect on the brain
- Patients with chronic disorders associated with abnormal intestinal patterns, leaky gut, and chronic low grade inflammation

REFERENCES

1. Kjeldgaard J, Cohn MT, Casey PG et al. Residual antibiotics disrupt meat fermentation and increase risk of infection. *MBio*. 2012 Aug 28; 3(5):e00190-12.
2. Berends BR, van den Bogaard AE, Van Knapen F, Snijders JM. Human health hazards associated with the administration of antimicrobials to slaughter animals. Part II. An assessment of the risks of resistant bacteria in pigs and pork. *Vet Q*. 2001 Jan; 23(1):10-21.
3. Vignaroli C, Zandri G, Aquilanti L et al. Multidrug-resistant enterococci in animal meat and faeces and co-transfer of resistance from an Enterococcus durans to a human Enterococcus faecium. *Curr Microbiol*. 2011 May; 62(5):1438-47.

CHAPTER 54

Two Great Gluten-Free Vegetarian Options

KEY POINTS

- Quinoa is one complete vegetarian food.
- Buckwheat bears no association with wheat and is gluten-free.

QUINOA

In addition to its fiber content, a high protein content of 15 percent makes it a very attractive protein source for vegetarians. Unlike some vegetarian sources, it contains all essential amino acids and is thus recognized as a complete protein source.

It is a rich source of vital minerals and vitamins, including magnesium, iron, omega fatty acids, and vitamin E.

Quinoa contains a variety of polyphenols, phytosterols, and flavonoids with possible nutraceutical benefits. Its physicochemical properties, including solubility, water-holding capacity, gelation, emulsification, and foaming, allow for its use in a variety of ways.

Quinoa is gluten-free.

> Quinoa is unrivalled in its qualities and nutritional ingredients. It has the potential to be used as a crop in NASA's Controlled Ecological Support Systems during long manned spaceflights (perhaps to Mars). A 1993 NASA report declared, "While no single food can supply all the life sustaining nutrients, quinoa comes close as any other in the plant and animal kingdom."

BUCKWHEAT

Buckwheat is not a grain but a seed. It is botanically characterized as a fruit. It originated in Southeast Asia 8,000 years ago and then spread across Asia to Europe.

The name buckwheat is a misnomer, since it is not related to wheat. The name owes its origin to its triangular seeds and that it is used like wheat.

Buckwheat is also used for honeybees, and its nectar for bees yields dark-colored honey.

UNDERAPPRECIATED NUTRITIONAL VALUE OF BUCKWHEAT

Long considered a nutritional powerhouse, buckwheat yields essential nutrients, including high-quality protein containing all the essential amino acids.

Crude protein content of buckwheat has been reported as high as 18 percent. According to Dr. Saturni and colleagues from Italy, protein comprises 10.9 percent of the dry mass of buckwheat, which is comparable to 11.7 percent of wheat. Dr. Alvarez-Jubete and colleagues reported 11.7 percent protein in buckwheat.

The biological value of the protein has been reported to be as high as 90 percent. Biological value of protein is a measure of the percentage of protein consumed that ultimately gets used or incorporated into proteins made inside the body.

Many experts consider it to be healthier than rice, wheat, and corn, because of its nutritious value, including higher quality protein content and low glycemic index.

In addition to high protein content, buckwheat is a rich source of antioxidants and vital minerals like zinc, iron, and selenium.

HOW IS BUCKWHEAT CONSUMED?

- The groats can be eaten raw or cooked.

- Buckwheat may be consumed as porridge, noodles, and pancakes.
- Buckwheat is one of the sources for gluten-free beer, used in lieu of barley.

In India, when people are on grain-free fast for religious reasons, it is customary to consume buckwheat foods instead, since it is not a grain.

POTENTIAL HEALTH BENEFITS

Brain function

Buckwheat extracts improve memory and cognition in animal models of Alzheimer's disease.

Obesity and atherosclerosis

Dr. Durendić-Brenesel and colleagues have demonstrated reduced weight gain as well as cholesterol- and atherosclerosis-lowering effects of buckwheat in animals.

Cancer prevention

Dr. Zeng and colleagues from the Biotechnology and Genetic Germplasm Institute in China recommend its use as part of cancer prevention strategies.

Arthritis

Animal studies from the Tongji Medical College in China have documented that buckwheat helps suppress arthritis in animals, along with reduction in inflammation.

Liver diseases

According to Dr. Lee and colleagues, components of buckwheat protect against liver damage via its antioxidant and anti-inflammatory activities in rats.

Lowering high blood pressure

Results of studies from Shinshu University in Minamiminowa, Japan suggest that fermentation of buckwheat sprouts yields potent antihypertensive compounds.

Gastrointestinal problems

Buckwheat compounds have been used to treat abdominal pain and dysentery in traditional Chinese medicine. Dr. Liu and colleagues from the Department of Liver Disease, The Affiliated Hospital of Nanjing University of Chinese Medicine in China have demonstrated that buckwheat extracts reduces inflammation, leaky gut, and susceptibility to pain in animal models of irritable bowel syndrome.

REFERENCES

1. Vega-Gálvez A, Miranda M, Vergara J et al. Nutrition facts and functional potential of quinoa (Chenopodium quinoa willd.), an ancient Andean grain: a review. *J Sci Food Agric.* 2010 Dec; 90(15):2541-7.
2. Lee CC, Shen SR, Lai YJ, Wu SC. Rutin and quercetin, bioactive compounds from tartary buckwheat, prevent liver inflammatory injury. *Food Funct.* 2013 Apr 30; 4(5):794-802.

CHAPTER 55

Fecal Transplantation

KEY POINTS

- Stool from a healthy person is delivered into the gut of unhealthy person.
- Total stool transplantation is frequently used for drug-refractory recurrent *C. difficile* colitis.

Altered flora has been implicated in many gastrointestinal as well as many non-gastrointestinal disorders. Fecal transplantation is getting increasing recognition for its therapeutic benefit.

DISORDERS WITH POTENTIAL BENEFIT FROM FECAL TRANSPLANTATION

The role of fecal transplantation is fairly well established for recurrent *C. difficile* colitis. There are also reports suggesting its use in a variety of other disorders. However, data from randomized controlled trials is lacking.

- Irritable bowel syndrome
- Ulcerative colitis and Crohn's disease
- Celiac disease
- Obesity
- Diabetes
- Rheumatoid arthritis
- Parkinson's disease

FECAL BACTERIOTHERAPY OR TRANSPLANTATION

This involves transfer of the entire bacterial flora from a healthy donor to the sick recipient.

PROTOCOL

- Protocols/recipes vary. I am not aware of any randomized controlled trials to examine most issues related to fecal transplantation.
- Single as well as multiple sessions have been used.
- Blended stool is administered via an enema or colonoscope.
- More recently, stool has been administered via a nasogastric (NG tube) into the stomach and even in capsules taken by mouth.
- No adverse effects have been reported with fecal administration, irrespective of the method of administration.

PRE-REQUISITE STUDIES IN DONOR

- Healthy donor with normally-formed stools.
- While some experts require the donor be a close relative, others suggest the opposite. There is a lack of studies to determine which strategy is better.
- No antibiotic use within at least the last six months.
- Absence of bacterial, protozoa, and viral pathogens in stool.
- Complete blood count and comprehensive metabolic profile.
- Exclude hepatitis A, B, and C, HIV, and sexually transmitted diseases.

REFERENCES

1. Vrieze A, de Groot PF, Kootte RS et al. Fecal transplant: a safe and sustainable clinical therapy for restoring intestinal microbial balance in human disease? *Best Pract Res Clin Gastroenterol.* 2013 Feb; 27(1):127-37.

2. Borody TJ, Campbell J. Fecal microbiota transplantation: techniques, applications, and issues. *Gastroenterol Clin North Am*. 2012 Dec; 41(4):781-803.

CHAPTER 56

Rising Autism and Chronic Pain Syndromes:
Does the Gut Hold the Key?

KEY POINTS

- Prevalence of autism has been rising by leaps and bounds without a reasonable explanation.
- Unhealthy gut and a disordered gut-immune-brain axis provide a unifying framework of causation of autism and chronic pain disorders.

AUTISM SPECTRUM DISORDERS

HISTORICAL PERSPECTIVE

First described by Dr. Leo Kanner in 1943, autism or autistic spectrum disorders including the classic autism is a heterogeneous group of neurobehavioral disorders with wide ranging clinical manifestations, ranging from communication and behavioral dysfunction to social difficulties on top of normal language skills and sometimes even extraordinary talents.

> "These characteristics form a unique 'syndrome,' not heretofore reported," he wrote based on initial observations, "which seems to be rare enough, yet is probably more frequent than is indicated by the paucity of observed cases."

RISING PREVALENCE ESTIMATES

Caused by a combination of genetic and environmental factors, the prevalence of autism has been rising by leaps and bound in recent decades. Initial estimates from 1966 suggested a prevalence of 4.5 per 10,000, rising to 19 per every 10,000 persons in the early 1990s.

Subsequent estimates suggested that it has been rising to epidemic proportions, with about one in every 110 kids affected. A recent study from the Centers for Diseases Control found a 23 percent increase over just a two-year period. The number affected with autism stood at one in 88 in 2008. But is this rise in prevalence real?

AUTISM PREVALENCE CONTROVERSY

Data is not strong enough, allowing many scientists to question the "rising tide" of autism. Others appear to be more realistic, in my opinion.

> According to Dr. Thomas Insel, director of the National Institute of Mental Health in Bethesda, Maryland, "This whole idea of whether the prevalence is increasing is so contentious for autism, but not for asthma, type 1 diabetes, food allergies — lots of other areas where people kind of accept the fact that there are more kids affected."

EXPLAINING THE RISING PREVALENCE OF AUTISM

The dramatic and continued rise in the prevalence of autism cannot be merely explained by increased awareness and diagnosis at an early age, use of broader clinical criteria for diagnosis, and the inclusion of kids affected with mental retardation.

Inability to explain the rising tide of autism based on what we know thus far suggests that some as yet unidentified factor or factors may be at play and research to find these factors needs to be undertaken at war footing. How the environmental factors affect the brain and the resulting problems continues to baffle modern science. Theories on causation abound. It is interesting that most of the money spent on autism research has been spent on exploring genetic factors, while only small fraction is devoted to environmental issues. The paucity of concrete facts makes it ripe for speculation.

ISSUES OF INTEREST

- Is the brain dysfunction of autism primary (occurring on its own) or secondary?
- Is the problem mainly in brain or are the brain effects secondary?

Other factors implicated in autism include age of parents, seizure disorders, problems with immune system and endocrine/hormonal system, and dysfunction of the mitochondria that are responsible for respiration at cellular level.

> Some of the fascinating facts that have come to light include the fact that that even some scientists may fulfill the criteria for autism. The risk of autism in a child increases when one or both parents have a scientific/engineering background.

DISORDERED GUT PROVIDES UNIFYING FRAMEWORK

A disordered gastrointestinal system may ultimately affect the central nervous system in various forms. Invoking the gut at the core of the disorder may provide a unifying framework for better understanding of autism and its multiple diverse manifestations. The range of presentations may vary based on the qualitative and quantitative differences of the digestive factors involved.

PRUDENT GUT-FOCUSED APPROACH TO AUTISM

While science on this issue is in its infancy (and the issue is mired in passionate debate), what is a parent to do? Should you wait for results from randomized controlled trials to establish the truth? That could be a long wait.

In my opinion, it would be pragmatic to target the gut factors, including intestinal bacteria, digestive enzymes nutrition, and leaky gut for therapeutic intervention. Already, parents claim and many studies have substantiated that gluten-free casein-free diet is of benefit. The majority of the patients are taking probiotics. A consultation with a practitioner of integrative medicine might be a valuable investment.

SYMPTOM-BASED OVERLAPPING CHRONIC PAIN SYNDROMES

Irritable bowel syndrome (IBS) is a prototype of functional gastrointestinal pain disorder, where the disorder is a symptom complex of which chronic pain is a prominent component.

It is common to have non-GI related pain symptoms with IBS. These include:

- Sleep disturbance in 25-75 percent of IBS patients
- Urinary/bladder symptoms in 50 percent of IBS patients
- Heightened sensitivity to pain
- Food intolerances: According to Dr. Berstad and colleagues from Norway, coexistence of IBS, fibromyalgia and chronic fatigue is remarkable and points to a common disorder. Food hypersensitivity may be one instigating factor. They found bread, milk, and fruits to be common instigators.

Results of their studies showed that patients with perceived food sensitivity are likely to have the triad of IBS, fatigue, and musculoskeletal pain like fibromyalgia. Dr. Berstad speculated that the cause may be an allergy with low-grade inflammation with the cluster of GI complaints.

- High levels of stress, including post-traumatic stress, anxiety, and depression. For example, 41 percent of TMJ disorder patients have depression.

- Female preponderance, suggesting the role of female hormones (especially estrogen) in increasing pain sensitivity.
- Pain treatment options are common to these entities and include use of antidepressants, cognitive behavioral therapy.

IBS co-exists with other symptom-based complex chronic pain disorders, including fibromyalgia, chronic fatigue syndrome (CFS), temporomandibular joint (TMJ) disorder, migraine headache, chronic backache, and urinary bladder problems like interstitial cystitis.

EXAMPLES OF CO-OCCURRENCE OF CHRONIC PAIN DISORDERS

- Fibromyalgia occurs in 20-32 percent of IBS patients.
- 50-80 percent of fibromyalgia patients have IBS.
- A significant portion of charges for hospitalization for fibromyalgia are related to GI procedures!
- In one study, the overlap of IBS with other syndromes was 16 percent for TMJ disorder, 59 percent for fibromyalgia, and 36 percent for CFS.

IS IT ALL ONE OR DIFFERENT DISEASES?

Dr. Beard, a neurologist, wrote over 100 years ago about "neurasthenia," describing patients with fatigue, pain, and exhaustion. He suggested that these patients had GI symptoms, poor appetite, poor sex drive, and sleep disturbances. It sure sounds like he's talking about patients with fibromyalgia, chronic fatigue syndrome, and IBS.

Frequently, a patient is defined to have the disease based on the specialist he sees.

> Dr. Wessley from the Guy's, King's and St Thomas' School of Medicine, London states that it is an artificial separation, and that the diagnosis that represents the patient's view is the best diagnosis. Multiple studies, including those by Dr. Chelimsky, indicate that interstitial cystitis is associated with other painful comorbid conditions like IBS, sleep problems, chronic fatigue, generalized pain, and migraine headaches. These co-occurrences mimic what we see in fibromyalgia and migraine, suggesting these are not primary disorders but part of an overall syndrome with different names given based on specialty of physician seen.

UNIFYING FACTORS FOR
THE CHRONIC PAIN SYNDROMES

- Disorders tend to occur in the same individual.
- Common mechanisms like functional brain changes and increased sensitivity to pain
- Therapeutic response to similar treatments
- All are deemed to be multifactorial, and the biopsychosocial model is invoked to explain diverse issues. It appears that they just have different expression of physical signs and symptoms to a varying degree, with some commonalities and similar mechanisms underlying pain syndrome.

FACTORS TO RECONCILE TO EXPLAIN
A UNIFIED FRAMEWORK

- Altered brain activation patterns: Different areas are activated in response to pain in healthy subjects versus patients with pain disorders like IBS, fibromyalgia, chronic fatigue syndrome, TMJ disorders, and interstitial cystitis. A common theme is abnormal autonomic nervous system, which is connected to the brain at one end and other organs at the other end.
- Abnormal activation of the immune system is seen in IBS, especially intestinal mast cells. Biochemical signaling molecules

released by these cells sensitize the nerves and lower the pain threshold.

- Immune activation may occur as a result of infection, abnormal intestinal bacteria and food sensitivities, as is seen in IBS.
- Fibromyalgia is also known to be preceded by infection, including various viruses and Lyme disease. There are similar reports of infection in temporomandibular joint disorder. An association with prior urinary tract infection is often reported in interstitial cystitis. Infections including viruses, bacteria, and mycoplasma have been associated with chronic fatigue syndrome.
- Dysfunction and maladjustment of hormonal-brain interactions is common. Most commonly, changes at the level of Hypothalamic-Pituitary-Adrenal (HPA) are reported.

Different genes have been implicated in causation of these disorders. However, they would be multiple and contribute only a minor component. Disease manifests when other environmental factors come into play in the right setting.

OVERVIEW OF A SIMPLIFIED COMMON PROCESS

- The process usually starts with an infectious GI problem, followed by post-infectious IBS. Added to that along the way are manifestations of chronic muscle pain, as in fibromyalgia and fatigue in chronic fatigue syndrome.
- The infectious agent disrupts the intestinal barrier, exposing gut immune cells to the bacteria and their toxins. The result is inflammation.
- Bacterial toxins then migrate across the leaky gut into the body and gain access to the brain. Injection of bacterial toxin in animals produces flu-like sickness and fatigue.
- The gut is the critical element for a unified framework.

> Inflammation, dysbiosis, and leaky gut can easily explain all the elements involved in chronic symptom-based pain syndromes and provide basis for a unified framework.

Inflammation

- Inflammation starting in the gut is the initial factor whether instigated by a particular food, allergy, or infection. A preceding infection is common prior to onset of IBS and is known as post-infectious IBS. Similarly, preceding infections have been implicated in other disorders.
- Food hypersensitivity to foods is common and can act as a trigger, especially when people eat food. Patients with these pain syndromes frequently feel better if they don't eat. A study by Dr. Berstad and colleagues from Norway indicated that as many as 71 percent patients with perceived food hypersensitivity fulfilled criteria for IBS plus chronic muscle pain plus fatigue. They speculated that allergy and low-grade inflammation, along with a diverse cluster of symptoms, might be results of intestinal dysfunction in response to foods.
- There is a significant high prevalence of gluten-related celiac disease in patients with IBS plus fibromyalgia, as compared to IBS alone. Many chronic pain patients report improvement with a gluten-free diet.
- Inflammation causes multiple changes in the brain in animals, including hormonal system originating with signals from brain (HPA axis), along with changes in neurotransmitters and hormone secretions.
- The immune reaction to bacterial toxin creates a sickness-like behavior as documented in animal studies. This includes anxiety, depression, and fatigue.
- The fatigue is likely related to inflammation in response to bacteria or bacterial products passing though the leaky gut.
- Fatigue is common in the autoimmune disease Sjogren's syndrome and is mediated via inflammation in brain cells.

- Dr. Fluge and colleagues from the Haukeland University Hospital in Norway successfully used immune-modulator drugs to heal chronic fatigue syndrome.

Leaky gut

- There is increased intestinal permeability or leakiness in IBS, which allows passage of bacteria and its toxic products across the leaky gut, interacting with nerves and also gaining access to the brain.
- According to Drs. Zhou and Verne from the Cincinnati VA Medical Center, the heightened sensitivity to pain in IBS is instigated by transient inflammation due to infection and/or leaky gut. This induces increased pain sensitivity and helps maintain heightened pain sensitivity via its interactions with the nervous system.
- There are increased levels of antibodies to the bacterial lipopolysacharide toxin, found in the cell walls of the bacteria, in patients with depression, suggesting intestinal bacteria passed through the leaky gut and activated immune cells to antibody reaction.
- Reports by Drs. Maes and Leunis from Belgium indicate that normalization of leaky gut in chronic fatigue syndrome is associated with clinical improvement.

Altered intestinal bacteria or dysbiosis

- Studies by Weinstock and colleagues from Washington University School of Medicine in St. Louis have shown that the majority of patients with interstitial cystitis have small intestinal bacterial overgrowth (SIBO).
- Bacterial overgrowth is common in IBS, and many patients respond to gut-selective antibiotics.
- Restless leg syndrome is seen in patients with IBS and responds to treatment of bacterial overgrowth.

- Activation of the immune system may occur due to preceding infection or due to bacterial overgrowth. LPS induces heightened sensitivity to pain in animals.

Combining the overlapping concepts of dysbiosis, leaky gut, and inflammation provides the roots for the unified hypothesis of the gut as a critical part of the gut-hormonal-immune-brain axis in the chronic pain syndromes.

ABDOMINAL MIGRAINE

Background

- Study by Dr. Kurth and colleagues reported 81 percent of migraine patients had GI symptoms, as compared to 38 percent in control population.
- Patients with migraines are more likely to have chronic abdominal pain.
- Frequent headaches occur in 50 percent of IBS patients, as compared to 18 percent in control.
- Similar to abdominal pain, a syndrome of abdominal epilepsy is also well-described.

FEATURES OF ABDOMINAL MIGRAINE

- Diagnosed mostly in children, but may be encountered in adults
- Midline abdominal pain for one to 72 hours, associated with a decrease in headache may occur in conjunction with reduced appetite, nausea, vomiting, and paleness. No other cause can be attributed to the symptoms, including no GI disorder.
- Pain triggers include foods like fish and alcohol.
- Strong family history of migraine and motion sickness.
- Diagnosis is delayed by an average of six years.
- Refractory to usual drugs.

Abdominal migraine needs to be considered in the differential diagnosis when episodic and recurrent abdominal pain and migraine features are seen.

REFERENCES

1. Heberling CA, Dhurjati PS, Sasser M. Hypothesis for a systems connectivity model of Autism Spectrum Disorder pathogenesis: links to gut bacteria, oxidative stress, and intestinal permeability. *Med Hypotheses*. 2013 Mar; 80(3):264-70.
2. Harris C, Card B. A pilot study to evaluate nutritional influences on gastrointestinal symptoms and behavior patterns in children with Autism Spectrum Disorder. *Complement Ther Med*. 2012 Dec; 20(6):437-40.
3. Kawicka A, Regulska-Ilow B. How nutritional status, diet and dietary supplements can affect autism. A review. *Rocz Panstw Zakl Hig*. 2013; 64(1):1-12.
4. de Theije CG, Wu J, da Silva SL et al. Pathways underlying the gut-to-brain connection in autism spectrum disorders as future targets for disease management. *Eur J Pharmacol*. 2011 Sep;668 Suppl 1:S70-80.
5. Wessely S, Hotopf M. Is fibromyalgia a distinct clinical entity? Historical and epidemiological evidence. *Baillieres Best Pract Res Clin Rheumatol*. 1999 Sep; 13(3):427-36.
6. Evans RW, Whyte C. Cyclic vomiting syndrome and abdominal migraine in adults and children. *Headache*. 2013 Jun; 53(6):984-93.

SEND FEEDBACK SO DR. MINOCHA MAY IMPROVE THIS BOOK!

I truly appreciate you taking the time to read The Seven-X Plan for Digestive Health. I would love to get your comments and suggestions.

If you enjoyed this book, please write a review.

If you liked the book, I would really appreciate if you would kindly write an honest review for it at www.amazon.com. This will help others know what they are getting and help them understand if this book is right for them.

Facebook: http://facebook.com/doctoranil

Twitter: http://twitter.com/dranilminocha

Email: physicianwriter AT gmail DOT com

Web site: http://minochahealth.typepad.com/

Dedication

This book is dedicated to my family: my loving parents Ram and Kamla, my siblings Kamal, Vimal and Rina, and the light of my life Geeta. Without their unconditional love and support, this book would not have been possible.

30108704R00259

Made in the USA
San Bernardino, CA
21 March 2019